The Overload System for Strength

A Modern Application of Old-School Training

Christian Thibaudeau
Tom Sheppard

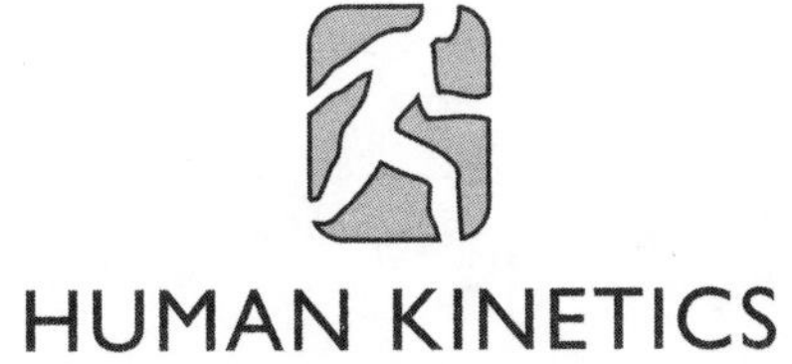

Library of Congress Cataloging-in-Publication Data

Names: Thibaudeau, Christian, 1977- author. | Sheppard, Tom, 1982- author.
Title: The overload system for strength : a modern application of old-school training / Christian Thibaudeau, Tom Sheppard.
Description: Champaign, IL : Human Kinetics, [2024] | Includes bibliographical references and index.
Identifiers: LCCN 2023015946 (print) | LCCN 2023015947 (ebook) | ISBN 9781718216044 (paperback) | ISBN 9781718216051 (epub) | ISBN 9781718216068 (pdf)
Subjects: LCSH: Weight training. | Muscle strength. | BISAC: SPORTS & RECREATION / Bodybuilding & Weightlifting | HEALTH & FITNESS / Exercise / General
Classification: LCC GV546 .T55 2023 (print) | LCC GV546 (ebook) | DDC 613.7/13--dc23/eng/20230425
LC record available at https://lccn.loc.gov/2023015946
LC ebook record available at https://lccn.loc.gov/2023015947

ISBN: 978-1-7182-1604-4 (print)

Acquisitions Editor: Korey Van Wyk; **Developmental Editor:** Laura Pulliam; **Managing Editor:** Kevin Matz; **Copyeditor:** Chernow Editorial Services; **Indexer:** Dan Connolly; **Permissions Manager:** Laurel Mitchell; **Graphic Designer:** Denise Lowry; **Cover Designer:** Keri Evans; **Cover Design Specialist:** Susan Rothermel Allen; **Photograph (cover):** David Laplante; **Photographs (interior):** Samuel Tessier, except photos on pages 51, 65, 95, and 205 courtesy of Tom Sheppard; **Photo Production Specialist:** Amy M. Rose; **Photo Production Manager:** Jason Allen; **Senior Art Manager:** Kelly Hendren; **Illustrations:** © Human Kinetics, unless otherwise noted; **Printer:** Sheridan Books

We thank Dave Tate and EliteFTS in London, Ohio, and Sport Évolution le Gym in Quebec City, Quebec, Canada, for assistance in providing the locations for the photo shoot for this book.

Human Kinetics books are available at special discounts for bulk purchase. Special editions or book excerpts can also be created to specification. For details, contact the Special Sales Manager at Human Kinetics.

Printed in the United States of America 10 9 8 7 6 5 4 3 2 1

The paper in this book is certified under a sustainable forestry program.

Human Kinetics
1607 N. Market Street
Champaign, IL 61820
USA

United States and International
Website: **US.HumanKinetics.com**
Email: info@hkusa.com
Phone: 1-800-747-4457

Canada
Website: **Canada.HumanKinetics.com**
Email: info@hkcanada.com

E8809

I'd like to dedicate this book to the generations of old-school lifters who paved the way with their passion, hard work, and willingness to experiment to always find better ways to get stronger and more muscular. I also want to dedicate this book to my wife, Geneviève, as I intend to not be killed in my sleep or in a freak lawnmower incident.

—Christian Thibaudeau

I dedicate this book to my father, Kevin, who sadly left this world before this book was ever finished. The world doesn't have enough heroes like him, and I was lucky enough to call him Dad. Rest in peace.

—Tom Sheppard

CONTENTS

ACKNOWLEDGMENTS

I would like to thank Naomi, my wife, who has always supported me in everything I do and who continues to push me past my own self-doubts and insecurities. Nothing great can ever be achieved without someone even greater behind you supporting you along the way.

I thank my eldest brother, Damian, for being the person who reached out to me at one of my lowest points and dragged me to the gym. It began the obsession that would define my life. Without you, I probably wouldn't be here.

Also, a special thank you to Dave Tate and EliteFTS for their support in allowing us to use their facility for much of the photography for this book.

Last but not least, I would like to thank my coauthor. You have propelled my career to levels I thought I would never reach. Your trust in me and guidance have opened up so many possibilities that I can likely never truly repay you. But, more importantly, you've become a close and dear friend in the process. Thank you.

—Tom Sheppard

INTRODUCTION

Ever since I started taking strength training seriously, I have continuously found ways to combine two of my biggest passions: inventing ways to increase strength and muscle size through the study of its history. I have always been attracted to what the old-school lifters—from the 1920s all the way to the 1970s—did to get stronger and bigger. They were not afraid to try new, outside-the-box methods and did not confine themselves to popular training ideas just because everyone else subscribed to them.

There was no social media (and very little actual media presence) in those days. Serious lifters didn't give a damn whether a method looked cool, was marketable, or would be socially acceptable. There wasn't much, if any, research being done on serious strength and hypertrophy training, which meant that serious lifters did not wait for numerous peer-reviewed studies to tell them that a method they wanted to try would work. There was also little arguing over minutia or armchair quarterbacking over what successful lifters did.

They found out the old way if something worked: They tried it.

Unsurprisingly, most of the effective strength-building methods come from those old-school lifters. Science is just now proving these methods to be effective (even though lifters have known for decades). I am not against science. Quite the contrary. It can help us understand why certain methods work and maybe help us better use the tools at our disposal. The fact remains that the ultimate test of a training approach is whether it works in the trenches and if it stood the test of time.

Would you rather use a method that has consistently helped people obtain strength and size over and over but is yet to be supported by scientific findings, or something that has been proven in experiments (often with beginners or less trained individuals) but has yet to be used in the trenches to produce real, hardcore results? That's why I've always gathered inspiration from legends of the strength game to develop my arsenal of methods.

I especially love to research lifters from the 1950s and earlier. Why? There are two main reasons:

- Lifters in the low-tech era had to be incredibly imaginative to develop effective training methods. The 1930s to late 1950s were also the first boom period of strength training. At this point, squat racks and stands didn't even exist. Neither did benches. These old-school lifters would probably think, "Why would I go to the gym to lie down?" Everything had to be based around big, basic lifts out of necessity. There was no option to be a coward and skip your squats in favor of leg extensions; it didn't exist.
- Lifters from that era were not using steroids. While testosterone injections started being used by athletes in 1956 (this was pretty much limited to Russian lifters and throwers), it was not until the early 1960s that testosterone and synthetic steroids began to be used more commonly by athletes. And even then, the dosages were extremely low. In fact, during the late

> 1960s, bodybuilders were arguing whether it would be safe to go from 5 milligrams (mg) of Dianabol per day to 10 mg. Compare that to today's bodybuilders who use between 1,000 and 3,000 milligrams per week of various steroids—sometimes more. Despite the lack of steroids or modern equipment, old-school lifters were able to build superhuman strength that rivals or even exceeds what many lifters are doing today with their heavy use of performance-enhancing drugs. Note that this is not an anti-steroids book, but it takes the position that methods that worked great for natural lifters are more likely to be effective across the board.

This book is influenced by the methods and training of some of the strongest men who ever lived. Guys like Paul Anderson who squatted 1,200 pounds (544 kilograms), push-pressed 560 pounds (254 kilograms), military-pressed 435 pounds (197 kilograms) or more, bench-pressed over 600 pounds (272 kilograms), and deadlifted 1,000 pounds (454 kilograms) with special hooks. Bob Peoples deadlifted 725 pounds (329 kilograms) at a body weight of 175 pounds (79 kilograms) in the 1940s. Herman Görner deadlifted 840 pounds (381 kilograms), did a 730-pound (331 kilograms) *one-hand* deadlift and clean and pressed 390 pounds (177 kilograms) in the 1920 and 1930s. And Anthony Ditillo could press 405 pounds (184 kilograms) overhead and do a 350-pound (159 kilograms) behind-the-neck press from a dead-start.

I also am greatly influenced by the worth of strength-training authors like Harry Paschall, who wrote for the pioneer magazine *Strength & Health* in the late 1940s and 1950s and was an advocate for heavy lifting, including a lot of heavy partial lifts, over the "pump" style that started to become more popular with the advent of the Weider publications.

And that's just to name a few.

What all these men, and most of the strongest men from that era, have in common was the belief that to build superhuman strength, you had to move the biggest weights possible. While full-range lifts were very important and the true measure of a champion's strength, the total weight moved was more important than the range of motion. In fact, many strongmen contests or shows used partial lifts. A good example is the back lift, in which a strongman would lift a platform held on his back while he was bent over, hand on a bench. He would use a small bend in his legs and arms to push the platform up a few inches. French Canadian strongman Louis Cyr, for example, did 4,337 pounds (1,967 kilograms) in this manner in the late 1800s.

And, unsurprisingly, the training of the strongest old-school lifters included a lot of partial lifts. The reason was that these partial movements allowed them to use a lot more weight and thus would contribute to making them stronger over the full range of motion. They didn't understand why (I will cover the science behind the overload system in chapter 2), but they knew that overload exercises made them stronger, period. As such, they developed tons of methods that allowed them to use heavier weights than they could over the full range. Partials, heavy holds, or even negative-only reps. Their core principle was simple: *Practice handling heavy loads and you'll get stronger.*

They also did plenty of full-range movements or even exercises with a longer range than the competition lifts. For example, Bob Peoples invented deficit deadlifts: deadlifting with a longer range of motion than the regular deadlift to complement his use of heavy partials.

As you will see, partial lifts are a fantastic tool for several reasons, but not everyone can fully transfer the gains from partial lifts to the full-range movements. That's why full-range lifting as well as special methods to facilitate the strength transfer from partial movements to the full-range lifts need to be an integral part of a program that will work for everyone.

This is what this system is about.

I am not going to lie. This is, first and foremost, a program to get you to gain strength at the fastest rate possible. If you do it properly, you can expect rapid and dramatic strength gains. However, it is not strictly a plan to get you strong. While strength and human performance are my true passion, I also like to be jacked and tanned! As such, a program that would add a huge amount of weight on my lifts but leave me looking the same would be of no interest to me. For that reason, I am not interested in developing a system that will not also allow me to build muscle and look more impressive, even if it means getting a lot stronger.

While this is far from a bodybuilding plan, it still uses plenty of hypertrophy work to support the neurological methods that are the cornerstone of the system. After all, improving neurological efficiency only allows you to use a greater proportion of the strength than your muscles can already produce; it will always be limited by the actual amount of muscle you carry. If you want super strength, you also want to increase muscle mass.

Another benefit of this program will be an increase in muscle density and firmness. In fact, if you are lean, this will be one of the most noticeable effects of this training style. Increased neurological efficiency is the most important element in increasing muscle tone (i.e., how hard the muscles look, even at rest). And overload work is the best way to develop that. When you do overload work, you also stimulate the fast-twitch muscle fibers more. These fibers typically lie in the superficial layer of the muscle tissue, and developing them will further increase that carved-out-of-stone look.

The scope of this program still makes use of isolated high-rep and low-load work. This type of work serves two main purposes:

- Increasing muscle tissue to boost strength potential
- Developing the tendons (which respond better to high reps and accentuated eccentrics), which will help increase your strength potential while reducing the risk of injuries

This system will use a combination of partial overloads, heavy holds, heavy eccentrics, and high-rep isolation work to maximize your strength and body.

The goal of this book is to first open your eyes to how some of the strongest individuals in history have trained, because many of these methods have been lost and are rarely seen nowadays. Then it moves on to the movements that will form the foundation of this system, including an in-depth chapter on the technical points of each main lift to ensure that you are performing them correctly. Next, the book will delve into the science of why and how these methods work and how to program them effectively before finally showing you how to put it all together and build your own overload system program. I hope that with this information, you are able to broaden your knowledge and experience with what are now seen as unconventional training methodologies and, of course, get super strong and jacked in the process.

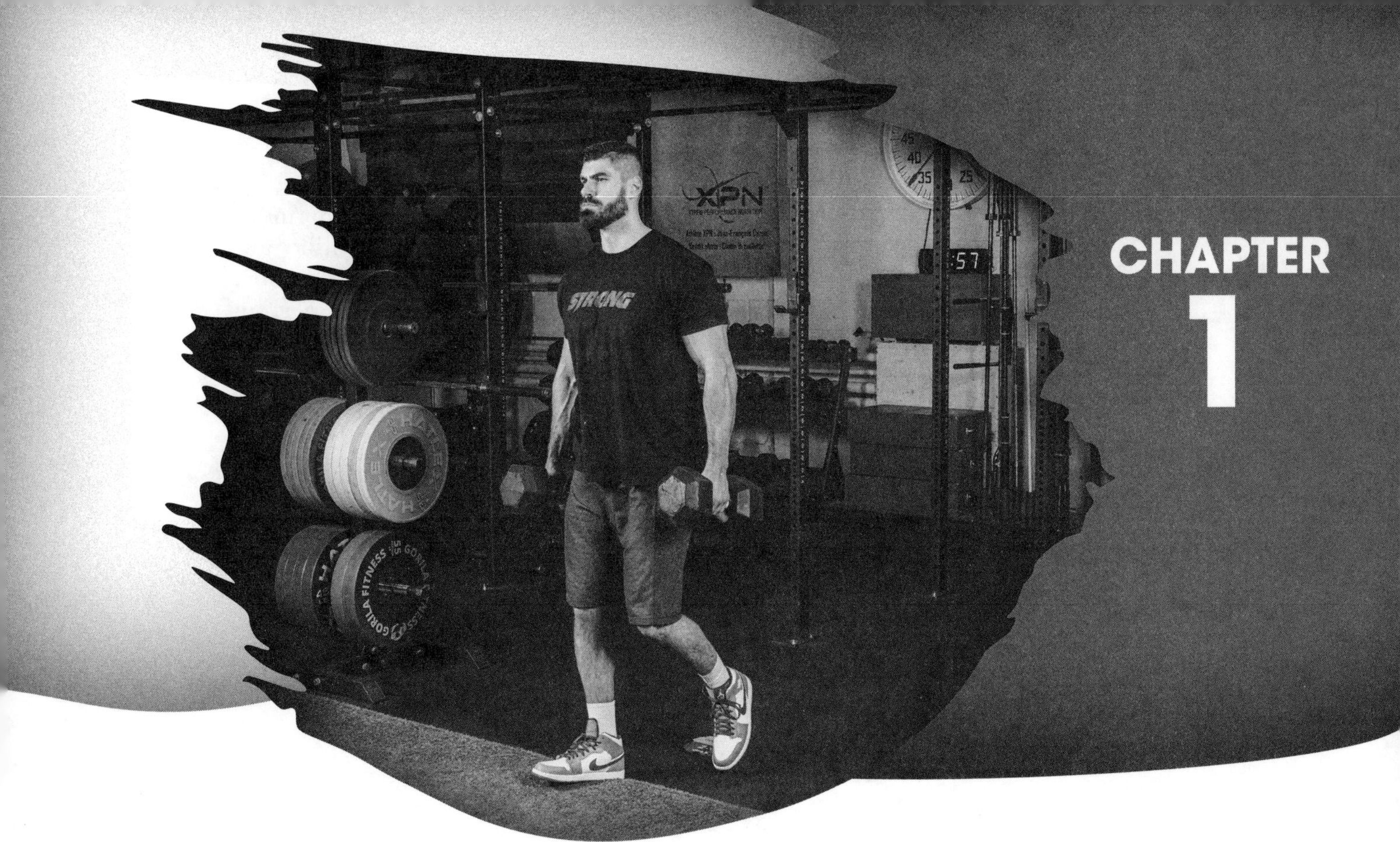

CHAPTER 1

The Overload System Methods

The overload system pays homage to old-school strength training that was all about lifting heavy stuff in as many different ways as possible. It was how strength training was done before the water became muddied by the widespread use of performance-enhancing drugs (PEDs), before people made up exercises just to look cool on Instagram, and when people were happy to focus on working brutally hard with minimal equipment in the pursuit of superhuman strength. The overload system is about providing a very strong stimulus for the nervous system in order to achieve the fastest strength progression. Let's take a closer look.

What Is the Overload System?

The overload system is a training system that uses a variety of training methods that would now be viewed as novel. But, in reality, most of the methods in this system have been around for decades. They simply went out of fashion as the strength-training world diversified.

The core, or motor if you like, of the overload system is providing a very strong stimulus for the nervous system. This is what will lead to the fastest strength progression.

Training strategies that are a common feature in this plan are the progressive range of motion and neurological carryover training method from Paul Anderson; supramaximal partial lifts espoused by Bob Peoples, Anthony Ditillo, and Harry Paschall; functional isometrics promoted by Bob Hoffman; and eccentric overloads. These methods have the strongest effect on maximizing the nervous system's capacity to increase force production.

These overload methods are also effective at inhibiting the muscle's protective mechanism—the Golgi tendon organs (GTOs)—allowing you to use a much greater proportion of your strength potential. They also include properly selected assistance work to fix weaknesses either in the range of motion of a lift itself or in a muscle involved in a lift. After all, a chain is only as strong as its weakest link. And, finally, we will also include high-repetition work on (mostly) isolation exercises with the dual purpose of increasing muscle mass and tendon resilience.

Because of the wide array of methods and types of training used, this system is just plain fun and exciting. This is not something to be dismissed, as the more you enjoy your training program, the more motivated you will be to train, and the better results you'll get.

What Are the Methods of the Overload System?

In chapter 2, we will thoroughly cover each method used in the overload system. But for now, let's take a broad look at the key methods and why they are effective at increasing strength and muscularity.

Progressive Range of Motion

Progressive range of motion, also known as neurological carryover training (NCT), is an integral part of this system. NCT involves using a progressively greater range of motion on the main lift as the program progresses.

This is a method developed by Paul Anderson to boost his squat and deadlift. What Anderson did was dig a hole in his backyard and place a loaded barbell (or a bar attached to loaded barrels for squats) over the hole. Every few weeks he would fill in the hole a little, which effectively increased the range of motion of the lift. He would use a load that was 20 to 30 pounds (9 to 14 kilograms) heavier than what he could currently lift over the full range of motion and started with a partial movement (one-third of the range, roughly) and perform as many repetitions as he could with that weight.

Every few weeks he would increase the range of motion while keeping the same weight, still attempting to get as many reps as possible. In the first position he might get 12 to 15 reps, and every time he increased the range, he would lose a few repetitions. The goal was to work all the way to a full-range movement while being able to do 1 to 2 reps with the weight, which exceeded his starting maximum by 20 to 30 pounds (9 to 14 kilograms).

This worked for four main reasons:

- It provided an overload that trained the nervous system, muscles, tendons, and skeletal structure to handle a certain weight. Because the overload was conservative, it facilitated positive adaptations. Essentially, you got your body used to handling a certain weight, and as it became more comfortable with that weight, you gradually increased the range of motion.

- It gave you a lot of repetitions with the load you wanted to adapt to. Sure, most of these repetitions were over a partial range of motion, but your body was still under the full load. The higher number of repetitions along with the more conservative overload made it easier to get your body to positively adapt and adjust to the load. The high number of repetitions was especially important for strengthening the tendons and skeletal structure.
- It inhibited the GTOs, which can be thought of as the sensors in your tendons. Their job is to evaluate how much tension is present on the muscles and whether that tension is dangerous (e.g., if it is excessive and there is an increased risk of tearing your muscle or tendon). If the GTOs deem the tension excessive, they inhibit muscle force production to protect against injury. Now, the GTOs are overly protective. As a result, "normal" (not weight-trained) individuals might only use 30 percent of their muscle strength potential. A well-trained individual might be able to use 50 to 60 percent and a world-class lifter 80 percent or more. Overloads speed up that inhibition. And a more conservative overload might be even more effective in that regard, at least for nonelite individuals.
- It gave a psychological boost by getting you used to the feeling of a very heavy weight.

Heavy Partials

When we say heavy partials, we are referring to performing a segment or a portion of the main lift with a load that is at least near maximal (compared to what you can lift on the full lift). An example is performing sets of 3 to 5 reps on a top-half squat with 95 percent of what you can lift for one rep on the full squat.

Heavy partials fall in the same category as the NCT method discussed previously. The main difference is that we do not gradually increase the range of motion; rather, we select the starting point that will provide the greatest benefit for the lifter. In general, the greater the range of motion, the easier it is to transfer the gains to the full movement. An effective strategy is to start slightly below the lifter's sticking point, to strengthen that weak point specifically (there is almost a 100 percent strength transfer for up to 10 degrees in joint range of motion, so you don't need to start exactly at the weak point).

This method leads to even higher tension produced by the muscle, which can potentially lead to more rapid increases in strength. It should also provide a more rapid inhibition of the GTOs and give you an even greater psychological boost.

However, for individuals with less of a strength-oriented background, the overload from heavy partials can actually be too much to lead to maximal positive adaptations. It's kind of like catching some sun to get a tan: If you go out for too long under sunlight that is too strong, you might get burned. More is not always better and, in some cases, can cause regression rather than progress.

Heavy partials are very useful and effective, but they are to be used with individuals who already have a good amount of experience with strength training and who have already used NCT or functional isometrics before.

Functional Isometrics

Functional isometrics is a training method that involves performing a partial range of motion using two sets of safety pins in a power rack. The pins are set to encase the desired range of motion. The bar starts on the lower set of pins and is lifted until it makes contact with the second (upper) set of pins.

Functional isometrics were developed by Dr. John Ziegler (who also contributed to the development of Dianabol) and then popularized by Bob Hoffman. Ziegler was the doctor to the U.S. weightlifting team, and Hoffman was the coach and sponsor of the team. Ziegler had two lifters train almost exclusively with isometrics or functional isometrics (along with one Olympic lifting workout): Louie Riecke and Bill March. Both made spectacular progress, going from average lifters to the top of the national ranking. *Full disclosure*: It was later found that both Riecke and March used Dianabol also, which diminished the desire to include functional isometrics as some lifters believed it was the drugs that were the primary agent in the progression. However, while 5 milligrams of Dianabol a day certainly helped (an anabolic dosage more than 10 times lower than what many *bikini competitors* use), we are not talking about a huge anabolic boost here.

Another reason isometrics didn't catch on among the masses was that it required special equipment (a power rack) that was not widely available at the time. The equipment was sold by Hoffmann, who owned York Barbell, but it was far from being a mainstay.

Finally, a lot of lifters disliked isometrics because they didn't see the weight move, and in many cases, they didn't use a weight, just a bar that they pulled against pins. This was less the case with functional isometrics, which included a very short range of motion and the use of heavy weights.

I (Christian) personally began using isometrics in 2001 when weightlifting coach extraordinaire Pierre Roy included them in his programs. The work of track-and-field coach Jean-Pierre Egger, who coached shot-putter Werner Gunthor (you can find his training videos on YouTube; if you want to see a freak, look no further!), further confirmed my passion for isometric and eccentric work. Both have been a staple in my programming ever since.

I especially like functional isometrics, as opposed to the more traditional overcoming isometrics in which you push or pull against an immovable object (e.g., a bar pulling and pushing against pins). Functional isometrics allow you to actually move a weight, thus measuring progress. I also believe that the movement, albeit small, facilitates transfer from the isometric to dynamic movements. In a functional isometric exercise, you pull or push a loaded barbell from one set of safety pins to a second one placed a few inches higher. When you contact the second set of pins you hold the weight there for 6 to 9 seconds. You can either work up to the heaviest weight you can keep in contact with the pins for the desired time or do multiple reps and sets.

There are several ways of using functional isometrics, and we will cover them more in depth in chapter 2. You can even use them to train the full movement, in which case you need to use two to three positions. Alternatively, you can use them to fix a weak point or strengthen a specific range or as an overload. In both of these uses, you only use one position.

Eccentric Overloads

This method involves loading the eccentric portion of the lift supramaximally, either by using special tools, such as weight releasers, or by only performing the eccentric portion of the lift (i.e., lowering a bar down to pins only). Emphasizing the eccentric portion of a lift has several benefits that will help you get stronger and bigger and reduce the risk of injury. In chapter 2, we take a deeper look into the methods of the system.

I also began using eccentric overloads in 2001, when Pierre Roy was including them in his programs. Then, just like isometrics, I became more familiar with them after reading the work of Jean-Pierre Egger. Charles Poliquin also taught me to see eccentric strength as a form of "strength potential": the higher your eccentric strength was, the more room you have to gain concentric strength and the more rapidly you could progress.

An eccentric overload consists of either executing exclusively the eccentric, or lowering, portion of a movement (e.g., starting a deadlift from the top and lowering it slowly to the floor) or using a greater load for the eccentric phase of a movement, either by using a tool like weight releasers or by lowering the load by yourself and having a partner help you with the lifting part.

Typically, you would use loads of 90 to 120 percent of your lifting maximum. When using 90 to 100 percent of your lifting maximum, multiple reps per set are done (typically 3 to 5 reps); when going above 100 percent of your max, we use either single repetitions or clusters (a set consisting of several singles performed with 20 to 45 seconds of rest). With very strong athletes I've used as much as 140 percent of their lifting max, but that was done after years of training with accentuated eccentrics.

Eccentric overloads are performed with anything from a controlled to a super-slow tempo, but typically I prefer a speed of 4 to 5 seconds down. The duration itself is not that important; rather, it's making a certain load as demanding as possible by being forced to control the load as much as you can.

Dead-Start Lifts

Here we are referring to movements that either naturally start from a dead-stop position (with no momentum) or, in most cases, where we set up a lift to begin from pins from a specific position of a lift. Some movements are naturally done from a dead-start lifting portion (where there is zero movement on the bar): the deadlift being the best example. But we can also include the strict military press in there.

Be aware that when training the deadlift or strict military press, we want to start every repetition from a dead-start if the goal is to maximize 1RM strength. When you use a touch-and-go (or even bounce-and-go) method on the deadlift or military press, as opposed to starting each rep from a stationary position, you will notice that the first rep is much harder than any of the subsequent reps. It's not unusual to have a lifter struggle with that first rep on deadlifts, only to get 5 to 6 more reps using the touch-and-go method.

The touch-and-go method is thus effective for muscle growth, but an overreliance on it will fail to improve the start of the movement as more of the reps will use a combination of the stretch reflex and a rebound to get the bar moving, thereby decreasing the contribution of muscle contraction in the start position.

That's the main benefit of lifts from a dead-start, even when used on exercises in which you don't actually start your reps from a dead-start: You are forced to increase the reliance on muscle contraction to get the bar started. It thus has a large impact on your strength at the beginning of a movement. It is also good for reducing the risk of injury by making your muscles stronger when they are elongated, making them more resistant to tears.

Note that our system already uses a lot of dead-start exercises simply because we have adopted methods like NCT and heavy partials. These always start from a dead-start, but we will also use them on full-range movements like the Anderson squat, bottoms-up bench, and full-range overhead press from pins.

Loaded Stretching

Loaded stretching involves placing a muscle into a lengthened position while supporting an external load. This is different from traditional stretching and can bring with it many benefits that other types of stretching do not provide. The first person to use loaded stretching for something other than increasing range of motion might have been 1968 Mr. World, Chuck Sipes, who used the dead lats hang (hanging from a chin-up bar with a heavy dumbbell attached to his waist) as his main lats-building exercise.

More recently, strength coach Jay Schroedder used loaded stretching for almost 50 percent of the volume in his training system. When Schroedder was training NFL physical freak Adam Archuleta in the early 2000s, the workouts were a combination of loaded stretching, plyometric and absorption drills, and heavy lifting (often combined with electrical muscle stimulation). In the modern bodybuilding world, loaded stretching has been a staple in the training system of Dante Trudel and Dr. Scott Stevenson. I have personally been using loaded stretches since 2003, and they are included in my 2005 book *Theory and Application of Modern Strength and Power Methods*.

Loaded stretching consists of performing a stretch while the target muscles are under a high level of tension, normally through the use of a weight. An example could be going down to the low point of a dumbbell fly and holding it there for anywhere from 45 seconds up to 3 minutes (Schroedder uses extreme durations of 2 to 3 minutes per set, while others recommend a 45 to 60 seconds mark). The load used has to make the selected duration challenging. If you can easily complete the prescribed duration, use a heavier load next time. In chapter 2, we will discuss why loaded stretching is so effective.

In the overload system, loaded stretching's main use is to strengthen the muscles while they are in their elongated position (something that the main methods tend not to focus on) and thickening the tendons to increase strength potential while reducing the risk of injuries.

Clusters

Cluster training is one of the simplest yet effective strength methods you can use. Clusters simply involve taking a specific rest period in between the individual reps of a work set.

I've been saying for years that clusters are my favorite training method to rapidly increase strength. Clusters were likely invented by Carl Miller, who was both an international weightlifting coach and an excellent lifter himself. Clusters were developed in the late 1960s and consisted of doing a series of single repetitions with a short rest period of 30 to 60 seconds in between each rep.

A cluster series (set) could include anywhere from 2 to 6 repetitions using loads ranging from 87.5 percent up to 97.5 percent. The principle is that by taking short breaks between reps, you can lift more weight for a certain number of repetitions than if you do the same number of reps as a regular set. This would obviously be conducive to more strength gains.

Now, there are many other benefits to cluster training, which has recently been proven to be more effective for strength than regular sets, and there are several variations that you can use—all of which will be presented in chapter 2.

Very High Repetitions

A particularity of using high reps is that very little work is actually done in the traditional bodybuilding zone (8 to 12 reps per set). We either go low reps and heavy (5 reps or less) or use very high repetitions (20 to 30 reps per set, or more). Very high repetitions are superior to sets of 8 to 12 (and very low reps) to develop the tendons. However, if they are taken to failure, they are just as effective as the 8 to 12 zone when it comes to building muscle.

Because high reps use several methods that place a huge demand on the nervous system already, we want to minimize fatigue as much as possible; isolation exercises with 20 to 30 reps per set (or more) are less neurologically demanding than the heavier 8 to 12 reps per set.

We also want to accomplish as much as possible with the least amount of work possible. Very high rep sets are more effective at building the tendons, which is something we need on this system, both to maximize performance and reduce the risk of injuries. Additionally, because high reps are just as effective as intermediate reps if a set is taken to failure, we can get the same hypertrophy response. We can thus achieve two things we need with a single method or exercise instead of using two different types of stimuli, which would increase volume significantly.

The very high rep work is done mostly on isolation exercises. I share Louie Simmons' view of using assistance work to develop muscle mass and tendons while minimizing the neurological cost of the exercise. If you are already demanding a lot out of your central nervous system (CNS), the last thing you want is to use assistance exercises with a high cost on the CNS. After all, we are only using assistance exercises to build muscle and tendons. Strength is developed with the main lifts and methods.

Loaded Carries

Loaded carries are generally associated with Strongman training and appear in nearly all Strongman competitions. There are many variations you can use, but the premise is simple: Pick up a weight and move it. As long as I've been a strength coach (over 20 years), I've used loaded carries with athletes. Whether in the form of sled, farmer's walks, or (more recently) Zercher carries, I have always been a fan of loaded carries to get someone stronger, more stable, and better conditioned.

I personally started using sled dragging in 1999. I was still competing in Olympic lifting then, and I was trying to drop down not one but two weight classes to have a shot at qualifying for the World University Games. This was around the time I had started reading articles by Louie Simmons, and one that piqued my interest was an article about sled dragging to improve work capacity. What attracted me to sled dragging was that I saw it as a way to lose fat while (hopefully) correcting my main weaknesses: my glutes and hamstrings.

The problem was that I didn't have a sled, and they were hard to come by. So, I simply attached a strap to a couple of 45-pound (20 kilogram) plates and then to my weight belt, and I would walk around the gym for 30 minutes per day. I was able to drop down from 222 to 182 pounds (101 to 82 kilograms) in around 10 weeks. Sure, dieting had a lot to do with it, but the sled work certainly contributed. And my strength actually did not go down. In training, my snatch, clean and jerk, and squat remained the same. However, at the competition, I sadly blacked out standing up from a clean and didn't register a total. Despite that poor ending, sled dragging—and later, loaded carries—remained one of the main tools that I used.

To make a connection with old-school lifters, some of the best lifters of the 1940s, 1950s, and 1960s were physical laborers. Bob Peoples was a farmer (and thus likely did a lot of carrying), and Paul Anderson also had a farm. While they didn't program loaded carries in their plan, they certainly did them quite a bit.

When it comes to using loaded carries, you can use them four ways:

- *Short distance and heavy weight*: Here we are talking about 10 to 50 meters done with the heaviest weight you can use for that distance. This is, obviously, to maximize strength development.
- *Moderate distance and moderate weight*: Here we are shooting for distances of 60 to 100 meters done with a challenging weight, but one that you can do smoothly for the whole distance. This is favored for developing muscle mass, especially in the 60 to 80 meter zone.
- *Intervals with a moderate weight*: Here we go for a set duration rather than a distance: roughly 45 to 60 seconds of work and eventually shooting for a 1:1 work-to-rest ratio. At first, you will likely need to rest twice as long as you work; over time, however, as conditioning improves, you will be able to reach that 1:1 ratio. The load used should be challenging for the duration prescribed but not all-out, since you'll have 4 to 8 sets to do and you want to be able to do all of them with the same weight. This is mostly a conditioning and fat-loss approach, which is why it is not really used in this system.
- *Long duration and low weight*: This is the combination I use a lot when trying to get ripped—for example, carrying a 25- to 50-pound (11 to 23 kilogram) sandbag or weight vest (or sled, like I first did 20 years ago) for 30 to 45 minutes. While there will be some benefits when it comes to the core and some muscles, it is mostly a fat-loss tool, and as such it is not included in this system, but it can be if your main goal is leaning out.

Loaded carries are awesome because they strengthen muscles in a way that regular exercises don't and are, as such, complementary. I also find them to be the most effective method for developing core strength, which is one of the most important factors in being strong on the big basic lifts.

Specialized Training

Training specialization is the process of concentrating a large part of your training load on developing a specific facet of your training. Most commonly this is done to improve a specific lift or to focus on one or two (often lagging) muscle groups.

One thing that was a lot more common with old-school lifters was specialization on a few lifts or body parts. Sure, balanced overall training was important to build a strong overall base, but most high-level lifters included specialization work at some point in their career and even used a rotation of specialization programs for overall development. As examples, Bob Peoples' specialization was the deadlift, and for Chuck Ahrens it was overhead strength. A plethora of arm or chest specialization courses were sold at the time.

The fact is that specialized training absolutely leads to a faster strength and size progression than overall training. Doing more work, with advanced methods and more frequency for a lift (or muscle), will speed up progression. With one caveat: You can't exceed your body's capacity to recover from the systemic stress of training. A mistake people make when they concentrate on a muscle or a lift is that they do not decrease the amount of work for other muscles or lifts—they should still be trained, but to a lesser extent. This will lead to an excessive overall training stress, which will prevent optimization of the results from the specialized work.

The best example I can give you about how effective specialized training can be is an experiment I did with snatch-grip high pulls (i.e., using a wide grip and lifting the bar explosively up to the mid-chest or clavicle level). I was training at Biotest/T-Nation headquarters around 10 years ago. Tim Patterson, T-Nation's owner, walked in during my workout and said, "Wow, this is cool. It's violently explosive but also doable by most people. We should film it with a truly impressive weight . . . like 180 kilograms [nearly 400 pounds]."

Never mind that I had 110 kilograms (242 pounds) on the bar when he walked in and that even when I was competing in weightlifting with a 140-kilogram (309-pound) snatch, the most I used on high pull was 130 to 140 kilograms (287 to 309 pounds)! But Tim seemed to have his mind set about the project. So, for just over three weeks, all I did was explosive pulls. Six days a week I would do high pulls and low pulls (with more weight, only pulled to the sternum). I would do a small amount of bench-pressing once a week just to stay sane. Well, after that three-week period, I actually was able to do a 180 kilogram (397 pounds) high pull. Even though this story is only to illustrate the power of specialized training, the high pull will be one of the exercises used in this plan. It is, bar none, the best way to build the traps and upper back.

What Are the Exercises Used in the Overload System?

The exercises are divided into three main categories: main lifts, assistance exercises, and remedial exercises.

Main Lifts

These are the six foundational exercises that constitute the core of the program and that we will discuss in more detail in chapter 2. The premise of this system is to make you as strong as possible on these movements. These exercises are the deadlift, squat, military press, bench press, Pendlay row, and explosive pulls. These are the most common big lifts used by lifters around the world, but you are free to select different variations of these movements as your main lifts if you feel that they are better suited for your body type or your goal. For example, those with long legs (especially long femurs) will not get much quad loading from a regular back squat. Why? Because they will have a much greater degree of hip flexion in their back squat, making it more posterior chain dominant. In that case, an anterior-loaded squat, like a front squat, is a better choice for leg strength. Unless you compete in a strength sport, there are no lifts that you must perform, so feel free to adjust based on your individual needs. Just make sure you respect the broad categories we have chosen (squat pattern, hinge pattern, etc.).

Assistance Exercises

These are exercises that will directly improve a main lift because they are structurally close to those main lifts; we will cover these exercises in chapter 10. There are five components that make an assistance exercise structurally similar to a main lift. An assistance exercise doesn't have to combine all five components, but the more it has, the more effective it will be at directly improving the main lift. These components are

- same joints involved, moving in a similar way,
- same muscles involved, doing the same function,
- same range of motion,
- same contraction types, and
- same rhythm.

When we say "same," it doesn't have to be exactly alike. For example, in a front squat the hips, knees, and ankles do not move the exact same way and reach the same angles as in a back squat (unless you have very short legs with a very long torso or have long tibias and short femurs, in which case it can be very similar to performing a high bar squat). However, the front squat is far more similar to the back squat when it comes to joint action than a leg press or hack squat, for example, because in the latter two examples, the hips move linearly.

Remedial Exercises

These are movements that target a specific muscle, or muscles, involved in the main lift. Remedial exercises are more often isolation or machine exercises, but if a lower stress multijoint movement is what gives you the best mind-muscle connection with a specific muscle, they can be used, too.

The goal of these exercises is to build and strengthen muscles, not train movements. It doesn't mean that they are not effective. Far from it. Remedial exercises are often the best way to fix a lagging muscle group and thus a weak point, and they do so with a lot less neurological stress than assistance exercises. The Westside Barbell Conjugate System is based mostly on the use of remedial exercises. This is often lost on people who look at that system: They see the max effort work and the dynamic effort work, but the use of remedial exercises, which constitutes 80 percent of their volume, is one of the keys to the system.

Note that we will not cover remedial exercises in this book because they would basically include every isolation and machine exercise known!

In the overload system, the main lift and assistance exercises are trained heavy while the remedial exercises are trained more "bodybuilding style," with 10 to 20 repetitions and even as many as 40 to 50 reps if you want to focus on developing tendons or preventing injuries.

The main lift is trained the heaviest and with the lowest rep range and typically includes more sets than the other movements in the plan. The assistance exercises still use heavy weights and low reps but not to the same degree as the main lift, especially when the main lifts are trained for sets of 1 to 3 reps. Typically the assistance exercises will be trained for sets of 5 to 8 reps (in this system). There are also generally slightly fewer sets per exercise on the assistance movement versus the main lift. The remedial exercises use the lightest weights, the highest reps, and the smallest number of sets. It is not unusual for me to program remedial exercises using the heavy-duty style of one set to total muscle failure; rarely do I program them for more than three sets (usually one to two work sets with one warm-up set, if necessary).

Now that you have been introduced to the methods involved in the overload system, hopefully you can see why it is different from any other training system out there. This is why we were excited for this book: It involves a whole bunch of fun and interesting methods that really aren't being used anymore. In chapter 2, we will go through how to use these methods in more detail and how to put them together into our overload system to create your own training program.

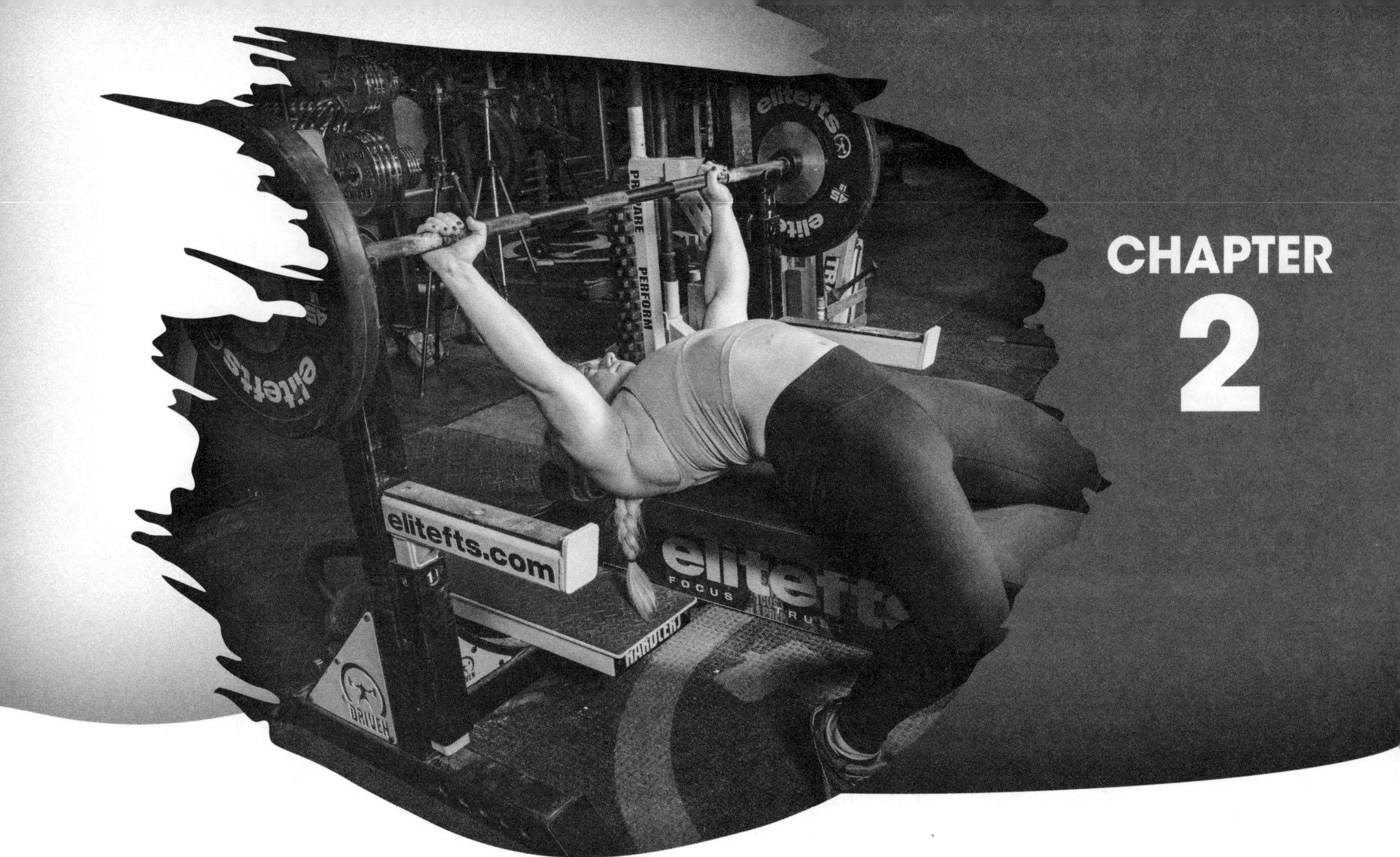

CHAPTER 2

Science and Application of the Overload System

Strength is a multifactor trait; it has many contributing factors. This is why we need to use several different methods that target different mechanisms if we truly want to build maximal strength. In this chapter, we will address what factors lead to the ability to express strength and how the overload system is set up to target all of these factors.

How to Get Stronger

To better understand why the overload system is so effective, and the reason behind the selection of the methods used in this system, we must talk about the various factors that can increase your strength and, to some extent, your muscle mass.

Getting stronger can actually be accomplished through several different paths. That's why you have strong people who can have completely different looks. You have massive muscular lifters who are strong, almost skinny wiry lifters who can lift a lot of weight, thick lifters, and lean and hard ones. There really isn't one type of body that is required to be strong. That might be one of the reasons why training for strength is so cool: While not everyone can develop the huge muscles of bodybuilders (especially drug-using bodybuilders), everyone can get significantly stronger. Throughout history, there have been the more compact and big-boned (not to say rotund) strong lifters, like Louis Cyr (5 ft 9 in. and as much as 330 pounds [150 kilograms]), Paul Anderson (5 ft 10 in. and as much as 360 pounds [163 kilograms]), Doug Hepburn (5 ft 9 in. and as much as 300 pounds [136 kilograms]), or Anthony Ditillo (5 ft 6 in. and as much as 300 pounds [136 kilograms]).

And you also had the mesomorph lifters who were muscular on a big and wide body and seemed to be born to be strong. This body type included Hermann Görner (6 ft 1 in. and over 265 pounds [120 kilograms] in lean condition); George Hackenschmidt, who actually invented the bench press and hack squat (a lean 225 pounds [102 kilograms] on a 5 ft 10 in. frame); Steve Stanko, who at 5 ft 11 in. and 225 pounds (102 kilograms) was both a member of the U.S. national weightlifting team and a Mr. Universe winner; and John Grimek (5 ft 8 in. and 215 pounds [98 kilograms] in lean condition), who was also a member of the U.S. national weightlifting team and a Mr. Universe winner. Heck, you even had ectomorphs (lanky, thinner, with long limbs) develop elite strength, with Bob Peoples (5 ft 9 in. and 165 pounds [75 kilograms]) being a prime example.

The point is that strength can be increased by optimizing several systems; everybody can significantly increase their potential, whereas not everyone can become huge. With the overload system, we are aiming to maximally develop all the facets that contribute to strength, with the goal being to get every individual as strong as they are capable of being regardless of their body structure.

Muscle Mass

All else being equal, bigger muscles are capable of producing more force than smaller ones. As such, increasing muscle mass will get you stronger. However, not everyone is as strong as they look (we will see why in the nervous system subsection). You do have large and muscular bodybuilders who don't lift heavy. That might be because of an inefficient nervous system, excessively conservative protective mechanisms, lack of joint stability, or simply a choice of training style.

However, anybody who gains muscle will get stronger provided that the other factors contribute to strength do not lessen. The way I like to explain it is to say that your muscle mass represents your strength *potential*. The bigger your muscles are or get, the higher your potential to produce force is. Whether you are strong or not is a matter of being capable of using a large proportion of this potential. How much of your potential you can use depends on several factors, including neurological efficiency, level of protective inhibition, joint stability, and technical efficiency. Having big muscles is like having a large factory with lots of employees: it certainly should allow you to be more productive, but to do so your employees must work hard and work well together.

Neurological Efficiency

The nervous system, in large part, dictates how much of your strength potential you can use. The nervous system controls how many muscle fibers are recruited, how fast they twitch (firing rate is a *huge* part of strength production), how coordinated the fibers within a muscle work together, and how synergistically the muscles involved in a movement are recruited.

Let's get back to our "muscle = factory" analogy. If the factory and the number of employees you have represent your muscle mass, the various neurological factors refer to how well your employees are working. Being able to recruit a lot of muscle fibers and make them twitch rapidly (high firing rate) represents how many of your employees actually show up to work and how hard they work. If you have lots of employees but they are lazy, you won't live up to your production potential. If your employees work hard but the workers at a similar workstation do their own thing and don't work well together, you still will not live up to your production potential. It's the same thing with your muscles: *Intramuscular coordination* is how coordinated your muscles fibers are when doing a movement. The better their coordination is, the more of your potential you can use.

And even if your employees work hard and work well together, you could still come up short of your potential if the various workstations are not in sync. This is called *intermuscular coordination* and refers to how well the various muscles involved in a movement are working together.

As you can see, if you want to use a large proportion of your strength potential, you must optimize your nervous system. When it comes to producing high levels of force, you must be frequently asking your body to produce a lot of force. Strength is a skill. You can have the body necessary to be strong, but if you don't practice heavy lifting, you will never reach anywhere close to your full potential.

Protective Mechanisms

Continuing the factory analogy, even if you do have a lot of employees who work hard and well together, you could still come up short of your production potential. If the supervisors are extremely worried for the safety of their workers, they could impose several security protocols and limit the production speed to reduce the risk of injuries among the employees. This would, of course, limit production in the name of safety. And it's a good thing. Just like we don't want any serious work-related injuries, we don't want to pull or tear a muscle or tendon because we are producing more force than is safe for our body. But when a factory's supervisors are overly conservative, they could very well limit production potential for no good reason.

It's the same thing with your body. The muscle protective mechanisms (mostly the Golgi tendon organs) are extremely conservative in the normal human body. They allow the average person to use (under normal circumstances) 30 to 40 percent of their muscle strength potential. That's why under situations of high adrenaline, you can produce a lot more force than you normally would: the adrenaline doesn't suddenly add muscle to your body; it inhibits the protective mechanisms and allows you to use more of your strength potential.

Now, the more experience you have with producing force (either from training or physical work) and the more force you are asked to produce, the less conservative your protective mechanisms become. Weight-trained (think "bodybuilding style") individuals might be able to use 50 to 60 percent of their muscle potential; strength training (more focused on heavy lifting) will increase that percentage even more. In fact, elite strength athletes are likely able to use 80 to 90 percent of their potential.

While any type of weight training will gradually reduce the sensitivity of the protective mechanisms, the heavier you go, the faster and more effective the process is. The caveat is that if the heavy lifting leads to trauma or injury, it could backfire and have the opposite effect. Overload exercises are thus more effective at inhibiting the protective mechanisms because they use more weight than you can use on the full-range movement. And even though you are using more weight, if you are using good mechanics, the risk of injury is actually lower because most muscle or tendon injuries occur when the muscle is in a lengthened position.

Stability

This is actually another part of the body's protective mechanisms. The more stable a joint is, the more of your strength potential your body will allow you to use. On the other hand, if a joint is unstable, you will be limited in how much force your muscles will be able to produce. To quote the great Fred Hatfield, who squatted 1,014 pounds (460 kilograms) at age 45, "You can't shoot a cannon from a canoe."

I see two main types of stability: passive and active.

Passive Stability

Passive stability is created by having, and pardon the scientific lingo, *lots of stuff* around a joint to create a compression. The compression puts pressure around a joint and stabilizes it. It is *kinda* like wearing knee wraps around your knees to make them more stable in order to lift more.

What is this "lots of stuff" I speak of? It could be intramuscular glycogen, water, and fatty acids blowing up a muscle to make it bigger and press more against the joint. It could be water outside the muscle, or it could even be fat.

By the way, the main reason that you lose strength on multijoint movements when dieting down is because of this loss of passive stability. When you do a fat-loss phase, you reduce calories and (most likely) carbohydrates. You often decrease sodium intake (not necessarily voluntarily, just by eating less sodium-dense foods). The result is that you lose a little bit (and eventually a lot) of that "lots of stuff." You decrease intramuscular glycogen, water, and fatty acids; retain less extracellular water; and lose fat around the various joints.

Active Stability

Active stability is when you create a more stable joint by contracting the muscles surrounding the joint. We often talk about "stabilizer muscles," which is really a misnomer because there is no such thing. Stabilizing (or fixating) is a muscle *function*, and every muscle is capable of doing that function. Furthermore, a muscle can stabilize in one movement but act as a prime mover in another one. Heck, it can even stabilize in some parts of the range of motion and be a prime mover or synergist in another part!

That's why movements seen to be working the stabilizers (e.g., isolated rotator cuff exercises) really do have a limited impact on improving your strength potential unless these muscles are inhibited or extremely weak to start with.

There are more effective ways of improving active stability during heavy lifting.

- Isometric work or stato-dynamic work. This type of workout increases the recruitment of the synergistic and antagonist muscles to create more stability.
- Lifting under conditions that require a greater effort to stay stable (e.g., tall kneeling overhead press, hanging band technique, loaded carries). Note that

making the object you are lifting less stable is more effective than making the base less stable.

- Eccentric work. When done by focusing on controlling the load (going down slowly), you develop the capacity to maintain tension throughout the range of motion, increasing stability. Plus, an eccentric overload activates the motor cortex more than other types of lifting, which will lead to faster motor learning and a more durable motor pattern.

Tendon Thickness and Resilience

It has long been known that tendons play a huge role in producing strength. Even the old-school lifters instinctively knew this to be true. They might not have known all the reasons why, but they knew that thick, resilient tendons were a huge part of being strong. In many old-school training books, they were typically referred to as "sinews," and getting them strong was a big part of many programs.

There are many reasons why thicker and more resilient tendons are important for strength production. One reason, first and foremost, is because tendons attach the muscles to the bones that they are moving. We tend to think of lifting as moving a bar (or another source of resistance), but in reality, what we are doing is moving our skeletal structure to produce movement while we are holding an external load. Essentially, your muscles move bones, which creates movement and allows you to complete a lift. The heavier the weight you are moving is, the more force the muscles must create to be able to "pull the bone" and create movement. The more force is produced, the greater stress the tendons are under.

As I explained earlier, the body has protective mechanisms in place to prevent it from tearing itself apart through voluntary actions. I mentioned the Golgi tendon organs (GTOs) that are situated, as the name implies, in the tendons. When the GTOs sense that there is too much tension and force applied to the tendons, they will trigger an inhibitory mechanism that will prevent further force production. It can even go as far as promoting relaxation (loss of force production) through its action on the inhibitory neuron. This mechanism is extremely conservative in a normal individual and is easily triggered by tension or by a rapid and forceful stretch. As you become more experienced with lifting, especially heavy lifting, you will develop some desensitization of the reflex.

Another way of reducing this reflex is to make the tendons thicker and more resilient. Thicker and stronger tendons can withstand a lot more tension and also stretch to a lesser extent. Having thicker, stronger tendons has an obvious positive impact on strength production, but so does having stiffer tendons. A tendon that is more easily stretched will transfer less force from the muscle to the bone because it will dissipate some of that tension through the stretch. To illustrate, attach a rope to a weight. Put the weight on the floor and try to yank it up by forcefully pulling on the rope. It should not be an issue at all. Now try to do the same with an elastic band instead of a rope; it will be a lot harder to get the weight moving. The stretchier the band is, the harder it will be to move the weight. Not to mention that stiffer tendons have a stronger stretch reflex, which can also contribute significantly to force production.

Some people are born with naturally thicker tendons, which gives them a mechanical advantage when it comes to building strength, but you can also develop the thickness of your tendons by using a combination of accentuated eccentric actions and high rep exercises, especially if the high reps work the muscle over the fullest range of motion possible or emphasize the portion of the range of motion where the muscles and tendons are stretched the most.

Adrenergic Sensitivity

This is also a neurological factor, but it is mostly peripheral rather than central. As a brief explanation, adrenergic receptors interact with adrenaline to either activate or inhibit a certain tissue. The beta-adrenergic receptors, when turned on, activate the tissue. For example, if you activate the beta-adrenergic receptors in the muscle, you increase the muscle strength, power, and speed potential as well as muscle tone. If the beta-adrenergic receptors in the heart are activated by adrenaline, your heart rate and heart contraction strength increase, allowing you to deliver more blood, faster. This is useful for physical activity because it sends more oxygen for energy production to the muscles as well as clears out the metabolites (waste products) of muscle contraction faster. If you bind adrenaline to the beta-adrenergic receptors in the brain, you become more motivated, driven, competitive, and aggressive. You also speed up motor programming and muscle fiber recruitment.

Another important thing to understand about receptors is that they can vary in their response to a hormone or neurotransmitter. If a receptor is *sensitive*, it will have a strong response, meaning that even a small amount of the hormone or neurotransmitter will elicit a strong response (and of course a large amount will lead to an even greater reaction). If a receptor is *resistant*, it will take a very large amount of the hormone or neurotransmitter to elicit a response.

What's even more important is that most receptors can be made more resistant (downregulation) or more sensitive (upregulation). The normal mechanism to achieve this has to do with the amount and frequency of stimulation of a receptor. The more often you bind a hormone or neurotransmitter to a receptor, the more it will start to downregulate (respond less and less to the hormone or neurotransmitter). This happens to an even greater extent if the amount of hormone or neurotransmitter is high. On the other hand, you can make some receptors more sensitive by reducing the frequency at which it is stimulated. The beta-adrenergic receptors are especially prone to downregulation. If they become less sensitive, your performance—both physical (drop in strength and speed, lower endurance and recovery) and mental—will drop considerably.

If you constantly "train on the nerve" (to quote weightlifting legend Alexeyev), the risk of downregulating the beta-adrenergic receptors is great. People who train all-out too often (or too often with a lot of volume) may start to see their performance degrade. They can even start to look worse as their muscle tone diminishes, making them look softer and smaller. This is all because they stimulate their beta-adrenergic receptors too much.

That also explains how deloading and peaking works for strength sports. It has very little to do with glycogen super-compensation. What happens is that the pre-contest training will downregulate the beta-adrenergic receptors to some extent. While the muscles are stronger, some of those gains are hidden by the fact that muscles are made less sensitive to adrenaline.

When you deload or do a peak week, you dramatically reduce training stress, which lowers adrenaline and allows you to upregulate (make yourself more sensitive through less stimulation) your beta-adrenergic receptors, which will make you more responsive to adrenaline and allow you to showcase more of the strength you have.

The take-home message is that doing too much, too often, too hard can make you weaker, and it is something that is extremely common among passionate lifters. As you can see, people can get strong several different ways, which explains why strength comes in all shapes and sizes.

We could have easily included technical mastery of the lifts as a way to get stronger. And it certainly is important to be able to demonstrate your strength in a specific lift. It is one of the reasons why Olympic weightlifters can lift two to three times their body weight from the floor to overhead in an explosive action. However, technical mastery does not really get you stronger. It simply allows you to apply the strength you have to complete a specific movement as efficiently as possible. While technical mastery is extremely important (which is why we have a whole chapter on mastering each of the basic lifts in this plan; see chapters 4 through 9), it is not a *physiological key* to get stronger.

With all of that in mind and a deeper understanding of the factors that can make you stronger, let's look at the effect of the various methods we will be using in this plan.

How the Overload System Methods Work

In chapter 1, we briefly outlined the various methods that are going to be used in the overload system. Now is the time for us to delve deeper into those methods: how they work, how to use them, and how they fit in to the overload system as a whole.

Progressive Range of Motion Training

This training, also known as neurological carryover training (NCT), uses three phenomena to its advantage.

- Supramaximal weights downregulate the GTOs to allow you to use more of your strength potential.
- The more force you have to produce, the more muscle fibers you recruit. If you reach a point where you are recruiting all the available fibers, then further force is produced by making the fast-twitch fibers twitch faster. This is called "firing rate," and it is the key to maximum voluntary strength production. The heavier you go, the more you increase it. Doing it over time will improve your nervous system's capacity to have a higher firing rate.
- Load habituation is a phenomenon in which the more you practice handling a certain load, the easier it becomes to lift and the less stressful it is on the body. In normal training, when your body is habituated to a load and it becomes easier to handle, you add weight to further challenge the body. For example, if you start with 200 pounds (91 kilograms) for 6 reps and it's hard, after a while it becomes a lot easier. If you graduate to 220 pounds (100 kilogram) and 6 reps, it will be the same level of difficulty as the original 200 pounds (91 kilograms) and 6 reps. With NCT, when you

start to be habituated to a load and it becomes much easier than it was the first few times you did it, you make the movement harder not by adding weight but by adding range of motion instead.

I also find that this method offers other benefits:

- If done properly (controlling the eccentric on each rep and respecting the proper mechanics of the movement), the overload done over a progressively larger range of motion dramatically increases active stability, which, as we saw earlier, will make you stronger.
- It gives you a psychological boost because you become used to the feeling of a certain weight. I find that when training for strength and using big weights, a lot of missed lifts occur not because the lifter lacked strength but because they were intimidated by the weight when they unracked it. This *psyches them out*, creating tension through anxiety and negatively affecting lifting technique. Practicing handling supramaximal weights, even if it's over a partial range of motion, will help you better handle the psychological stress of moving those loads over the whole range of motion.
- It allows you to work on technique. It's much easier to make technical adjustments to short-range movements, with less moving parts, than addressing the full movement right away. That's one of the reasons why most Olympic lifting coaches teach the snatch, clean, and jerk by segmenting the movement and gradually building up toward the full lift as the pieces are mastered.

To ensure this method works for you, when doing your partial reps, it is important that your body position and movement are the same as they would be at that point in the full-range movement. The most common example (which we mostly see during simple partial reps training) happens when someone is doing rack pulls from above the knees: They will wedge their knees and lower part of their quad under the bar. This brings the knees far forward, making the torso more upright, allowing them to leverage the weight up by doing something like a quarter squat. You can use a lot more weight like that (but it will not transfer to the full lift) or even when you simply move to below the knees. When I started doing heavy partials at age 20, I would use that *wedging* technique and could do over 1,000 pounds (454 pounds) from above the knees. The only thing was that my full deadlift was a mere 500 pounds (227 kilograms)!

Heck, I remember doing a Strongman competition (if I'm not mistaken it was in 2000, so I was 22 years old) and actually winning the train wheel deadlift against guys who were a ton stronger and bigger than I was. I was 5 ft 9 in. and 190 pounds (86 kilograms), and the next smallest guy was 6 ft 2 in. and 260 pounds (118 kilograms), with a few of the other lifters in the range of 280 to 320 pounds (127 to 145 kilograms). I actually beat a guy who could deadlift 780 pounds (354 kilograms) from the floor (I was doing 550 pounds [250 kilograms]) simply because I could wedge myself under the bar and he couldn't. While that's good for the ego, it will not help you get stronger over the full range of motion, which is the goal of partial lifting, or the progressive range of motion method of lifting.

The basic principle of this method is to start with a very short range on the selected lift. The starting position is on safety pins in a power rack or on blocks, and the initial height will be somewhere in the upper third of the range of motion. I personally believe that you should start with the smallest range of motion possible while still feeling like a lift. For example, in the bench press, I will start from a position that is around two inches from the lockout. The only downside with starting from a very short range is that it lengthens the time it will take you to reach the full range. However, that is actually a benefit as it gives you more time to get habituated to a weight.

You select a load that is 10 to 30 pounds (5 to 14 kilograms) more than your maximum on the full-range lift. How heavy you go really depends on your strength gain potential. For example, if you are already deadlifting 800 pounds (363 kilograms), I doubt that you will be able to add another 30 pounds (14 kilograms) in 6 to 8 weeks, whereas if you are deadlifting 400 pounds (181 pounds), it should be fairly manageable. It's better to be more conservative, anyway. Patience is the greatest attribute a strong person can have. In an ideal world, you should shoot for 12 to 15 reps in that initial position the first time you do it. If you can do more, by all means do, but if you only manage 7 to 11 reps, the load is likely excessive, and you will hit a wall before the end of the cycle.

The goal is to increase the range of motion very gradually (I'm talking about 0.5 to 1.5 inches). The more gradual the progression, the easier the strength transfer will be as you progress through the range of motion. If you go with smaller increases (0.5 inch), you can increase the range every two or three workouts. If you need to use larger increments (1.5 inches), then you will need to do more workouts for each position, four to six workouts ideally.

In a program, we don't have a choice but to write when to increase the range of motion. In reality, you should increase the range only when a certain position is significantly easier than it was. Let's compare that with weight increase in regular lifting: If you did 200 pounds (91 kilograms) and 6 reps, and it took you everything to complete that sixth rep, then going up to 210 pounds (95 kilograms) the next week is likely a bad idea and will lead to rapid stagnation. But when you work up to a point where 200 pounds (91 kilograms) and 6 reps is almost easy, then you are ready to progress. The same thing applies to range of motion training. Do not add range if you don't feel like you have had a progression. For example, if you did 14 reps with 300 pounds (136 kilograms) in your first session, 15 reps in your second session, 15 in your third session, I would say that you are not ready yet to move up in range. That's the art of training, and sadly it cannot be taught in a book.

Obviously, as you increase the range of motion, reps will drop down. It is unrealistic to think that you can start with 15 reps lifted for 2 inches and that after 6 to 8 weeks you'll be able to do the same 15 reps over the full range with the same weight. The method is powerful, but it has its limits! That's why we want to start at a point where you can get 12 to 15 reps in the first position. With a normal rep drop-off, this should allow you to reach 1 to 2 full-range reps at the end of your cycle.

Don't forget, it's perfectly fine to extend the cycle by spending more sessions at a certain range of motion level. I would rather have you take 2 to 3 more weeks to finish your cycle and be successful than force yourself to do it in 6 to 8 weeks and fail because you increased the range before you dominated a certain range of motion.

TRAINING PARAMETERS

PROGRESSIVE RANGE OF MOTION

- *Load*: 10 to 30 pounds (5 to 14 kilograms) more than your current full-range max.
- *Reps:* Variable depending on range.
- *Sets*: 1 to 3.
- *Effort level*: We don't want to go to real failure, as each rep must be done with good technique, but we do need to push ourselves. I'd say keep a rep in the tank.
- *Frequency:* 1 to 2 times per week per movement (I prefer 2).

Supramaximal Partials

The purpose of this method is similar to that of the progressive range of motion (PRM) method, but let's just say that it is the less elegant and more brutish version. The PRM method is more of a high precision method in which you are using a small overload and gradually working toward transferring the capacity to lift that weight over the full range of motion. Supramaximal partials do not share this transfer. Instead, it is simply about creating the greatest overload possible while maintaining a decent range of motion. As such, the starting position can vary depending on the lifter and the lift. We normally use either a low supramaximal partial (starting at around one-half to two-thirds of the range of motion) or high supramaximal partials (doing the last quarter, or even less, of the movement). What I find is that the lower you start, the easier it is to transfer the gains to the full range of motion. However, the higher you start, the heavier you go, the greater the psychological benefit is, and the more effective the exercise becomes to downregulate the GTOs.

Throughout my 20 years of using supramaximal partials, I have also learned that some people can more easily transfer gains made on partial movements than others. These people should use a higher starting position (shorter range of motion) to create the greatest overload possible. Those who are not as efficient at transferring gains made on partial movements should start lower and more likely start just above their weak point (mostly as a tool to strengthen their weak point).

There are several ways of using this approach. Chuck Sipes, who bench-pressed over 560 pounds (254 kilograms) at 220 pounds (100 kilograms) in the 1960s, used "free partials" on his bench press. This meant doing a regular bench press but lowering the bar only one-third of the way down before reversing and pressing it back up.

Anthony Ditillo started his partials from pins. More recently, with the Westside Barbell Conjugate System of training, you have people using boards placed on the chest for the bench press and a box to sit on for squat (they start from pins for the deadlift).

All three approaches work and have their pros and cons. The Sipes free partial method is likely going to transfer better to regular lifting because you are training the eccentric-to-concentric reversal, which you don't do in the other two methods (or not as well or as much). However, it is much harder to be consistent with the range of motion you use because you don't have a reference point for where you need to stop the bar. A lot of people will subconsciously start reducing the range of motion so that they can use more weight. A way to counter that is to use safety pins as markers, lower the bar until it almost touches the pins, and then lift up. This solves the issue, but it can be hurtful to your focus and affect performance for a while.

The Ditillo pin press-pull partials method is the one I personally use the most because you can reset properly on every repetition and because it is the only pure concentric method (where the concentric is not preceded by loading of the muscles and eccentric action or the activation of the stretch reflex). As such, it is a superior method to improve voluntary contraction of the muscles. It is also easy to keep using the same range of motion or to adjust it upward or downward precisely to get the desired training effect. The main drawback is that people subconsciously fail to control the bar properly when they are lowering it back down to the pins. Special attention should be paid to returning the bar slowly and under control to the pins. The complete lack of eccentric or concentric transition (you pause and release tension when the bar is on the pins) also makes it harder to transfer the gains to a regular lift.

The Westside board press and box squats are a middle-of-the-road solution. When the bar is on the boards or when you are seated on the box, your body is still under load. However, when you use pins, it becomes unloaded. If the pause on the boards or box is less than 2 seconds, you still get a stretch reflex (albeit a small one) and train the eccentric-to-concentric transition (less than with the Sipes method but more than with the Ditillo approach). Because you are lowering the bar to a board or sitting down on a box, you can easily regulate the range of motion. I actually like the board press, but I find the box squat potentially hazardous if someone is not technically efficient and doesn't control the bar properly. Although there will be individual differences, I find that you can use the most weight (for the same range) with the partial from pins, followed by the Westside box approach, and finally, the free partials.

Supramaximal partials are much less complex than the PRM method. You simply want to increase the amount of weight you handle over time. However, adding weight should not come at the expense of altering the technique to leverage more weight up; your positions and actions should mirror that part of the range of motion during full-range lifts. I find that to get the most out of partial repetitions, you need to use slightly higher reps than you would with full-range strength work yet use a rep range that will still allow you to load significantly more weight than your maximum on the full-range lift.

I do believe that accumulating a sufficient amount of mechanical work in a set is necessary to maximize both size and strength, and I also believe that the nervous system needs to be able to produce force for the duration of a true maximal effort for the training set to be transferable. For example, a true maximal effort on the bench press might last 3 to 4 seconds (including the eccentric, transition, and concentric phases) and the squat up to 5 seconds. If you do 1, 2, or even 3 partial repetitions, you might not put the muscles under tension for the 4 to 5 seconds minimum you need to make sure that you can keep producing high tension for long enough to complete a full maximal effort—it's always best to have some reserve. It's not a muscle or energy thing. It's mostly about being able to maintain a strong neural drive for the duration of the max effort.

Gymnastic coach Carl Paoli once told me during a session that in gymnastics, when you train for a strength-based skill (iron cross, maltese, etc.), you typically use a duration that is three times what you will need in a routine. I find this to be fairly accurate for partial lifts, too. As such, I feel that supramaximal partials are best performed for sets of 4 to 8 repetitions (depending on the range). This falls in line with Chuck Sipes' method. You can use 2 to 3 reps for short periods of time to work on your capacity to increase you peak force potential, but most of your training on supramaximal work should fall in the range of 4 to 8 repetitions. The shorter the range, the more reps you should do. Why? First, because each rep has a shorter duration and, second, because even when doing 6 to 8 reps on a one-quarter or one-eighth range, you will be able to use a lot more weight than your max on the full lift, whereas if you do a half-range movement, you probably won't be able to use a weight that constitutes an overload if you have to do 8 reps.

With supramaximal partials, you do want to add weight over time, but you should use an old-time Strongman mentality and consider your sets as practice: You want to dominate every rep in your set. Going to failure on partials might actually delay the downregulation of the GTOs. Failing is seen as a dangerous situation by the body, especially when handling supramaximal loads, whereas if you dominate each rep in a set, you tell your body that this load is not dangerous.

The goal is to *add weight over time*, but only do so if you know that you will be able to dominate every repetition. That is the beauty of supramaximal partials: even if you have to stick to the same load for 4, 5, or 6 weeks (or more), it still works because it's still an overload versus your full-range poundage.

TRAINING PARAMETERS

SUPRAMAXIMAL PARTIALS

- *Load*: 40 to 100 pounds (18 to 45 kilograms) more than your full-range maximum (depending on movement, range, and number of reps).
- *Reps*: 4 to 8 with occasional work for 2 to 3 reps for a week or two.
- *Sets*: 2 to 5, often done ramping style (gradually adding weight until you reach your top weight for your last set).
- *Effort level*: You want to dominate each repetition. Only add weight when you know that you will be able to do that.
- *Frequency*: 1 to 2 times per week for a lift (I prefer 2).

Functional Isometrics

I (Christian) have been a huge fan of isometric training since around 2003. My first experience seriously using isometrics occurred after I had stopped training for Olympic weightlifting for two years. It was a period during which I focused mostly on "bodybuilding-type work." I read Bob Hoffman's books on overcoming isometrics (basically pushing or pulling against the pins in a power rack with an empty bar) and on functional isometrics, which combined a very short-range movement with an isometric. This is achieved by using two sets of safety pins a few inches apart from one another. You start the loaded barbell on the lower set of pins and press it into the second set of pins and hold it there while pressing and pulling as hard as you can. Because Hoffman was a weightlifting (Olympic lifting) proponent, the system was originally marketed for lifters, not bodybuilders. I decided to try it while refocusing on the Olympic lifts to see how well it would work.

I would do functional isometrics three times a week (I found that pure isometrics did not motivate me as much, and there was no feedback regarding progression) and snatch, clean, and jerk and squat once a week (which was the original recommendation), and I regained my previous best performance level in less than a month, then actually achieved a snatch and squat PR a few weeks later: I snatched 315 pounds (143 kilograms), whereas my previous best had been 291 pounds (132 kilograms), and squatted 550 pounds (250 kilograms) times 5 reps and 600 pounds (272.5 kilograms) for a single, whereas my previous max had been 550 pounds (250 kilograms) for a single rep. As you can imagine, I was easily convinced of the power of functional isometrics! But in my typical fashion, as soon as I find out how well something works, I wanted to try something new!

To understand why functional isometrics work so well, you must first understand the benefits of pure isometrics—that is, isometrics where there is no movement. There are two main forms of pure isometrics:

- *Overcoming isometrics*: producing force while there is no movement but while attempting to lift the immovable resistance (e.g., pushing or pulling against pins)
- *Yielding isometrics*: producing force while there is no movement, attempting to prevent the weight from falling down (e.g., holding a barbell at the mid-range of a curl)

Functional isometrics are a combination of a partial movement (more often a supramaximal partial) over a few inches, ending with an overcoming isometric. Overcoming isometrics are effective for strength because they increase four important things:

Muscle fiber recruitment: During a maximal overcoming isometric effort, you can recruit up to 10 percent more muscle fibers than during a maximal concentric and dynamic effort.

Fast-twitch fiber firing rate: On top of better fiber recruitment, if you try to produce as much force as humanly possible during an overcoming isometric action, you can reach a higher firing rate in the fast-twitch fibers. This is likely the most important muscle factor in reaching a very high level of strength, and you need to train it to improve it.

Recruitment of the synergistic muscles: The muscles that assist the prime movements in a lift have been shown to be recruited to a greater extent during a maximal isometric action than a maximal concentric action by an average of 13 percent. This can, over time, train your nervous system to better use these muscles during a regular lift, which will obviously increase your strength.

Recruitment of the antagonist muscles: Antagonist muscles, those that oppose the prime movers (e.g., biceps in a bench press), also get recruited to a greater extent during a maximal isometric effort. The initial reaction would be to think that this would actually decrease strength because the antagonist would resist more, making it harder to lift. In reality, it actually makes you stronger because the reason for this increased recruitment is to increase active joint stability. Ironically, being able to increase the activation of the antagonist muscles at certain phases of a lift (e.g., activating the hamstrings more when you are at the half squat position) will make you stronger because as the body feels more stable and better braced, the protective inhibition will not be turned on as easily and you can use a greater proportion of your strength potential.

Maximal overcoming actions thus train the nervous system to be more efficient at motor tasks that will be useful for you to increase overall strength production. The main drawback is that pure isometric actions have specific effects:

The strength gained occurs mostly at the joint being trained. There is some carryover for up to 15 degrees, but the further you get from the train angle, the lesser the transfer will be.

The strength gained in purely isometric actions are harder to transfer to dynamic movements. The muscle recruitment pattern is different between isometric, concentric, and eccentric actions. As such, improving the neurological components involved in force production in one type of contraction doesn't necessarily transfer well to other types. Some people are more efficient at doing it than others, though. That's why I prefer the use of functional isometrics instead of pure overcoming isometrics.

The fact that you initiate the set with a concentric action makes the gains more transferable to a dynamic movement. It also increases the strength transfer range. What I like the most about functional isometrics is their effectiveness at strengthening a specific portion of a lift. They can also almost perfectly mimic the sticking point of a lift. Essentially, a sticking point occurs when the barbell speed slows down at a specific position in the range of motion. As lift speed and momentum decreases, you require a lot more effort to be able to push through, and if the momentum stops completely and speed drops to zero, you miss the lift. Functional isometrics stimulate and train the nervous system to be able to grind and produce an even greater neural drive when the bar reaches that sticking point and the momentum is killed.

From the previous discussion, you probably already understand the usefulness of functional isometrics to fix a weak point, and it is indeed the main use for this method in my system. Another is to fill the range of motion gap, if you are using the PRM method, for instance, and are not yet in the low ranges. In this case, I will often use functional isometrics in the low portion of the movement to make sure that it will be strong once you reach a full range of motion lift.

I should also mention that functional isometrics were originally designed as a stand-alone training system to be used as the only training method to gain strength over the full range of motion. This required the use of three positions per lift. It is not something I use, or if I do, it is extremely rare. I find it more effective to combine lifting and isometrics, using isometrics to strengthen a specific range only.

The original recommendations were to hold the bar against pins (trying to push or pull on them as hard as you could) for 8 to 12 seconds. If you could not keep the bar in contact with the pins for 8 seconds, you decreased the weight; if you could hold more than 12 seconds, you had to add weight. I generally agree with these recommendations because this method stays in the phosphagen energy system (which is what you want for intense neurological work), and it is long enough to train the nervous system to maintain a maximal neural drive to be able to grind through a sticking point.

I sometimes recommend 6 to 9 seconds, but really anything in the zone of 6 to 12 seconds will work just fine. As I explained, I personally prefer to use only one position, either to train a neglected range or to target a weak point. If you are using functional isometrics to fix a weak point, the second (highest) set of pins should be just below or at the sticking point (and the lower set of pins about 2 to 3 inches lower than your sticking point).

TRAINING PARAMETERS

FUNCTIONAL ISOMETRICS

- *Load*: As much as you can use for the prescribed duration.
- *Reps*: 1 rep of 6 to 12 seconds per set.
- *Sets*: 3 to 4, but only the last set is a maximal effort.
- *Effort level*: The last set is an all-out effort. In the first 2 to 3 sets, you work up to your top weight.
- *Frequency*: 1 to 2 times per week for a lift (I prefer 2).

Isometronics

This is essentially an advanced form of functional isometrics. I tend to prefer functional isometrics to strengthen a weak point and isometronics to strengthen a specific range, but only once the lifter has experience with regular functional isometrics. In an isometronic set, you also use two sets of safety pins that are set up exactly the same way as for a functional isometric set. Just like with functional isometrics, you press and pull the bar from the lower set of pins up to the higher set of pins. The main difference is that with isometronics, you actually do several reps going from pin to pin, and you do not hold against the higher set of pins, except for the last repetition. This was a favorite of Anthony Ditillo, who used it extensively on pressing and deadlifting movements.

The best use for isometronics is to strengthen a range of motion that is neglected by other methods or to strengthen half or a third of a movement. While it will work to strengthen a sticking point, it is not as effective as functional isometrics for that specific purpose because the load used will be much smaller (it will normally be around 70 to 75 percent of your maximum).

I also find isometronics to be an effective tool to stimulate muscle growth. You do 4 to 8 partial repetitions (depending on the position in the range of motion and the length of the range you select). On the last rep, you push against the higher set of pins and try to keep the bar in contact for as long as possible. Normally you want to use a weight with which you can do your planned reps and be able to hold for about 6 seconds on the last rep. To finish the set, you attempt to do

TRAINING PARAMETERS

ISOMETRONICS

- *Load*: While it will vary depending on the position being trained, in our system it is more often used for the lower half of the range of motion, so 70 to 75 percent of the full-range max is a good starting point.
- *Reps*: 4 to 8 plus a 6-second isometric and an attempted last rep.
- *Sets*: I would only recommend one all-out work set. You can take a few sub-maximal and gradually heavier sets to work up to the work set poundage.
- *Effort level*: The last set is an all-out effort.
- *Frequency*: 1 to 2 times per week for a lift.

one last repetition after the isometric. There is a good chance that you will not be able to get it, but you push and pull as hard as you can, trying to get it, for up to 6 seconds. As you can see, it's a very demanding method!

Supramaximal Holds

This is technically a form of functional isometrics in that you will lift the bar over a short range of motion starting from safety pins (top quarter or top eighth of the range) and then hold the position for 9 to 12 seconds. It is a very short partial followed by a hold (yielding isometric). *Note*: There is also a powerlifting version where you don't really lift the bar. If you do it on a squat, you unrack the bar and just walk out as if you were going to squat it, and in the bench, you get a handoff by your spotter. This allows you to practice your walkout and handoff skills, which are often neglected when training for a powerlifting competition. A lot of lifters actually miss their lift because of a poor walkout or handoff.

The main use of this approach is really just to get the body and mind used to being under a huge amount of load. Your focus should be to keep everything as tight as possible when holding the weight. Lifting heavy is, first and foremost, dependent on the capacity to avoid *strength leaks*, and this is done by keeping the whole body braced and under tension when under load. Like with all supramaximal work, there will obviously be a positive effect on GTOs inhibition over time.

The first time I used supramaximal holds was when I did Dr. Fred Hatfield's 80 days powerlifting program. As a sidenote, I'm proud to have been involved with Dr. Hatfield as a contributor of articles to his website some 23 years ago and also having published a website with his son Fred Hatfield II. Dr. Hatfield (Dr. Squat) was one of the first to apply science to training. He was a great teacher and also one heck of a lifter, with a 1,014-pound (460-kilogram) squat at 45 years of age! Chuck Sipes was also a big proponent of very heavy holds. He actually treated them like an exercise with multiple sets. However, Sipes was known for his inhumane training volume (he would do 3 full training sessions per day, training for up to 5 hours a day). Not everyone can take as much punishment as he did.

The main differences between the way Sipes and Hatfield used supramaximal holds was the intent and the load used. Sipes used it as a strength-building tool, going as heavy as he could for 6 to 9 seconds. That was sometimes 150 to 200 pounds (68 to 91 kilograms) more than his full-range maximum! To do that, Sipes lifted the bar from pins over one-eighth of the range of motion, then he would hold. Hatfield used supramaximal holds simply to get the body used to handling a bit more weight than his maximum, to prepare for handling bigger weights in competition without being surprised by the load. He would use around 5 percent more than his current maximum and hold for 6 seconds. On squats, Hatfield would walk the bar out, and on the bench he would *unrack* it himself from the rack and bring it to the start position of the bench (he didn't use the method on deadlifts). Basically, he also used the holds to train the walkout and get into the starting position of a competition bench.

The Sipes method was seen as an exercise in itself, and you would normally work up until you reached your top weight, whereas in the Hatfield method you would just do 1 to 2 holds after your work sets on squats or bench, so there was no reason for a gradual load ramp-up. I personally use the Sipes method more often but normally stick to the Hatfield method with competitive powerlifters. Just understand the difference and when each is the best tool to use.

TRAINING PARAMETERS

SUPRAMAXIMAL HOLDS

Sipes Method

- *Load*: Working up to as heavy as you can.
- *Reps*: 1, holding for 6 to 12 seconds.
- *Sets*: You gradually work up to the heaviest weight you can hold for the prescribed duration (only do a single set at the top weight).
- *Effort level*: The last set is an all-out effort.
- *Frequency*: 1 to 2 times per week for a lift.

Hatfield Method

- *Load*: 5 to 10 percent more than your max on the full-range movement.
- *Reps*: 1, holding for 6 to 12 seconds.
- *Sets*: 1 to 2 after your work sets on the full-range lift.
- *Effort level*: Focus on the quality of the walkout and the solidity of the position.
- *Frequency*: When you train the target lift heavy, or heaviest, in your microcycle.

Clusters

Cluster training is my go-to method for rapidly increasing strength. It never fails. Clusters consist of rest periods between all the reps in your set. One set becomes a series of single reps with very short rest periods in between. While you can do clusters with any type of loading and rest intervals, the traditional cluster requires you to use a load of around 90 percent of your 1RM (which is normally your 3RM load) and to do 4 to 6 reps with that weight. You would do so by resting anywhere from 10 to 20 seconds between reps, depending on the exercise. A set could look like this:

Unrack the bar and do rep 1.

Rack the bar and rest 15 seconds.

Unrack the bar and do rep 2.

Rack the bar and rest 15 seconds.

Unrack the bar and do rep 3.

Rack the bar and rest 15 seconds.

Unrack the bar and do rep 4.

Rack the bar and rest 15 seconds.

Unrack the bar and do rep 5.

Rack the bar (end of set).

Several factors explain why clusters can influence strength gains:

- You recruit and fatigue the fast-twitch muscle fibers.
- You develop the capacity to make the fast-twitch fibers twitch as fast as possible. This is called a high firing rate.

- You build muscle mass.
- You desensitize the GTOs.
- You become more psychologically comfortable with the lift.

You achieve maximum fast-twitch fiber recruitment when the load on the bar is around 80 to 82 percent of your maximum at that moment. Sure, you can get there by using lighter weights and using fatigue to increase the relative load of the bar, but by using clusters with 88 to 90 percent of your max, you are recruiting all those fast-twitch fibers from the get-go. As a result, you won't have any reps that simply drain energy.

It is not enough to recruit the fast-twitch fibers. The real strength gains will come from improving your capacity to use a high firing rate. This is a motor skill, and motor skill acquisition depends not only on the number of repetitions done with the skill emphasized but on the ratio of "good" and "bad" reps. The closer you are to your maximum strength, the higher the firing rate. Firing rate increases the most when you need even more force and you can no longer recruit more fibers. At 90 percent, you have a very high firing rate from the start. If you do 5 cluster reps with 90 percent, you'll get 5 reps with a very high firing rate and no reps with a low firing rate. From a motor-learning standpoint, that's golden. Now compare that to doing 10 reps with 70 percent. Because of fatigue, you will still end up with 5 to 6 reps where the fast-twitch fibers are maximally recruited and probably 3 reps with a high firing rate. But you also get 5 reps with a lower firing rate. From a motor-learning perspective, this is vastly inferior. It's like trying to play golf and doing 30 great swings, 20 suboptimal ones, and 50 bad ones. Chances are you won't improve rapidly.

Clusters are also very good at building muscle. Hypertrophy has a lot to do with the number of maximally effective reps. A maximally effective rep is one where you are recruiting as many fast-twitch fibers as possible. Since these have the greatest growth potential, it's all about stimulating them as much as possible. As we just saw, when the load represents 80 percent of the max weight you can lift at that moment, you will be recruiting the max number of fast-twitch fibers you can recruit. You can get there by using less weight because each rep fatigues you. As you are fatiguing, your strength will go down (by 2 to 4 percent per rep), so the weight on the bar is relatively heavier compared to what you can lift.

Relative load refers to how much of your strength potential a load represents *at that precise moment in time*. If we start with 80 percent on the bar, then the relative load before we initiate the first rep is 70 percent, as we have not accumulated any fatigue yet. But let's say we have performed 3 reps with that load. If our max force output fatigues at 3 percent per repetition, then by the time we have performed 3 reps we have also accumulated 9 percent fatigue. This means that the relative load has now risen from 70 percent to 79 percent (see table 2.1).

As you can see, by rep 5, you would have maximally effective reps. That gives you six maximally effective reps in the set. Now let's look at a cluster set in table 2.2. Because of the rest period you'll have some recovery, so fatigue is a bit slower.

Clusters allow you to get as many growth-producing reps as you normally would in a higher-rep set, without having to waste energy doing reps that don't contribute to growth.

TABLE 2.1 Relative Load and Fatigue: Straight Set

Rep	Weight on bar	Fatigue level	Relative weight
1	70%	0%	70%
2	70%	3%	73%
3	70%	6%	76%
4	70%	9%	79%
5	70%	12%	82%
6	70%	15%	85%
7	70%	18%	88%
8	70%	21%	91%
9	70%	24%	94%
10	70%	27%	97%

TABLE 2.2 Relative Load and Fatigue: Cluster Set

Rep	Weight on bar	Fatigue level	Relative weight
1	90%	0%	90%
2	90%	1.5%	91.5%
3	90%	3%	93%
4	90%	4.5%	94.5%
5	90%	6%	96%
6	90%	7.5%	97.5%

Because all the reps in a cluster will be above 85 percent of what you can lift at that moment (it will range from 90 to 100 percent at the beginning of the rep), not only are you recruiting all your available fast-twitch fibers from the start, but each of those reps has a high firing rate. The better you are at having your fibers twitch fast, the higher the firing rate. This means you will be able to produce more force.

Developing the capacity to have the fibers fire at a high firing rate is a motor skill. It's not only the number of reps with a high firing rate that counts, but the ratio of reps with a high firing rate to reps with a normal one. In a cluster of 6 reps, all 6 reps have a high firing rate. That's awesome for motor learning. In our 70 percent set above, you'll have 3 reps with a firing rate comparable to what it is during a cluster, 5 reps with a low firing rate, and 2 reps with a moderate firing rate. From a motor-learning standpoint, this is vastly inferior to clusters because of the inferior ratio.

What if we compare a set of 5 cluster reps and a regular set of 5 reps? In the regular set, you also have no wasted repetitions and do all the reps with a pretty high firing rate. This is true; sets of 5 repetitions are awesome for strength and size, but clusters are just a little bit better because of the higher average load. In a cluster, you use around 90 percent of your max, and with regular sets of 5 reps, between 80 and 85 percent. While fatigue evens out the relative load at the end of the set, the heavier weight still has a greater mechanical load than the lighter one, which will cause more muscle damage. In a cluster with 90 percent versus a set of 5 reps at 82 percent, you still have 3 more reps with a very high firing rate (the closer you are to a 100 percent effort, the higher the firing rate). With 82 percent, it will take you 2 to 3 reps to reach a relative load of 90 percent like you have in the cluster.

Finally, during a cluster set, peak power, force, and velocity are better maintained from rep to rep, which makes for more quality reps and better motor learning. For all these reasons, clusters are my favorite strength-building method. This method builds as much muscle mass as regular sets of 8 to 12 repetitions because of the number of maximally effective reps. Clusters train the nervous system as well as the max effort method, maybe even better because of the higher number of reps.

The most popular cluster recommendations, which were popularized by Charles Poliquin, are actually not optimal for most people. Strong individuals or people with a high ratio of fast-twitch fibers will have trouble with the parameters, especially the 15 to 20 seconds between reps recommended by Poliquin. The inability to recover between reps and sets means it will be difficult to be able to use more weight than you would for a normal set of that number of reps.

That's why I prefer to use one of the original versions, developed by international weightlifting coach Carl Miller. The Miller accumulation cluster uses 87.5 to 92 percent of your maximum for a target of 4 to 6 repetitions, but instead of the 15 to 20 seconds of rest recommended by Poliquin, it uses 30 to 45 seconds between repetitions. The Miller intensification cluster uses up to 92.5 to 97.5 percent and shoots for 2 to 3 repetitions per set, with 40 to 60 seconds of rest between reps. I personally recommend doing 2 to 3 sets of clusters, with the last one being an all-out effort (getting as many reps as possible, even if that means going above the prescribed number); the second set is hard, but you should still dominate each rep, and the first work set is about an 8 on a 10-point rating of perceived exertion (RPE) scale. In this system, a lot of the work sets for the full-range main lifts are done either as clusters, waves, or pyramids.

Accentuated Eccentrics

Most competitive athletes are weaker eccentrically in comparison to their concentric strength. This is because, in the training of athletes, the eccentric phase of the movement is rarely focused on (same for isometric actions) and the various types of muscle action have different recruitment patterns. As such, it is possible to greatly increase concentric strength while only gaining a moderate improvement in eccentric strength.

Ideally, we would want maximum eccentric strength (the maximum amount of weight you can lower under control and with solid technique) that is at least 40 percent higher than your maximum concentric strength. For example, an athlete who can squat 400 pounds (181 pounds) should be able to lower 560 pounds (254 kilograms) under control (controlling the weight all the way to the low position) either by using weight releasers or doing pure eccentrics lowered to the safety pins of a power rack.

An athlete who can bench press 315 pounds (143 kilograms) should be able to lower 440 pounds (200 kilograms) to their chest, controlling it the whole way.

Few athletes have that level of eccentric strength. Yet some elite strength athletes who have used eccentric training methods—shot-putter Werner Gunthor, for example—have reached an eccentric-to-concentric ratio as high as 2:1 (200 percent)! Gunthor, who had a body weight of 290 pounds (132 kilograms) on a 6 ft 7 in. frame, looked like a hurdler of 175 pounds (79 kilograms) when doing plyometric drills. (Note: Gunthor's coach Jean-Pierre Egger has been my greatest influence on how I work with athletes.)

In reality, the higher your eccentric-to-concentric ratio is, the greater your potential to further increase strength. I like to see eccentric strength as strength reserve. If you can lower 560 pounds (254 kilograms) under control, it means that your muscles are physically capable of producing enough force for the muscles to handle that weight.

It also means that your GTOs, the protective mechanisms that prevent you from using all your muscle strength potential, are permissive enough to allow your body to lift 560 pounds (254 pounds). I have already spoken about the importance of GTOs when it comes to maximal strength development, so I won't bore you by going into detail on this again. But this is one of the main reasons why most elite weightlifters aren't more muscular than lower-class lifters.

Other benefits of training eccentrically are that the eccentric muscle action tends to stimulate muscle growth mostly in the distal portions of your muscles; the parts of the muscles closer to the tendons will receive more growth stimulus and the tendons themselves will also be strengthened more. This has three positive effects:

- It reduces the occurrence of musculoskeletal injuries. In fact, the higher your eccentric-to-concentric strength ratio is, the less likely you are to tear a muscle.
- By thickening the tendons, you can store more elastic energy during explosive actions; that elastic, or potential, energy can be used in subsequent concentric action to produce more force (making you stronger and more powerful).
- Thicker tendons allow you to produce more force without inhibition.

It is my belief and experience that emphasizing the eccentric is the nuclear weapon of strength gains and performance improvement. It leads to very rapid changes in force production, and as such, it should be included in the training of every athlete.

One of the reasons that emphasizing the eccentric is so effective is that the fast-twitch fibers are preferentially recruited during an eccentric action (especially an eccentric overload). During an intense eccentric action, fewer muscle fibers are recruited, even though you are stronger, but it is mostly fast-twitch fibers that are recruited. As such, these fibers are under a greater load. The amount of force required to control the weight is divided over fewer total fibers; therefore, each recruited fiber has to produce more force. This represents a very strong stimulus for both growth and strength improvement.

When it comes to concentric strength (e.g., regular lifting strength), lifting heavier weights is more effective than lifting light loads. The same applies to eccentric training. Lowering maximal loads under control is more effective at building strength than lowering moderate loads more slowly or for more reps. However, maximal lowering, just like maximal lifting, requires preparation work; you cannot simply jump right into it. If your muscles, tendons, and nervous system or your technical efficiency is not up to par, you risk injuries and you won't be able to fully benefit from the heavy methods.

Even though the maximal (eccentrics with 90 to 100 percent of your maximum concentric strength) and supramaximal (eccentrics with 105 to 140 percent of your max concentric strength) are the most effective for athletes who require rapid and drastic increases in strength, the lighter methods using slow eccentrics for more reps are required to prepare the body for the rigors of the heavy methods. In this chapter, I will focus on the eccentric overloads. Slow eccentrics, which are used in the program too, are simply regular exercises performed with a slow eccentric or lowering phase (5 to 6 seconds normally).

For these methods, the average intensity is the average of the eccentric and concentric load used. For example, if you use 100 percent of your concentric maximum on the eccentric and 70 percent on the concentric, the average intensity would be 85 percent. I see no reason to load more than 120 percent of your concentric 1RM on the eccentric. The risks outweigh the potential benefit. If you developed great eccentric strength and if 2 reps with 120 percent on the eccentric, lowering the bar in 3 seconds, is no longer challenging, then slow down the eccentric to 4 to 5 seconds per rep. If 2 reps with 120 percent done in 4 to 5 seconds becomes too easy, then increase the reps to 3 or 4.

Near-Maximal Eccentrics (Average Intensity 80 to 85 Percent)

With this method, we use either weight releasers or a power rack. We want to use 90 percent of your concentric maximum during the eccentric phase and 70 percent on the concentric phase. If you are using weight releasers, it is pretty straightforward: Put 70 percent on the bar and an extra 10 percent per releaser. If you are using the power rack, you lower the bar to the safety pins and your partners remove some weight. To make it simple, load the bar with 70 percent, put collars on, then add 10 percent per side outside the collars. In both cases, we need to use a cluster approach (resting 15 to 20 seconds between reps to allow the partners to either put the weight or releasers back on). Rack the bar between reps. Perform 4 to 6 reps per set (RPE of 8 to 8.5). The eccentric phase is performed under control (3 to 4 seconds) for the whole range of motion. You lift with as much speed as you can.

Maximal Eccentrics (Average Intensity 85 to 90 Percent)

This is exactly like the preceding method in application, only the loading differs. You use an eccentric load of 100 percent of your maximum concentric strength (your 1RM on a lift) and 75 to 80 percent on the concentric. If you are using releasers, you load the bar with 75 to 80 percent and add an extra 10 to 12.5 percent per releaser. If you are doing the set in a power rack, you load 75 to 80 percent, put collars on, and add an extra 10 to 12.5 percent per side outside the collars. The eccentric is done under control (3 to 4 seconds) for the whole range of motion, and you perform 3 to 4 reps per set.

Supramaximal Eccentrics (Average Intensity 90 to 95 Percent)

Again, this is the same application as the previous two methods, only the loading is now 105 to 110 percent on the eccentric and 75 to 80 percent on the concentric. (There is no need to go heavier than 80 percent on the concentric for any eccentric method since that is not what we are trying to emphasize.) The eccentric is done a bit faster (2 to 3 seconds) compared to the other methods, but it is still under control all the way, and 1 to 2 reps are done per set.

Advanced Supramaximal Eccentrics (Average Intensity 95 to 100 Percent)

Same approach still, but now the eccentric load is 115 to 120 percent (the concentric stays at 75 to 80 percent). This is obviously a very advanced approach and should only be used when the athlete has already built significant eccentric strength. The eccentric duration is 2 to 3 seconds under control the whole way, and 1 to 2 reps are done.

TRAINING PARAMETERS

ACCENTUATED ECCENTRICS

Obviously, this varies depending on the method that you use. The more intense methods will obviously require the use of less overall volume. Since all of these methods use a cluster approach, I program them in essentially the same manner that I would clusters. I use the average intensity (i.e., the average of eccentric load and concentric) as the loading parameter. The only difference is that I lower the volume a little to take into account the extra neurological stress of the heavier eccentric (and also the instability added by the weight releasers if you are using them). If you go back to the earlier section on clusters, you can use the Miller cluster methods as a good guide.

Stato-Dynamic Method (Paused Lifting)

Stato-dynamic refers to combining static and dynamic work within a set. In plain terms, it means including pauses somewhere in your reps or set. There are multiple possible applications of the stato-dynamic method.

Pre-Fatigue Stato-Dynamic

Here you start your set with an isometric hold in a key position of the lift. It is normally at the position of highest tension. On movements like a bench press, military press, squat, and deadlift, it is usually performed at the mid-range point of the lift; in exercises like rows and pull-ups, the peak contraction position is preferred. This is held for 10 to 30 seconds (depending on the goal), and the normal reps are immediately done after the hold. This method is used mostly to improve lifting technique by better programming a key position in the lift or to improve mind-muscle connection. It uses the lightest weights of all the stato-dynamic methods (60 to 70 percent of maximum). This method is useful for preparing the body to lift heavy weights safely rather than to directly build strength as such, and 4 to 8 reps can be done after the hold.

Intra-Rep Stato-Dynamic

In this version, you include 1 to 3 holds on each repetition. The duration of each hold depends on the number of holds:

- *1 hold per rep* = 4 to 6 seconds
- *2 holds per rep* = 3 to 4 seconds
- *3 holds per rep* = 2 to 3 seconds

The holds can be performed during the concentric or eccentric phase as follows:

- *Holds during the concentric:* This method is best used with *only one hold* just above or below the weak point of the lift to strengthen it by forcing your muscles to do the job without relying on momentum. You must overcome inertia, thus improving your capacity to contract your muscles at that part of the range of motion.
- *Holds during the eccentric:* This method is best used with 2 to 3 holds throughout the range of motion to improve your capacity to maintain posture and tension throughout. It is effective for lifters who lose either posture/positioning or tension when lifting heavy.

The number of reps will vary depending on why you are using the method:

- *For strength*: 2 to 5 reps
- *For hypertrophy*: 4 to 8 reps

Post-Fatigue Stato-Dynamic

Here you perform your regular set, and at the end of your set, you hold a certain position for as long as possible. This is effective to both increase hypertrophy stimulation and to strengthen a key position in the lift. I like to use either the position of highest tension or the stretched position (when it's doable and there is still tension in that position). The former will be better for strength development; the latter is a bit more effective for hypertrophy. The biggest benefit, though, is improving active mobility and preventing injury (see the upcoming section on loaded stretching).

Stato-dynamic methods can be used on the main lift or on the main assistance exercise. They are most effective in lifters who have problems maintaining tension and posture throughout a lift or someone who has an inconsistent lifting technique. A stato-dynamic method can also be a good way for strong lifters to give their body a break because it forces them to use less weight on the bar compared to their regular lifts while still providing a strong stimulation.

Very High Repetitions

In the book *Science of Sport Training*, Thomas Kurz wrote about the benefits of very high repetitions per set (20 to 30 or even up to 50+) on developing the tendons. I personally first learned about very high repetitions from Louie Simmons and Westside Barbell. I then learned (and this detail attaches this method to the underlying theme of the book) that Eugene Sandow used the approach quite a bit in the 1800s.

As we saw earlier, having thick and resilient tendons is a prerequisite for developing superstrength. It is also very important to minimize the risk of injury from constant heavy lifting. While heavy lifting and supramaximal work are effective at downregulating the tendons' protective mechanisms, it's lighter work with very high reps that is best suited to thickening the tendons. This is probably because tendons receive less blood flow than muscles and require a lot more mechanical work to be stimulated to develop. High reps are used for remedial exercises. These are mostly isolation movements focusing on the development of one main muscle working around one joint.

To get the best results possible both for the development of the muscles and tendons, we also want to use exercises where the muscle can be worked over the fullest range of motion possible while still being under tension in that stretched position. Stretching the tendons and muscles is a big key to development through mechanical stress.

Just because your main goal might be to get brutally strong doesn't mean that everything you do should be done heavy for low reps! In this system, we already have *a lot* of heavy work. And not just heavy, supramaximal heavy! The nervous system and muscles already receive all they need (and more) to develop superstrength with the main lift work, the partials, holds, and functional isometrics. Not to mention that the main assistance work is done with fairly low reps and heavy weight too (typically 5 to 8 reps per set). There is no sense and very limited benefit to continuing to pound the body with heavy loads on the remedial exercises. These remedial exercises are here to develop specific muscles and your tendons, and higher reps with a concentrated effort are better for that purpose.

You may also think that you can't build muscle with 20 to 30 reps per set, but you can.

Using very high reps is straightforward and doesn't require much explanation. You want a continuous effort (so no rest, myo-reps, or muscle-rounds) to achieve the target number. One thing we can do, however, is finish a set with partial repetitions (in the portion where the muscle is lengthened the most) if you can't get to the prescribed number because of muscle fatigue or excessive burning (hydrogen ions and lactate accumulation). If these partials are done under control (not yanked) and in the portion when the muscle and tendons are lengthened, it will work for our purpose.

The repetition style is important, too. Think of contracting then stretching the muscle instead of lifting the weight. And focus on maintaining a good mind-muscle connection and quality muscle tension throughout the whole range of motion.

TRAINING PARAMETERS

VERY HIGH REPETITIONS

- *Load*: Around 50 percent of your 1RM.
- *Reps*: 20 to 30, using partial repetitions if necessary.
- *Sets*: 3, typically.
- *Effort level*: You want to reach failure but without resorting to compensation or momentum to get the reps in.
- *Frequency*: 1 exercise usually, for one or two of the main muscle groups involved in the pattern of the day.

Loaded Stretching

I hate stretching . . . hate it! It has always felt like a total waste of gym time and is as boring as hell, yet neglecting it can lead to big problems down the road. This is why I love loaded stretching: It doesn't feel like a waste of time because

I'm simultaneously building muscle and getting an amazing pump from it. Want to learn about this amazing method that will help you add new muscle to your body while also making you bulletproof? Then read on!

First, a little history. The concept of stretching a muscle while simultaneously contracting it to build muscle is nothing new. Chuck Sipes was hanging from a chin-up bar with a weight attached to his waist as his primary lat builder back in the early 1960s. John Parrillo was intensely pushing fascial stretches to build muscle as early as the 1980s. He used 28 different loaded stretches to help build muscle. Dante Trudel, inventor of the popular DC training bodybuilding method, became an early proponent of loaded stretching for bodybuilding and was the first to popularize the use of heavy weights to load stretches. Successful bodybuilding experts like John Meadows and Dr. Scott Stevenson are also big proponents of loaded stretching for maximum growth. In the performance world, Jay Schroedder became a huge advocate of long-lasting loaded stretches not only to build muscle but also to work on proper muscle recruitment patterns. At about the same time, Tony Schwartz wrote a chapter on this type of training in my book *Theory and Application of Modern Strength and Power Methods*. All that being said, we must not forget that this type of training actually originates from the training of gymnasts and likely dates back more than 60 years.

The concept is simple: Put a muscle (or several muscles) in a stretched position while also contracting it hard. Basically, you are stretching a tensed muscle. This type of training can increase size, strength, and performance and help prevent injuries. Plus, it gives very rapid results!

Loaded stretching works with any exercise in which the target muscle reaches an elongated position at the end of the eccentric portion: flies, dips, push-ups, hands-on blocks, split squats (feet on blocks), overhead dumbbell triceps extensions, overhead squats, Romanian deadlifts, chin-ups, and so on. The concept is simple: Slowly go down to the end of the eccentric portion of the movement (where the target muscle is stretched) and try to hold that position as long as tolerable. As you fatigue, your range of motion will increase because you cannot hold the position anymore (owing to muscle fiber fatigue), but you still try to maintain the position. It then becomes a really slow eccentric. You stop the set when the burn is unbearable.

Loaded stretching is so effective because it stimulates several different pathways to elicit a positive response through many mechanisms. Here, I will address each of these pathways and how they help us reach our goal of being as strong and jacked as possible.

Loaded Stretching and Hypertrophy

Loaded, or tensed, stretching is effective at stimulating muscle growth. Here are the reasons why it works.

mTor Activation

First, you need to understand what mTor is (a protein/enzyme) and what it does (plays a key role in regulating cellular proliferation). It works basically like a switch, whereas protein synthesis (muscle building) is the light. To be even more precise, mTor is like a light switch with intensity settings; the more you turn it on, the more light is being produced. Same thing with protein synthesis; the more you turn on mTor, the more muscle you will build.

Loaded stretching significantly activates mTor because it combines the two types of contractions that have the greatest impact on mTor: accentuated eccentrics and placing the muscle under load in the stretched position. However, to make these types of muscle actions effective at activating mTor, you need to use a significant external load. A general guideline is that if you can hold a position for longer than a minute, the load is insufficient

Occlusion Effect

When a muscle is contracting hard, blood flow to that muscle is restricted. The same thing happens when a muscle is stretched. So loaded stretching, which combines both conditions, significantly restricts blood flow to the muscle. This has two effects: First, it prevents the disposal of metabolites (e.g., lactate and hydrogen ions), and second, it deprives the muscle of oxygen. Both of these conditions lead to the release of local growth factors that can help with hypertrophy—specifically, IGF-1 and its splice variant MGF, which are the most anabolic hormones in the body involved in cellular growth and muscle cell growth, respectively.

Reactive Hyperemia

When the body senses that the working muscles lack oxygen and can't get rid of the accumulating metabolites (because blood to the muscles is restricted), it will try to divert more blood flow to the working muscles to increase cardiac output. If you maintain the stretch and contraction, blood flow continues to be restricted. When you finally release the muscle tension, there is a hyper-compensation in terms of the amount of blood that flows to the muscles. If that blood is loaded with nutrients (pre-workout nutrition), then you can shuttle more nutrients to that muscle, which can also contribute to protein synthesis. Furthermore, when loaded stretching is performed at the end of the workout, you can get more growth out of the heavier work you performed before the stretch, and you will also recover faster from your session.

Fiber Recruitment and Fatigue

If you use the proper load, you will reach full muscle fiber recruitment very early in the set, and this is amplified by the lack of oxygen (due to blood flow restriction). The body will naturally turn to the glycolytic fast-twitch fibers when blood flow is restricted to a muscle, since these fibers do not require as much oxygen to do the job. As such, you will recruit the growth-prone fast-twitch fibers early in the set, and you will also be able to fatigue them to a significant degree. Even though the fatigue was not imposed by a dynamic exercise, it still represents a mechanical stimulus for growth.

Note that you reach this level of fatigue while using up a lot less glycogen, which means a lower cortisol response than with regular training or a less significant increase in cortisol production over what you previously released during the workout.

IGF-1 Receptor Sensitivity

Loaded stretching also has a powerful impact on the sensitivity and responsiveness of the IGF-1 receptors. This basically means that not only does it increase IGF-1 release, but it also makes your receptors more sensitive to it. It is a biochemical hypertrophy bomb!

TRAINING PARAMETERS

LOADED STRETCHING FOR HYPERTROPHY

- *Timing:* Either at the end of the workout for the muscles that were trained or after you are done training a muscle.
- *Duration:* 45 to 60 seconds per set. If you can hold for longer than that, the load is insufficient for maximum growth.
- *Exercise selection:* Isolation for the targeted muscle or muscles.
- *Sets:* For maximum hypertrophy, we are shooting for a total time under loaded stretch of 2 to 3 minutes for a muscle. This means anywhere between 2 and 4 sets of 45 to 60 seconds.
- *Rest period:* The goal is incomplete recovery between sets. We want to still have some residual fatigue as well as some metabolites still present in the muscle when we initiate the next set. I recommend starting with a work-to-rest ratio of 2:1. So, if your set lasted 60 seconds, rest for 30 seconds before the next one.
- *Advanced variation:* Those with experience performing loaded stretching can use a more advanced version done at the end of a lifting set. Here, you perform a lifting set for the target muscle (this needs to be a lift where the target is placed in a stretched position under load), and then at the end of the set, you perform a loaded stretch for max time. It is more difficult to do load stretching this way because you are in a greater state of fatigue (both from a muscular and postural standpoint), but this is also what can make training this method so effective.

Loaded Stretching and Performance

This type of training is not only effective at building muscle, but it is also a great tool to make you a better athlete, either by improving eccentric and isometric strength or by improving muscle recruitment.

More Efficient Changes of Direction

In sports, the eccentric and isometric strength actions are very important yet undertrained. If you lack eccentric strength, your absorption phase (when changing direction or sprinting) is longer, and a lot of the potential energy dissipates (strength leaks). This makes the switch from eccentric to concentric a lot slower, and you lose a significant amount of power. If your isometric strength is lacking, there is a delay between the end of the absorption phase and the switch to the concentric phase, once again making the switch slower and less efficient.

Loaded stretching increases rigidity during the eccentric and isometric actions; in addition, it teaches the body not to rely exclusively on the stretch reflex to perform a change of direction. This makes the movement faster and more efficient. Even though it is an isometric action (the slowest of all muscle actions), it actually has a significant impact on explosiveness.

Fast-Twitch Fibers Recruitment

Loaded stretching increases your capacity to recruit fast-twitch fibers. I know it sounds weird since we are talking about exercises devoid of movement (so much less speed), but it actually greatly helps explosive movements! When the body is deprived of oxygen (put in a hypoxic state), it tends to rely on the fast-twitch fibers. So, using loaded isometrics, which are hypoxic in nature, forces an earlier recruitment of the fast-twitch fibers and keeps them turned on for longer. It basically becomes a motor-learning session for fast-twitch activation and work.

Muscle Recruitment Programming

Another element of loaded stretching (or any other long-duration isometrics) is that you can focus on a specific muscle recruitment pattern. For example, you can hold the bottom position of a DB press by creating a co-contraction of the upper back and pressing muscles; the pressing muscles will be turned on automatically by the load, but you can focus on firing the upper back. Since there is no movement to coordinate, it is much easier to focus on the muscle contraction, and because it will be maintained for a long time, the programming is fairly rapid.

TRAINING PARAMETERS

LOADED STRETCHING FOR PERFORMANCE

- *Timing*: At the end of the workout to avoid fatigue that could affect dynamic performance.
- *Duration*: 30 to 45 seconds per set if the focus is on eccentric or isometric strength; 75 to 90 seconds for motor programming.
- *Exercise selection*: Multijoint exercises to focus on position and proper recruitment pattern.
- *Sets*: A total of 90 to 120 seconds for strength and 3 to 4 minutes for motor programming. So, 2 to 4 sets.
- *Rest*: Complete rest if strength is the goal, so a 1:1.5 or 1:2 work-to-rest ratio. For motor programming, a 1:1 ratio.
- *Advanced variation*: Another advanced method that those with experience with loaded stretching could use is pairing a loaded stretching mini-set with explosive movements. For example, iso-dynamic contrast: 15 second loaded stretch/1 explosive movement/15 second loaded stretch/1 explosive movement/15 second loaded strength/1 explosive movement. This is a very advanced method that requires the athlete to have excellent positional strength and movement quality because performing explosive movements in a fatigued state can be hazardous otherwise.

Loaded Stretching and Injury Prevention

Of course, as a stretching method, this training does work great to improve mobility. More importantly, it improves mobility while the muscles are contracted, which is what you need for most sports. This is important both for performance improvement and for injury prevention. Here's why.

Strengthening the Muscles in Their Elongated State

The body will always look for the most economical way to do things. As such, it has learned to use the stretch reflex whenever a muscle has to produce force from an elongated state. This is good, and we need that protective mechanism. However, it also makes the muscles more prone to injuries because over time, the nervous system becomes less efficient at producing actual contractile force in a stretched position. Let's say you are playing a sport and suddenly and forcefully stretch a muscle, but your muscle is weak in the stretched position. The reflex alone will not hold you up, and you are at greater risk of tearing that muscle. If you focus on keeping the target muscle tensed, loaded stretching programs your nervous system to become efficient at contracting a muscle when it is elongated. This has a positive effect on both performance and injury prevention.

Making Tendons Thicker and Stronger

Loaded stretching will increase tendon thickness and resiliency as well as create distal muscle hypertrophy, both of which make the muscle and tendons less likely to tear. From a performance standpoint, thicker tendons allow you to store more elastic energy, and stronger tendons allow you to make better use of that stored elastic energy during subsequent concentric actions. So, thickening the tendons will not only make you less prone to serious injuries but also stronger and more explosive.

Increasing Dynamic Mobility

In sports, active (when the stretched muscle is tensed and contracted) and dynamic (when you are moving) mobility are key, and they are not well correlated with passive stretching. Loaded stretching increases elasticity of the muscles while they are being maximally contracted, which will translate to an increase in active and dynamic mobility. This increased mobility will then transfer to better technical execution of many skills, as well as an important reduction in the risk of injuries. It also leads to a very rapid increase in range of motion in many movement patterns.

TRAINING PARAMETERS

LOADED STRETCHING FOR INJURY PREVENTION

- *Timing*: Can be done at the beginning of a session to improve mobility on a lift when you have limitations. Otherwise, it is best done in its own session or, if time is an issue, at the end of a session.
- *Duration*: Shoot for a total of 3 minutes under load and get there in as little total time as possible. So, start with a load you can hold for about 90 seconds at first.
- *Exercise selection*: Multijoint exercises or isolation exercises, depending on what needs to be fixed.
- *Sets*: Get to 3 total minutes in as little total time as possible (so short rest intervals).
- *Rest*: See above; short rest intervals.
- *Advanced variation*: For advanced loaded stretching for injury prevention, perform contrast sets where you do loaded stretch (75 to 90 seconds) with a set of lifting. For example, split squat EQI (loaded stretched), followed by back squat, push-up EQI, followed by bench press. You would rest 2 to 3 minutes between each exercise and perform 3 sets. This is an advanced method because the initial loaded stretch will help you to use a larger range of motion on the following exercise and place the target muscle under a greater degree of stretch while under load. This loading in an even more stretched position is fantastic for injury prevention (e.g., to prevent tears), but if done too early it can actually increase injury risk. The target tissues need to be prepared appropriately, and the athlete needs to have good enough movement control and technique to load the joint and muscle optimally in the stretched position.

So there we have it, all the supercool methods of the overload system laid out in all their glory. Hopefully, you now have a better understanding of not only why these methods have been chosen for this system but also *how* they are going to improve your performance. In chapter 3, we are going to start looking into the main exercises that form the foundation of the overload system before we then address each of them individually in depth from a technique and execution standpoint.

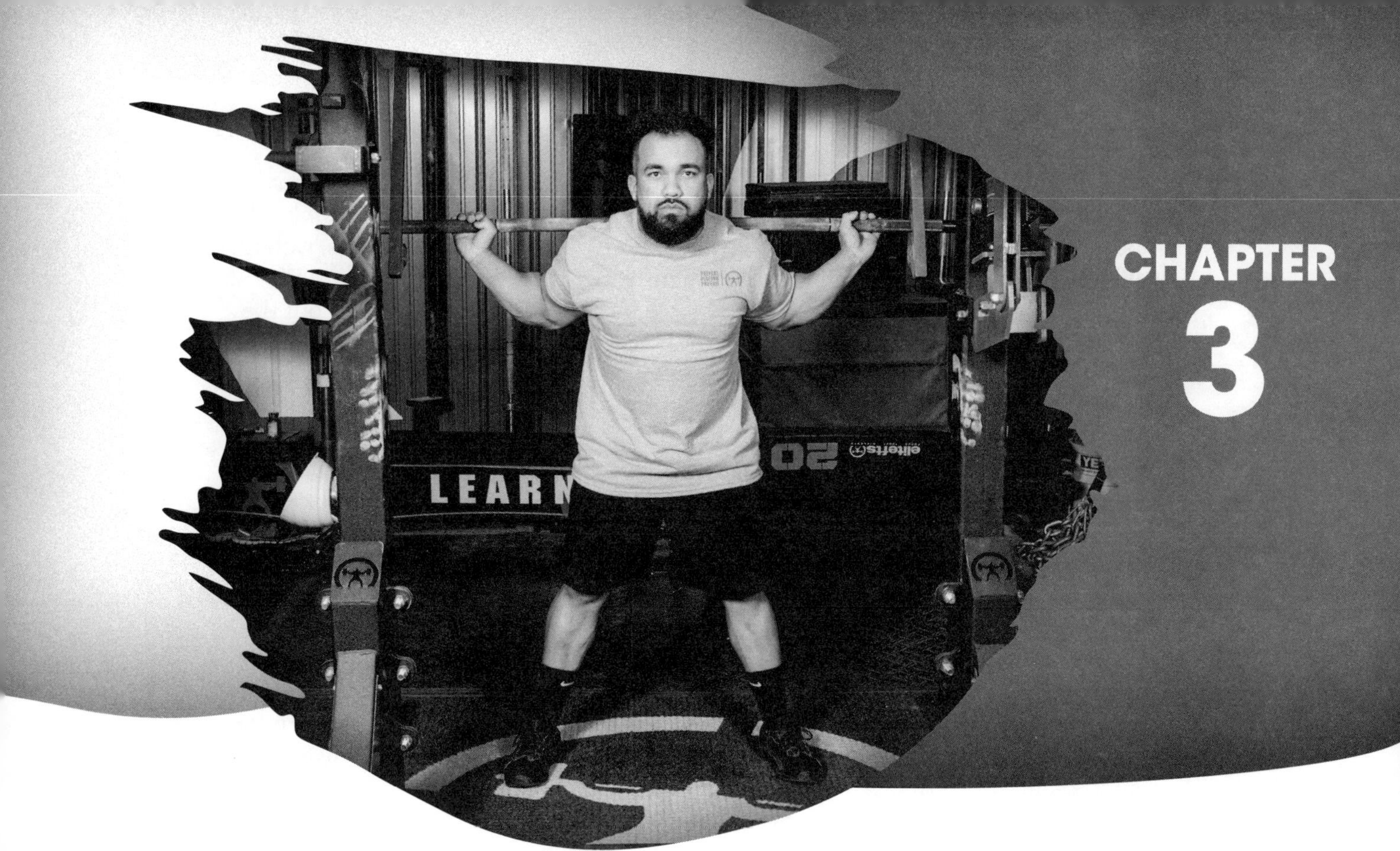

CHAPTER 3

The Overload System Foundational Exercises

Exercise selection is possibly the most important factor when it comes to designing an effective training program. Lifters have gotten results using all forms of set and reps, training splits, or loading schemes, but when it comes to building strength, the big barbell lifts are basically a constant among those who have built impressive levels of strength (this is especially true in the pre-steroid era). That's why it is so important that we cover these exercises in detail. Performing them correctly is going to be imperative to get the desired results from the overload system. Over the next few chapters, we will cover why we have chosen to focus on these specific exercises and cover each of them in detail to ensure that you are able to perform them effectively.

The Overload System and Old-School Progression Models

All the legendary lifters mentioned so far in this book built their physique and strength without the use of exercise machines or even pulley stations. They relied on a barbell, a power rack, a bench, and dumbbells. The core of their programs was big, multijoint movements: the deadlift, overhead press, bench press (starting in the 1950s), and squats. A lot of them also did explosive movements like the power clean or high pull (even the power snatch) since before the 1960s, weightlifting (as in Olympic lifting) was a strong influence on the training of most lifters. Some lifters did include more isolated movements, especially for arms, but they were just the icing on the cake. Getting stronger on these big basic lifts was the main training principle they abided by. Even beginners were often advised to do sets of 5 to 10 reps; none of that 12 to 20 reps to get started safely that we often see today (on machines, most of the time).

A popular system for beginners in the 1930s was the Milo course: Lifters would start a movement doing 5 reps per set for their first workout, then add 1 rep per workout with the same weight (three whole-body workouts per week) until they reached 10 reps per set. Then they would increase the weight, drop back down to 5 reps per set, and build back up. This was the original "double progression model."

Unsurprisingly, the overload system relies on the same approach. It is the approach that helped both of us (Christian and Tom) to get strong and less puny in the first place. Christian started out training for football and early on was mentored by a strength coach who had him do workouts that consisted of back squats, deadlifts, bench presses, military presses, power cleans, and barbell rows. The plan typically used three phases. In phase 1, 3 to 4 sets of 8 to 10 reps were performed (5 for power cleans). In phase 2, we switched to 3 to 4 sets of 5 reps (3 on power cleans); and in phase 3, we would use complex training, which consisted of combining a strength and a power movement in a compound set, as in this example:

Jump squats with 20 percent of the max squat × 5; 2 minutes rest; back squat × 3

Power clean × 3; 2 minutes of rest; deadlift × 3

Medicine ball throw overhead × 5; 2 minutes of rest; push press × 3

Medicine ball slam × 5; 2 minutes of rest; barbell row × 5

There were some variations, but that's what Christian did for the last four years that he was playing football. Immediately afterward, Christian moved on to Olympic lifting, which, as you can imagine, included even more work on the big basics. That went on for six years. Then it was a mix of powerlifting-type and bodybuilding training, but his size and strength were mostly built during those first 10 years of basic work.

As for Tom, he got in to lifting as a 114-pound (52-kilogram) 16-year-old (which at 5 ft 10 in. is what we class as excessively puny) with a background in long-distance running (forgive him for the sins of his previous life). His first three or four years of training revolved primarily around typical "bro"-style training—chest, back, arms, shoulders, and legs—with lots of exercise variation, high volume, and over time, lots of intensifying techniques (drop sets, forced reps, etc.). There was no real progressive overload or a huge amount of time spent under a heavy barbell. It should be no surprise, then, that these years didn't bring tremendous progress in terms of getting jacked or strong. To stay motivated, Tom decided to channel his lifting toward some type of competitive endeavor. Unhappy with the subjectivity of bodybuilding (and the necessity of wearing a thong), he decided to work toward competing in powerlifting. Needless to say, his training became far more streamlined around the "big three" and their accessory movements. This lower volume, lower rep approach started to bring Tom meaningful progress in his strength levels and physique. Tom has since gone on to be a successful competitor (including Junior World Records, Open European champion, and several British Championship wins) and a coach in the sport of powerlifting.

Christian's Best Lifts

My own training has always been slanted toward strength, except for brief bodybuilding periods thrown in there every year. While I never was a world-class strength athlete, I reached a decent level. Here are some of my best lifts; pretty much all were done at a body weight of around 205 to 215 pounds (93 to 97.5 kilograms) at 5 ft 9 in.

Back squat: 550 pounds (250 kilograms) x 5; 600 pounds (272 kilograms) x 1

Front squat: 485 pounds (220 kilograms) x 1

Frankenstein squat from pins: 405 pounds (184 kilograms) x 1

Zercher squat: 500 pounds (227 kilograms) x 1

Snatch: 315 pounds (143 kilograms, but only did 285 pounds [130 kilograms] in competition)

Power snatch: 264 pounds (120 kilograms) x 5 (blocks); 280 pounds (127 kilograms) x 1

Clean and jerk: 374 pounds (170 kilograms) x 1 (only did 352 pounds [160 kilograms] in competition)

Power clean: 330 pounds (150 kilograms) x 5 (hang); 341 pounds (155 kilograms) x 1

One-arm power snatch (with bar): 185 pounds (84 kilograms) x 1

Bench press: 415 pounds x 5 (188 kilograms); 425 pounds (193 kilograms) x 3; 445 pounds (202 kilograms) x 1 (done at a body weight of 225 to 228 pounds [102 to 103 kilograms])

Bench press from pins (bottom position): 425 pounds (193 kilograms) x 1 (also done at a body weight of 225 to 228 pounds [102 to 103 kilograms])

Military press: 235 pounds (107 kilograms) x 5; 275 pounds (125 kilograms) x 1

Push press: 315 pounds (143 kilograms) x 5; 345 pounds (156 kilograms) x 1

Shoulder press from pins starting just above head: 345 pounds (156 kilograms) x 1

Snatch-grip high pulls (to mid/upper chest level): 398 pounds (181 kilograms) x 1

Power shrug: 765 pounds (347 kilograms) x 3

Rack pull from just above knees: 1,000 pounds (454 kilograms) x 1 (gym); 845 pounds (383 kilograms) x 1 (Strongman competition; in this case, I was down to 187 pounds [85 kilograms] to qualify for a lower-weight class in a weightlifting competition)

Deadlift: not worth mentioning

Tom's Best Lifts

I won't go into detail, but I got into training out of necessity. So it was a case of finding what motivated me within the realm of training. Bodybuilding training and body part splits never did it for me; any form of training where the main premise was focusing on how you look just didn't sit well with me mentally.

Then came strength training. Being strong was something that really did appeal to me. It was objective, and it had a clear progression system and metric of success—things I can get on-board with. So, from here on in, this became my focus for my training. Although I still compete, competing has never been something I particularly cared about. I care far more about my own standards. I'm just as happy hitting a lift in the gym as I am on the platform, which certainly helps explains why, like Chris, I'm a terrible competitor. These are some of my notable lifts to date:

Back squat: 260 kilograms (573 pounds)

Front squat: 200 kilograms (441 pounds)

Bench press (raw): 205 kilograms (452 pounds)

Bench press (equipped, using a 3-ply bench shirt): 365 kilograms (805 pounds)

Deadlift: 310 kilograms (683 pounds)

Push press: 140 kilograms (309 pounds)

Snatch-grip high pull: 170 kilograms (375 pounds)

Pendlay row: 170 kilograms (375 pounds)

The Foundational Exercises

It is thus with good reason that the cornerstone of the overload system is doing big, multijoint, heavy compound movements. While science points out that you can build muscle with light weights and isolated exercises, the reality is a bit different. The most impressive physiques and the strongest people got there in large part by focusing on getting strong on the big basic lifts. I'm not necessarily talking about focusing on 1 to 4 reps strength work, but certainly I mean trying hard to add weight to the barbell whenever you can on the rep ranges you selected.

Except for genetic freaks and people who use lots of performance-enhancing drugs, I don't know many people who got jacked by only doing isolated or machine-based exercises. I am not saying that these exercises are without value. They are useful to fix specific weaknesses, but by their nature (only hitting a small part of the body), they carry some disadvantages that make it hard to maximize your muscle growth and strength gains if they are the focus of your training.

- Since they hit so little muscle mass, you need a lot of exercises and a lot of volume to get the same overall stimulation as you would from a few basic barbell exercises. This can both increase your training time and volume significantly and make it harder to recover from your training. It is my experience that one of the main reasons why "natural" people (those not assisted by PEDs) do not progress is that they do too much overall volume relative to their capacity to recover. If your training is centered more on minor movements, this will almost be a given.

- Isolated and so-called easy exercises provide a much smaller challenge to the nervous system, limiting how much it can improve. Making your nervous system better at recruiting fibers, making them twitch faster, and improving how coordinated they are is the key to getting stronger, but it's also very important for growth. Getting stronger allows you to use more weight even on your minor exercises, increasing muscle tension and thus mechanical stress and growth stimulus as a result. A main reason beginner and intermediate lifters fail to grow is that they are too weak to benefit from the minor exercises (because they won't be able to produce enough tension in their muscles), and these minor exercises are the focus of their training. The stronger you are, the more beneficial isolated work will become. First, consider that you will be strong enough and neurologically efficient enough to place a sufficient mechanical tension to promote growth. In addition, these smaller movements will allow you to get enough volume without overloading the central nervous system (which strong lifters already tax with their heavy work).

The foundations of this system are big compound lifts that recruit a lot of muscle mass at the same time, provide a strong neurological stimulus, and place the whole body under a high level of tension. Our main movements (or variations thereof) will be these:

- Deadlift
- Squat (or front squat)
- Military press
- Bench press
- Pendlay row
- Explosive pulls (power shrugs, high pulls, power clean)

Because of the methods we use, such as the progressive range of motion method and heavy partials, we will also do plenty of heavy partial range of motion work on these patterns.

In the next several chapters, we will take a closer look at how to perform these exercises properly. After all, and this is important, *doing* an exercise is not enough: You must do the exercise with the best possible technique to properly load the muscles, maximize your lifting performance, and reduce the risk of injuries.

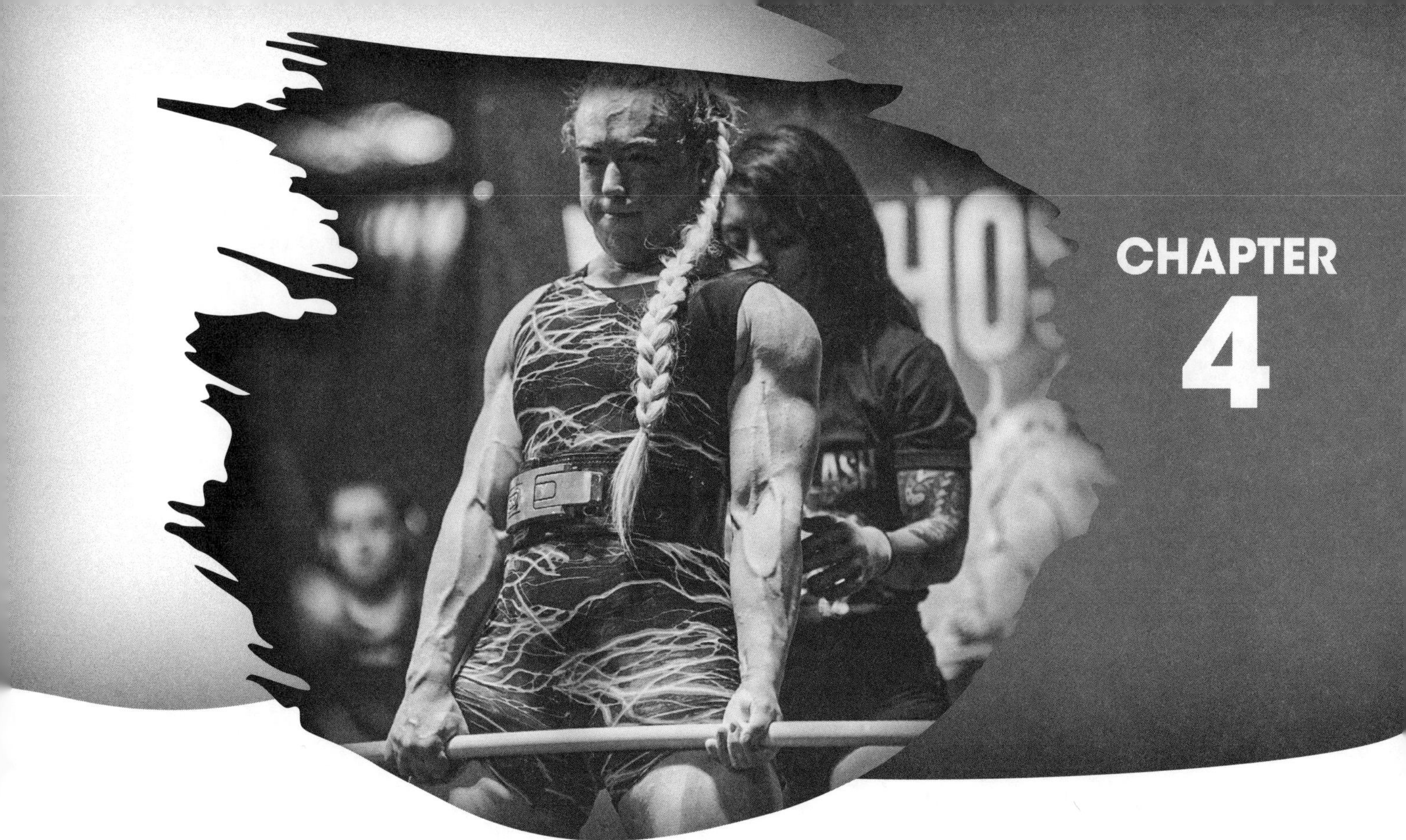

Deadlift

For a long time, how much weight one could lift from the floor was the most important feat of strength. As a result, the deadlift (in all varieties) became a central focus in strength training. For many, the deadlift is still regarded as the "king of the lifts" and rightly so. There is just something satisfying on a basic and guttural level about lifting a heavy load from the floor.

The deadlift is mostly a hip hinge movement. Where the squat pattern teaches us how to move primarily through the knee, the deadlift teaches us to move primarily through the hip. Although as we'll see, it is not *entirely* a hip-driven movement because the quads play a key role in the lift also.

The real key to a good deadlift is torso stiffness and rigidity. A properly executed deadlift will test the core musculature (i.e., abs and obliques, lats, upper and lower back muscles, among others) like few other exercises. If you can lock in your torso, then the lift itself is essentially a leg press, except in this scenario you are pushing the floor away as opposed to what happens in the leg press platform. In theory, it is that simple, if you can get the setup executed properly.

Lastly, even though the deadlift is often referred to as a "pull," do not think of it as a pulling exercise. That will only encourage a back-dominant, stiff-legged style of lift. The deadlift is a push exercise, as in *push* the floor away. The only pulling you should be focusing on is pulling the slack out of the bar (more on that later).

Setup

In this section, setup guidelines are included for the conventional, or proper, version of the deadlift (see figure 4.1*a*) as well as its heinous long-lost brother, the sumo deadlift (see figure 4.1*b*), where relevant.

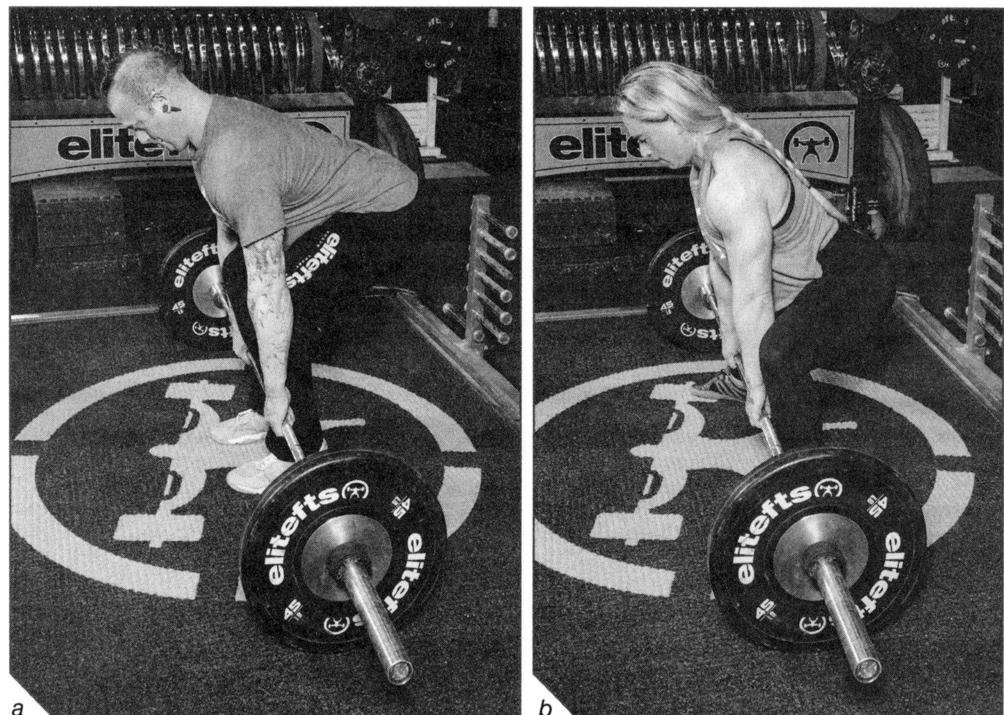

FIGURE 4.1 Setup for the deadlift: *(a)* conventional and *(b)* sumo.

Width of Stance

The foot placement for the conventional and sumo deadlifts is as follows:

Conventional

The simplest way to find your foot placement is to put your feet in the same position you would for a vertical jump. Subconsciously, you know this is the position in which you can create the most upward force. You may need to adjust slightly either way, but this is a good starting point. The other factor to take into account is the size of your torso. Those with bigger waistlines will benefit from having a wider stance so that there is enough space between their legs to fit their torso into with proper positioning. Those with slimmer waistlines can get away with a hip-width (or slightly narrower) stance. In terms of foot angle, the vast majority will be perfectly fine with a toe angle of 5 to 10 degrees. See figure 4.2*a* for an example of the foot position for a conventional deadlift.

Sumo

For anyone other than very advanced lifters, I like to go with the widest stance that allows you to have your knees vertically stacked over your ankles in the start position. This will vary because of a person's limb proportions, hip mobility, and other factors. Some lifters will benefit long term by going wider again to reduce the ROM, but for 90 percent (or more) of lifters, these guidelines will give you the optimal setup. Foot angle is relatively easy to work out; you want to angle your feet so that in the start position your toes point in the same direction as your kneecap. This simply means that your feet, knees, and hips are in optimal alignment at the start of the lift. See figure 4.2*b* for an example of the foot position for a sumo deadlift.

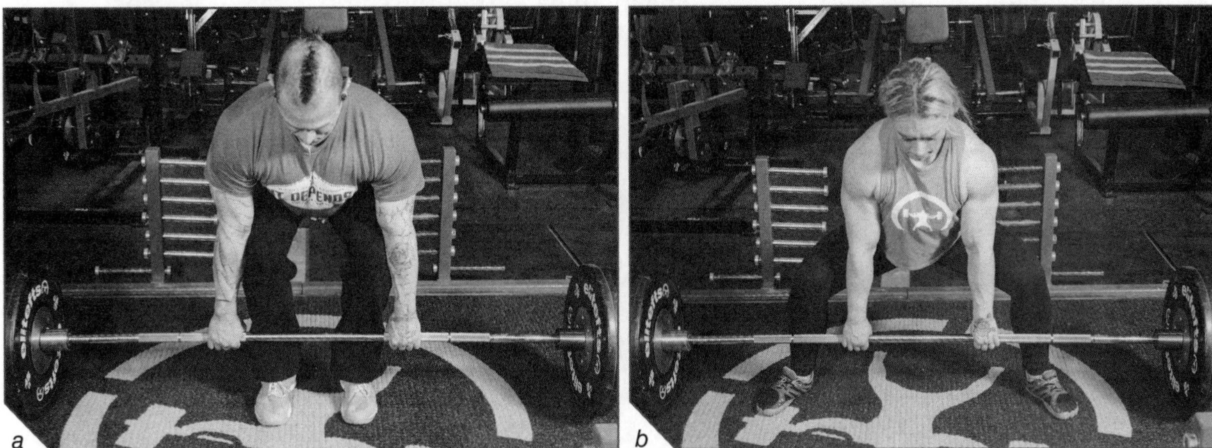

FIGURE 4.2 Foot placement for the deadlift: *(a)* conventional and *(b)* sumo. These are good starting placements for the majority of lifters.

Bar Placement

Regardless of stance, when setting up, the bar *must* be centered over the midfoot. The bar will start closer to the shin in a sumo deadlift simply because the feet are rotated outward more (minimizing the horizontal distance from the shin to the midfoot), but the principle remains the same.

Hip Height

If the foot placement is set correctly, then the correct hip height is easy to find. With your feet set in place, bend through the knee until your shin is against the bar (do *not* let the bar move). From this position, push your hips back and hinge down to the bar while twisting your knees away from each other. Once you have hip hinged enough to be able to grip the bar properly, then you have your hips in the correct position. Where your hips will be in vertical space, however, will differ between conventional and sumo as the levers are different. At the end of the day, the main advantage (for some) of sumo is that it reduces the hip extension demands by getting them closer to the bar. Here's what we are looking for in each stance.

Conventional

For a powerlifting-style deadlift, the hips should be set in the highest possible position while maintaining two criteria: the shin staying against the bar (and the bar not moving during set up) and the hips being lower than the shoulders. This position allows for the most hip-dominant movement that can move more load. It differs from a clean deadlift in which the hips are set purposely low to achieve a more upright position. The clean-style deadlift is less efficient for moving maximal loads, which doesn't matter for Olympic lifting because you'll never be performing a clean with a load anywhere near a max deadlift. See figure 4.3*a* for an example of proper hip height for the conventional deadlift.

Sumo

The most common mistake in a sumo deadlift is setting the hips too low and trying to squat the lift too much. The main benefit of the sumo is that it lessens the horizontal distance between your hips and the bar, lessening the demand on the hip extensors. If you squat too low when setting up, then your hips will sit back further from the bar and defeat the purpose of the stance. So, when setting up, focus on getting the front of the hip bone as close to the bar (in horizontal space) as possible, using the guidelines presented at the beginning of this section. See figure 4.3*b* for an example of proper hip height for a sumo deadlift.

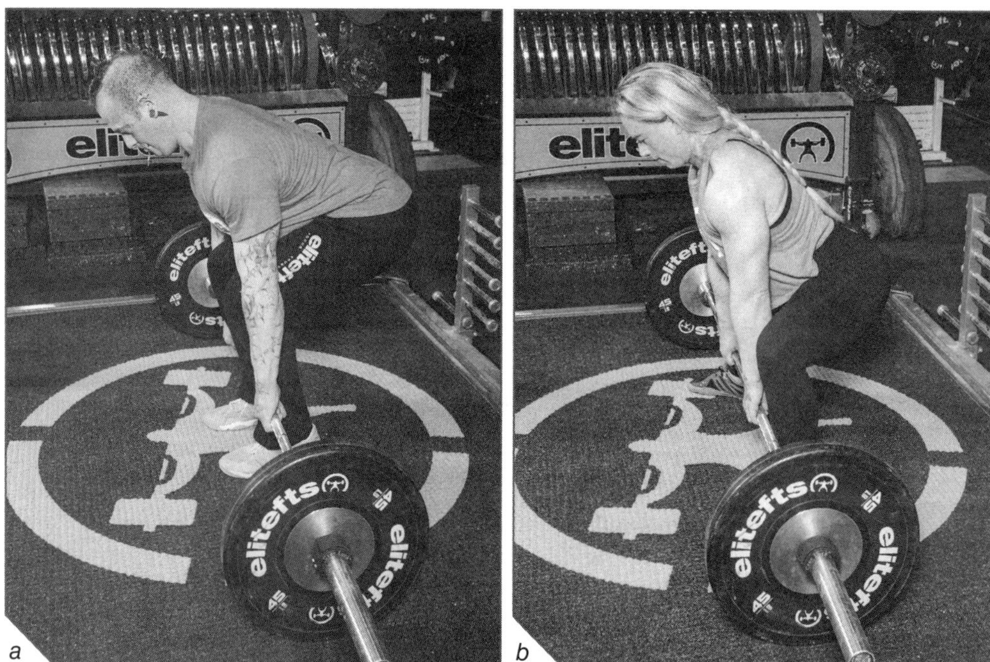

FIGURE 4.3 Proper hip height for the *(a)* conventional and *(b)* sumo deadlift.

KEY POINT

Many people are under the impression that you should try to set up so that your shoulders are *behind* the bar when deadlifting. This is incorrect and would mean you are essentially doing a stiff-legged deadlift from the floor. A better way to look at it is that your armpits should be directly over or slightly in front of the bar in the start position. Which setup is correct for you will depend on your proportions and choice of stance. As a general rule, though, we would expect to see the following:

- *Long limbs and short torso*—shoulders in front of bar, arms angled back
- *Short limbs and long torso*—shoulders directly over bar, arms vertical

Note that the sumo stance allows a more upright torso, in turn causing the shoulders to be slightly further back compared to a conventional stance.

Grip

Where you should grip the bar is going to be determined in large part by your choice of stance. The goal with our grip placement is always to reduce the range of motion as much as possible by having the arms as long as possible in vertical space. Think about how much further you need to reach if you do something like a snatch-grip deadlift; we don't want that.

Grip Placement

While it may seem simple, where you grip the bar is important. Let's walk through the grip placement for the conventional and sumo deadlift.

Conventional

Your grip needs to be as narrow as possible while still allowing enough room for your forearms to get past your knees when you set up. When in the start position, your forearms will be partially behind your knees. If your grip is too narrow, you won't be able to get your knees past your elbows, meaning you won't be able to get the bar against your shins. Going too wide will mean increasing ROM. See figure 4.4*a* for an example of proper grip on the bar for a conventional deadlift.

Sumo

Easy. Let your arms hang directly down. This is your grip width. You want your arms as long as possible, meaning we want a perfectly vertical line down from the shoulders to the hands on the bar. See figure 4.4*b* for an example of proper grip on the bar for a sumo deadlift.

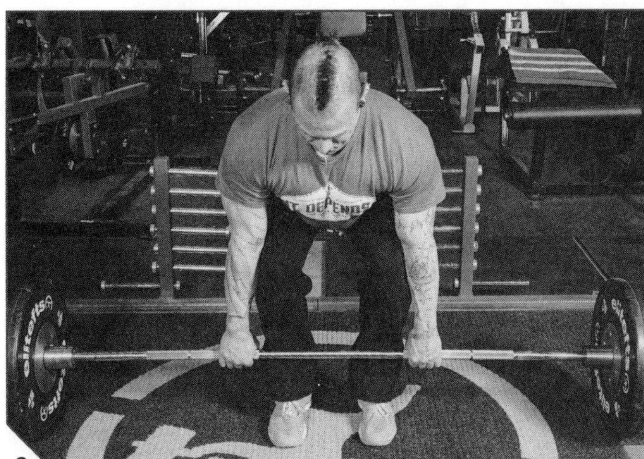

a

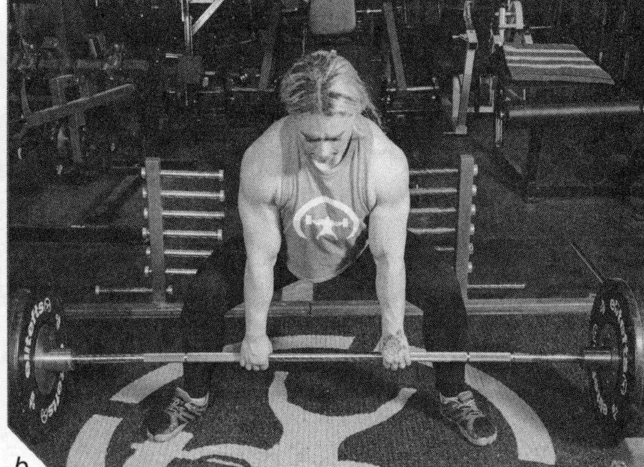

b

FIGURE 4.4 Deadlift grip: *(a)* conventional and *(b)* sumo.

Type of Grip

There are two options regarding the type of grip you can use for truly heavy or maximal deadlifts. Unfortunately, a regular (double overhand) grip simply isn't strong enough for when we are doing maximal lifts, so we need to change strategy. The vast majority of lifters use an under-over grip, mainly out of convenience. But as we will see, it isn't necessarily optimal.

Under-Over Grip

An under-over or mixed grip (one hand pronated, one hand supinated) is the most commonly used grip when deadlifting heavy. With good reason, the mixed grip stops the bar from rolling in your hands, making it much more secure. The downside, however, is that you then end up deadlifting crooked. Look at the length of your arms when pronated compared to supinated; the supinated arm is effectively longer because of how it is oriented in the shoulder joint. Over time, this crooked deadlifting can lead to an imbalance in which one hip will sit higher than the other. To avoid this, make sure you alternate your mixed grip (i.e., change which hand is pronated or supinated). You will always have a dominant mixed grip and a weaker mixed grip, so if you want to use mixed grip a lot, I suggest at least doing all warm-ups in your weaker mixed grip, then swapping over for your work sets. This should help avoid developing an imbalance. See figure 4.5*a* for an example of under-over grip.

Hook Grip

The hook grip, in which the thumb is wrapped around the bar and then is gripped by the fingers, is much more common in Olympic lifting circles. That's because it is a stronger grip that doesn't involve having to supinate one arm (which wouldn't work too well for clean and snatch). The hook grip is very strong and even gives you a mechanical advantage because it makes the bar sit lower in the hand (meaning you can start slightly higher, with less ROM). The downside: The hook grip hurts worse than standing on a plug. You need to hook grip regularly to keep the nerves in the thumb desensitized, otherwise you just go back to square one. Technically speaking, everyone would be better off using the hook grip for deadlifting; it gives you a mechanical advantage in the lift, it is potentially a stronger grip than the mixed, *and* it doesn't involve the risk of developing an imbalance like the mixed grip. This tends to be easiest to implement when you are a novice and the loads are light(er).

Sumo pullers especially can benefit from the hook grip because it makes the lockout smoother. Sumo pullers can miss deadlifts at lockout because the hands have to drag over the quads to finish the lift. This is then exacerbated by the thumb of the pronated hand (if using mixed grip) protruding and catching even more so. The hook grip effectively makes the hands smaller when they are being clenched more *and* removes the protruding thumb, as the grip is set over it. See figure 4.5*b* for an example of hook grip.

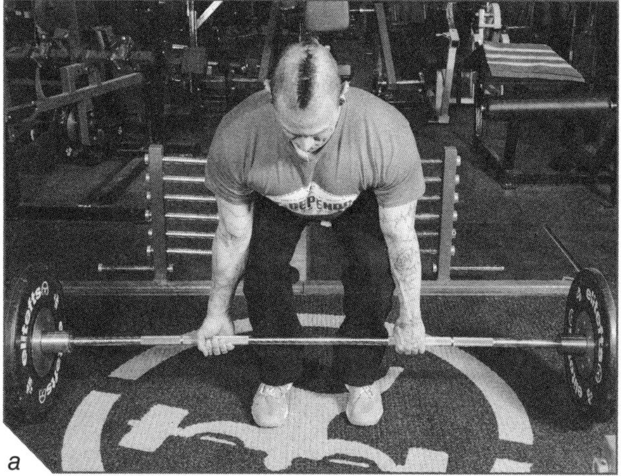

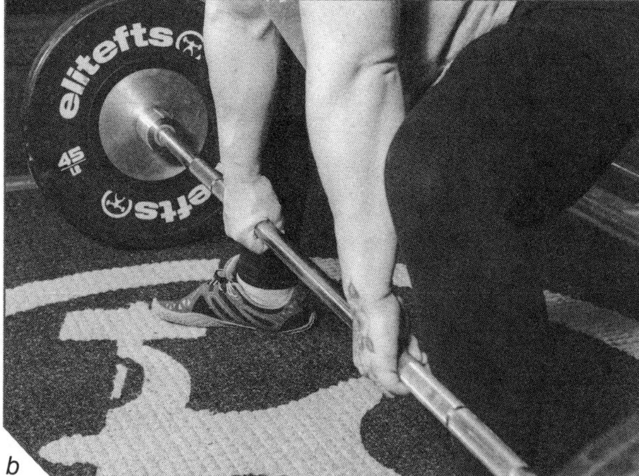

FIGURE 4.5 Types of grips for the deadlift: *(a)* under-over and *(b)* hook.

It is also worth mentioning that some people (especially women) with smaller hands may struggle to get an advantage from the hook grip as their hands are too small to wrap around the bar enough. If this is you, then you may be stuck with the mixed grip, I'm afraid.

Setting the Upper Back

Creating adequate tension in the upper back and lats is an absolutely crucial stage of the setup and a big determining factor in whether the lift will be successful. This part of the setup, along with adequate bracing, is what will maintain your spinal alignment throughout the lift. The vast majority of deadlifts are missed due to a power leak somewhere in the torso; think about how much you can leg press compared to deadlift.

Lats

The lats play a huge role in torso rigidity, as well keeping the bar against the legs during the lift, especially for lifters with a short torso who start with their shoulders in front of the bar (think about the moment arm around the shoulder). When the lats are set correctly, they will help stabilize nearly the entire length of the spine as well as stop the bar drifting forward from your center of gravity.

There are two mechanisms that will ensure the lats are engaged properly during the lift.

The first is externally rotating your arm, which is a smart way of saying that once you have gripped the bar, twist your elbows back as hard as you can. Imagine you are desperately trying to snap the bar between your hands (causing more pressure on the pinkie finger side of your hands); this should result in your biceps facing forward more and your elbows being pointed behind you. You will also see the shoulders depress (pull down) into the body when you do this (see figure 4.6*a*).

The second mechanism is actively pulling the bar back in to the shins (see figure 4.6*b*). This is akin to doing a cable straight-arm pull-down; in fact, I like to

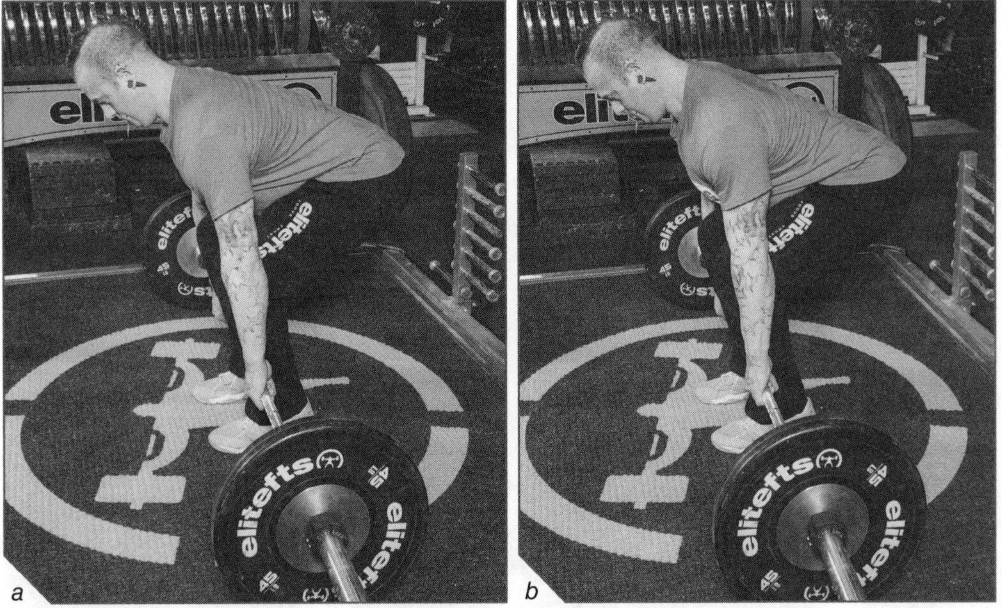

FIGURE 4.6 Setup *(a)* without lat tension and external rotation and *(b)* with external rotation and lat tension. Note in the second photo the elbow is more angled backwards and shoulders are set further back.

use these movements (with hips bent and a pause at the bottom) as a warm-up for the deadlift to get the lats firing the way we want. This pulling back motion needs to be consistent throughout the entire lift. If these two things are done correctly, the lats will be contributing what we need them to throughout the lift.

Upper Back

When I say upper back, I am referring primarily to the traps, rhomboids, and rear delts, the muscles responsible for shoulder retraction. The upper back muscles are used to stabilize and fix the thoracic spine in place. The downward force of the barbell will be pulling the shoulders forward into protraction, and it is the job of the upper back to stop that from happening.

The upper back is also responsible for pulling the slack out of the bar, which is a crucial part of the setup. If the slack is not pulled out of the bar, then when you go to initiate the lift, you are lifting only the weight of the bar until the plates catch, then the rest of the load hits you suddenly. This causes a very jerky start to the lift, often resulting in a loss of positioning.

Once you have done all the previous steps, you pull the slack out of the bar simply by contracting through the traps, rhomboids, and rear delts in a shrugging back motion. There will be some minor shoulder retraction through this process, but the main movement should be the bar flexing upward (how much will depend on the bar used and the amount of weight on the bar). Please note this is a purely shrugging *back* motion (not up); the shoulders should stay pulled down into the body through the action of the lats (see figure 4.7*a*).

A common flaw seen here is actually over-shrugging (see figure 4.7*b*) We only want enough retraction to pull the flex from the bar; that is, the goal is not to achieve a large retraction movement. Most of the work done here is isometric in nature. Shrugging the shoulders too far back does two things:

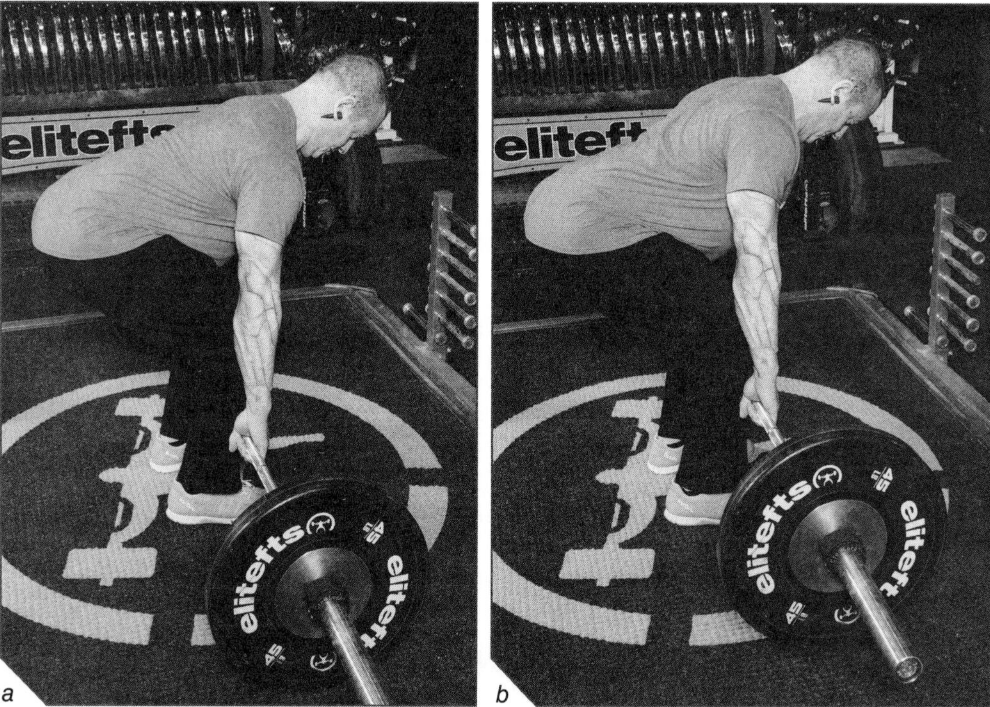

FIGURE 4.7 Setting the upper back with *(a)* the correct degree of retraction versus *(b)* the common mistake of over-retracting.

- Effectively shortens the arms, meaning you have to reach down further to the bar, increasing ROM.
- Puts the shoulder girdle and upper back muscles in a weaker position. A fully retracted shoulder position puts the upper back muscles far away from a neutral or resting length, which in turn is a position that is more difficult to maintain. Our postural muscles are strongest when held in positions around neutral, which is what we are aiming for here. If you start in an over-shrugged position, as soon as you initiate the lift, the postural muscles will get pulled forward out of retraction and often past neutral to a protracted position, provided there is any form of appreciable load on the bar, of course.

Head and Neck Position

The most common mistake you see with deadlifting is how the head is positioned. How often have you seen someone set up like a fishing rod for a deadlift and then hear someone else shout "Chest up." And what is the response? You probably would crane your head up toward the ceiling while keeping the same lousy spinal alignment (no cookie for you).

Listen, the spine is almost always at its strongest when it is neutral, and when I last checked, my spine went all the way up into my neck and my head. So, try this: Stand tall and look straight forward with your chin slightly tucked (neutral) (see figure 4.8*a*). Now hip hinge until your torso is at the same angle it would be at the start of a deadlift (see figure 4.8*b*). Make sure your neck and head move in tandem with the rest of your spine. Where are you looking now? At the floor just in front of your feet? Right, this is the position your head should be in when you start your deadlift.

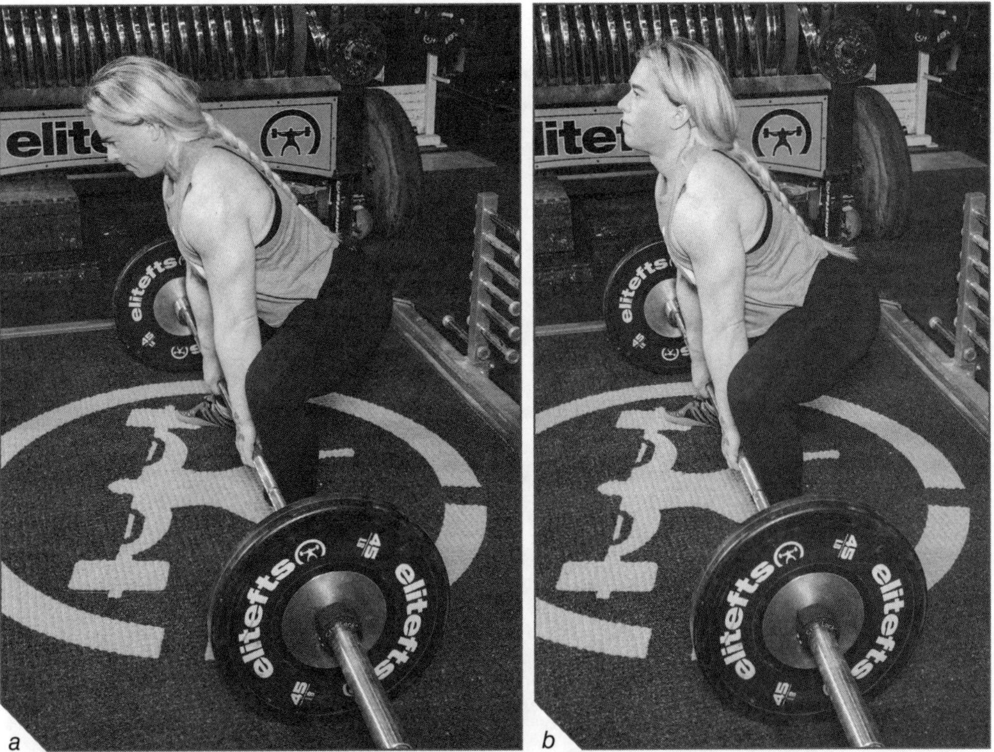

FIGURE 4.8 Deadlift setup with *(a)* correct neck and head position versus *(b)* an over-arched neck position.

Bar Path and Movement Pattern

A properly executed deadlift will have a vertical bar path, starting over the midfoot and staying aligned over it until it is locked out (see figure 4.9 for the full movement of a conventional deadlift and figure 4.10 for the full movement of a sumo deadlift). Any deviation from this path is simply costing you energy and

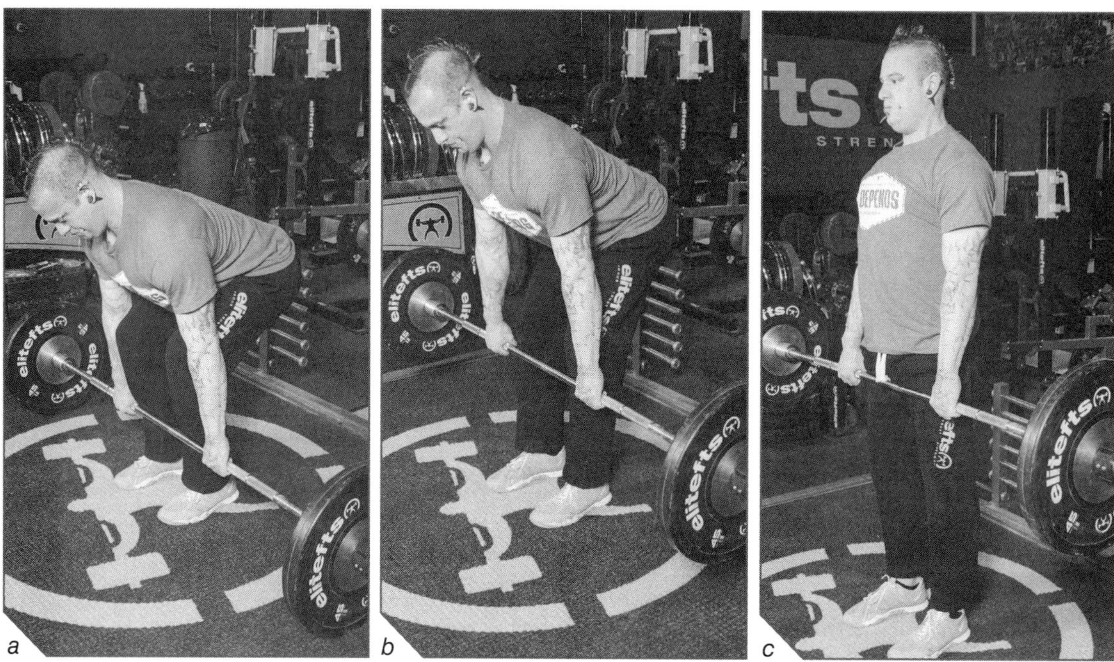

FIGURE 4.9 The segments of the conventional deadlift: *(a)* start position, *(b)* end of phase I, and *(c)* end of phase II.

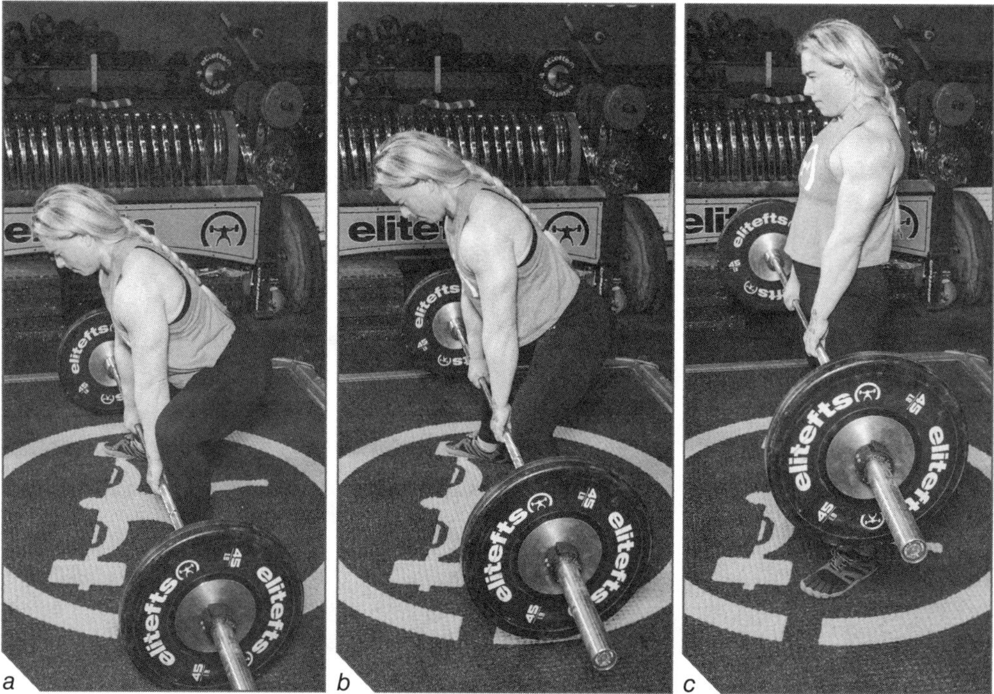

FIGURE 4.10 The segments of the sumo deadlift: *(a)* start position, *(b)* end of phase I, and *(c)* end of phase II.

leading you to be less likely to succeed in the lift. That's basic physics. This is achieved through two different phases of movement.

Phase I: Floor to Knee: Knee Dominant

Those keen observers in the audience will have pieced it together: "If the knees start over the bar, how can the bar move in a perfectly vertical path without hitting them?"

Well done; have a cookie. That's what phase I of the lift achieves: It gets the knees back out of the way of the bar. In summary, phase I gets the bar to the bottom of the kneecap, give or take, via the knee joint, while maintaining the torso angle (relative to the floor).

The quads primarily drive phase I of the lift; meanwhile the glutes, hamstrings, and lower back work in an isometric fashion to maintain the torso angle. To say it in smart language, during phase I, the bar is lifted by knee extension without concurrent extension through the hip. There, see how smart I can sound if I wanted to bore you to death? You're welcome.

The best way to monitor this movement is to watch a video of yourself deadlifting. If you perform phase I correctly, your hips and shoulders will rise in tandem until the bar gets to the knee. The shoulders will stay in front of, or directly over, the bar (depending on where they were in the start position) and you should find yourself in a position that looks suspiciously like the bottom of a Romanian deadlift. If you did that, then well done, have another cookie. That position is the exact position we want to put ourselves in for phase II.

Here's a quick recap on how to perform phase I correctly:

1. Set up perfectly (obviously, as outlined previously).
2. Initiate the movement by pressing down into the floor through the legs. Focus especially on driving your big toe into the floor and pushing your knees back out of the way of the bar, which will help you utilize your quads more.
3. Don't allow your hips to creep forward. Focus on using the quads and allow your chest and shoulders to stay over the bar throughout this phase.

KEY POINT

I can't stress this enough: Using the hips to move the bar from the floor is a great way to set yourself up for failure. It's essentially trying to do a supramaximal good morning from the bottom up. It is inefficient at best and, at worst, a recipe for disaster when one of your vertebrae decides to emigrate to the other side of the room, rather violently. Trying to extend through the hip from the floor only puts more shear stress on the spine while taking the load away from the muscles best situated to lift the load from that position—namely, the quads.

Phase II: Knee to Lockout: Hip Dominant

If you have made it this far, then you've successfully completed half of an acceptable deadlift. At this point, if you were to stop, it should literally feel like the load is hanging from your glutes and hamstrings.

Now, in phase II, the hips really take over the lift. Phase II of the deadlift is very simply the concentric portion of a Romanian deadlift, except you have some momentum at the beginning of the lift. This is why I like to use the Romanian deadlift as a gateway to the full deadlift. If you can't do a proper Romanian deadlift, then you cannot do a proper deadlift.

Phase II is all about bringing the hips and the bar together. During this phase, the torso angle relative to the floor does change as the hips extend forward, in turn making the torso more upright. As well as driving forward through the hip, it is also very important to forcibly pull the bar back toward the hip at this juncture, as the bar is often lost forward when going over the kneecap. In essence, we attack the gap between the bar and the hips from both sides; the hips drive forward toward the bar and the lats pull the bar back toward the hips. Doing both of these moves effectively locks the bar out as early as possible in the movement. When this isn't initiated correctly, the bar often drifts forward away from the legs, or the lifter is shifted slightly forward onto the toes, or both. Either way, the lift is often then lost.

Here's a quick recap on how to perform phase II correctly:

1. As soon as the bar reaches just below the knee (or ideally just before, taking into account processing time), aggressively drive the hips forward through the glutes and hamstrings toward the bar.
2. Simultaneously, use the lats to drag the bar back over the kneecap and the quads back toward the hip (imagine trying to pull the bar back through your thighs).
3. Upon completion, stand as tall as possible with your knee and hip joint locked out.

Lockout

Despite being the easiest part of the lift from a leverage point of view, it is still quite common to see lifters performing the lockout inefficiently. They might have a muscular weakness in some circumstances, or there may be other factors, like poor grip (grip starts to give way toward the end of the lift). Some lifters may partially "switch off" because they believe they've completed the hardest part of the lift and think the lift is now a given to be successful. Let's look at the two most common faults with regard to finishing the lift.

Leaning Back

It is common to see lifters lock out a deadlift by leaning back at the top of the movement (see figure 4.11). This is often due to a lack of hip strength or simply poor body awareness. In the locked-out position, you should be as tall and upright as possible; think about pushing your head up to the ceiling with your posture. Leaning back simply puts unnecessary strain through the lower back and indicates poor lifting mechanics.

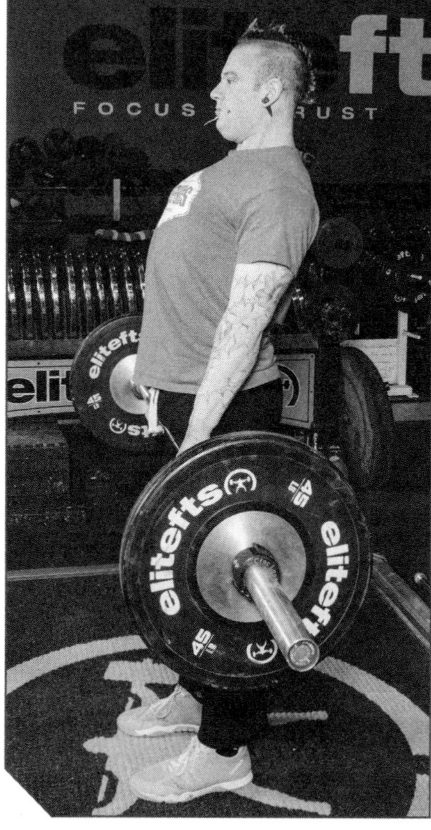

FIGURE 4.11 Incorrect lockout technique: leaning back.

Hitching

Hitching refers to the act of partly or fully supporting the weight of the bar on the legs (see figure 4.12). It is usually accomplished by re-bending the knee joint to give the bar a platform to rest on. While hitching is permitted in Strongman competitions, this is not a technique I would recommend for general lifters because it is not properly training the hip extension element of the deadlift. Even athletes on the competitive Strongman circuit ideally wouldn't deadlift this way all the time, as it would leave them with a strength deficit through their hip extension capabilities. Needing to hitch a lift simply illustrates that you are lifting a load that is too heavy or that you don't know how to use your hip properly to lock out the lift.

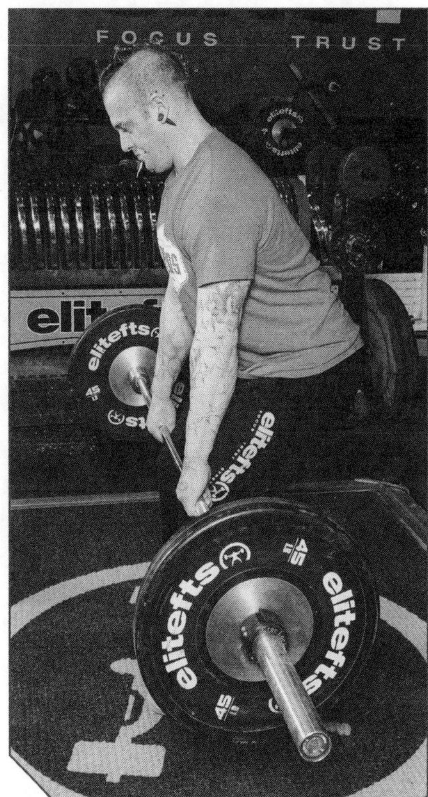

FIGURE 4.12 Incorrect lockout technique: hitching.

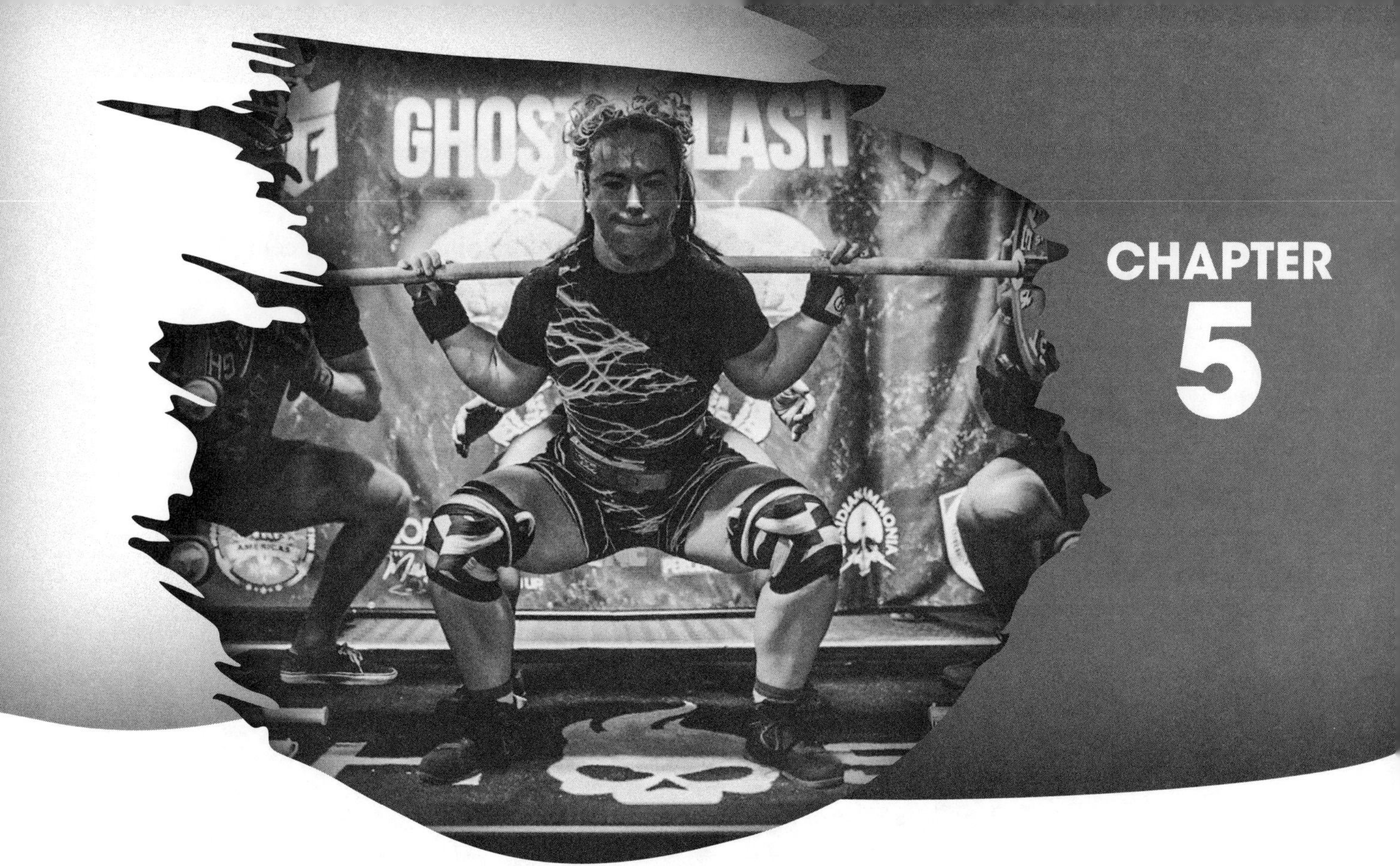

CHAPTER 5

Squat

Just to be clear, when I use the word "squat," I am referring to the back squat. The back squat is *the* squat, and all others are derivatives of it. So, in my opinion, the term "back squat" is irrelevant in the same way the term "squat clean" is.

No exercise divides opinions in lifting circles quite like the squat. It is the most avoided exercise in gyms worldwide while simultaneously having a cultlike following and devotion from other lifters. Listen, I'm (Tom) not going to lie. I'm not a lover of squats. However, it is an unavoidable fact that the squat is a key movement pattern and lift for anyone who wants to be impressively strong.

The squat is often overcomplicated, in my opinion. The squat teaches us to move primarily through the knee joint to move the hip vertically through space. Contrast this to the deadlift, which primarily has us move through the hip joint; it is about moving the hip horizontally through space. Once you get this distinction clear in your head, it becomes easier to stop making your squat look like a deadlift (or good morning) and your deadlift like a squat. In my opinion, the squat is possibly the best teacher (and test) of full-body tension. While the deadlift may be "the king" in some people's eyes, we have all seen plenty of heavy deadlifts that were completed with less than perfect mechanics. You will be much harder pressed to find any truly heavy squats that were completed with similarly faulty mechanics; it is simply less forgiving. It could be said that the deadlift has a little more room for a brute-strength approach while the squat in turn more heavily favors technical precision.

Setup

Since a beautiful squat requires good alignment and stability from the feet right up to the head and neck, that is how we will address the setup procedure. See figure 5.1 for the proper setup for the squat.

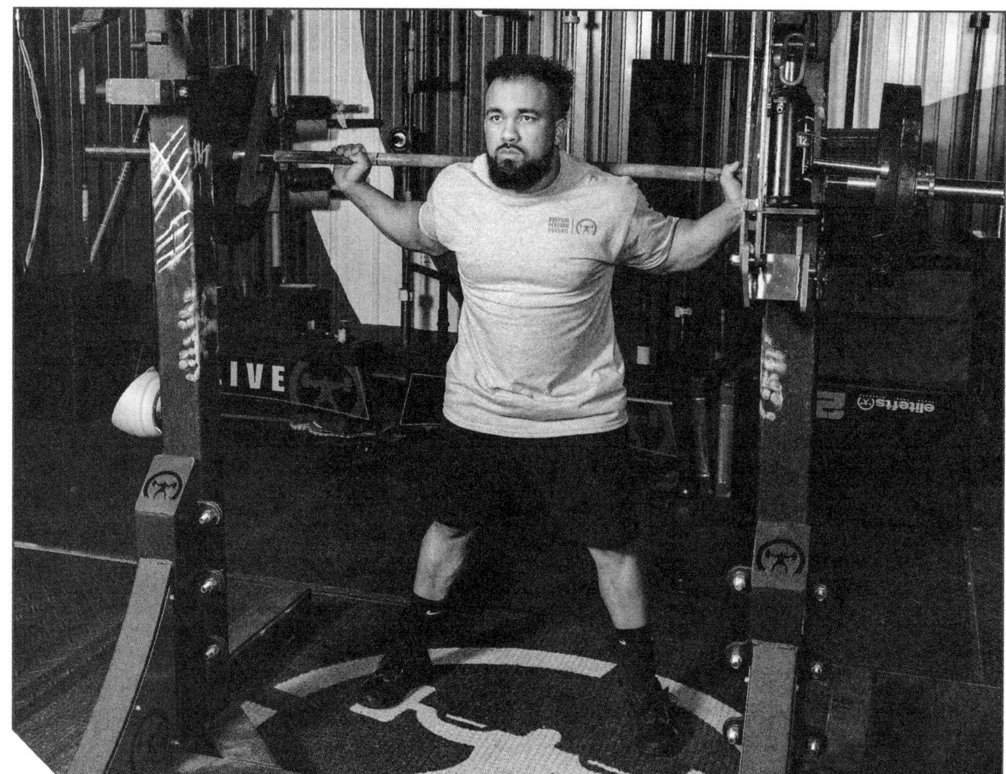

FIGURE 5.1 Setup for the squat.

Width of Stance

Width of stance can heavily come down to personal preference, but since this book is all about moving maximal poundage, that is the viewpoint I will address it from. Remember, we are also talking about the squat in the context of a real squat, one that is done to a depth in which the hip crease passes below the level of the top of the knee.

Assuming mobility isn't an issue, which it shouldn't be for any respectable lifter, then the stance width is going to depend on two main variables:

- *Your limb proportions:* All else being equal, the proportionally longer your legs are (specifically your femurs), the narrower a stance you will require. This is because long-legged, short-torso lifters require more forward knee travel to get to depth because of the extra hip flexion they will need to keep the bar over the midfoot.
- *Hip morphology:* The more outward-facing your hip sockets are (there are ways to test this), the wider a stance you can get away with. It means you can keep your femur centrated (fancy word, huh?) in the hip socket even with a wider stance.

With that being said, your strongest squat stance will be the widest stance that satisfies these two criteria:

1. *The ability to achieve proper depth (hip crease below superior part of knee) without a significant change in spinal alignment (i.e., butt wink):* I am not going to be one of those people who tells you that your squat is awful because you have a tiny bit of butt wink, but a large amount has a huge negative impact on your ability to brace effectively and is simply inefficient in terms of muscular alignment and recruitment.
2. *Being able to keep the knee joint at least stacked vertically directly over the ankle, or slightly outside, all the way through the movement:* In general, performing a loaded squat (or any squat really) with your knee joint inside your ankle joint is not a good idea. Yes, some elite, experienced lifters squat big numbers with a knee-inside-ankle stance (although in raw lifting, they are few and far between), but they have spent years learning exactly how much wiggle room they have and conditioning their soft tissues to the rigors of it.

See figure 5.2 for an example of an optimal squat stance compared to stances that are too wide or too narrow.

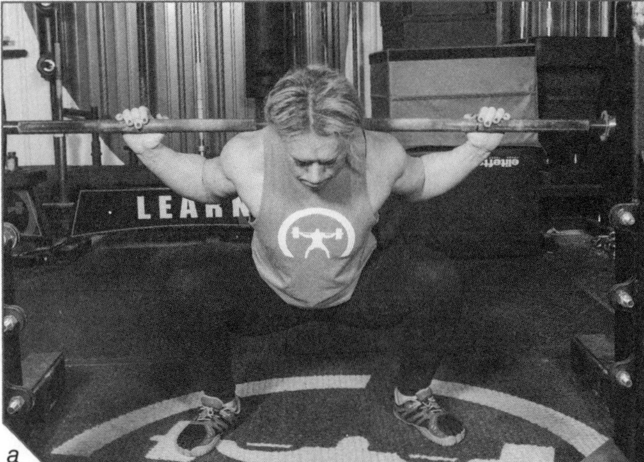

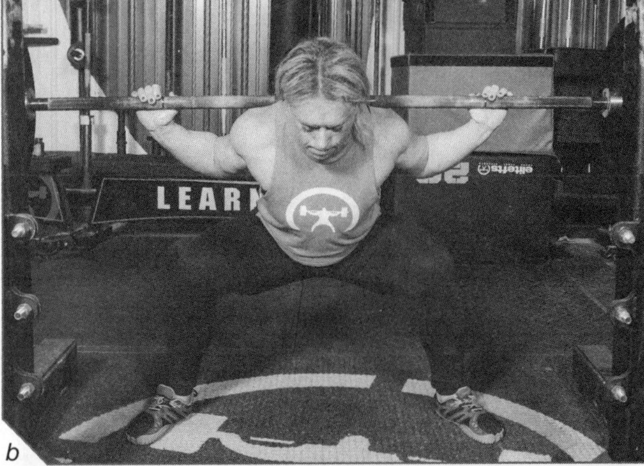

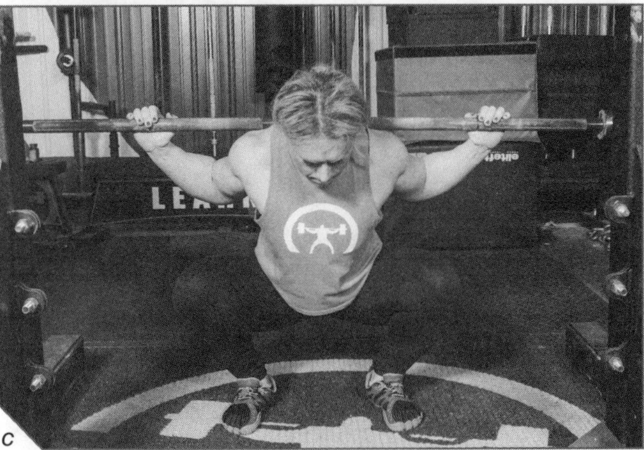

FIGURE 5.2 Comparison of squat stance widths: *(a)* optimal with knees stacked over ankles, *(b)* too wide where the knees are inside the ankles, and *(c)* too narrow where the knees are outside the ankles.

KEY POINT

A lot of people end up making life incredibly difficult with lousy walkouts. It literally burns my eyes when I watch someone walk out a heavy squat and then spend 2 minutes tap dancing around to try and find their stance. Listen, a walkout should consist of one step with each leg and then a slight readjustment of your feet, if needed. The simplest way to achieve this is to simply set up under the bar in your squat stance. Then all you have to do is step directly backward and voilà, you're good to go. Sound stupidly simple? Maybe. But then why do so many people get it wrong?

Foot Angle

Yes, I know we are technically working back down the chain here, but your foot angle will depend on your stance width, not the other way around. Your foot angle is simply the angle that allows your knees to track in the same direction as your toes throughout the lift.

This is easy. Set up and perform a squat and pause at the bottom. Ensure you are twisting your knees out through your glutes just like you would for a heavy squat. If your kneecaps and toes are pointing in the same direction, as shown in figure 5.3, then congrats, you have found your foot angle.

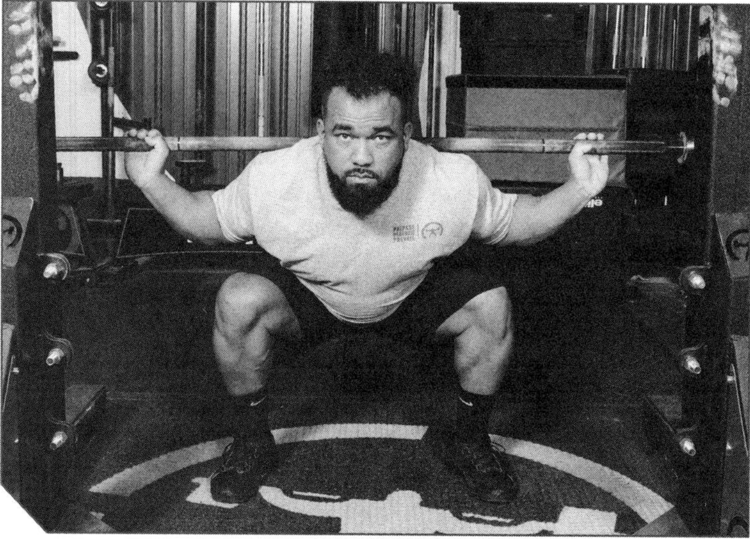

FIGURE 5.3 Proper foot position for the squat.

Hip Alignment

To set up and brace effectively for a squat, you must be standing in a position that allows your rib cage to be stacked directly over your pelvis (i.e., you must be standing tall and upright). This is the position in which the diaphragm and pelvic floor muscles are aligned in a manner that allows the highest degree of intra-abdominal pressure to be created. Once the brace is achieved in the stacked position, then the rib cage and hip alignment should be maintained throughout the entire movement (see figure 5.4). Any change in spinal alignment at this point is simply a power leak.

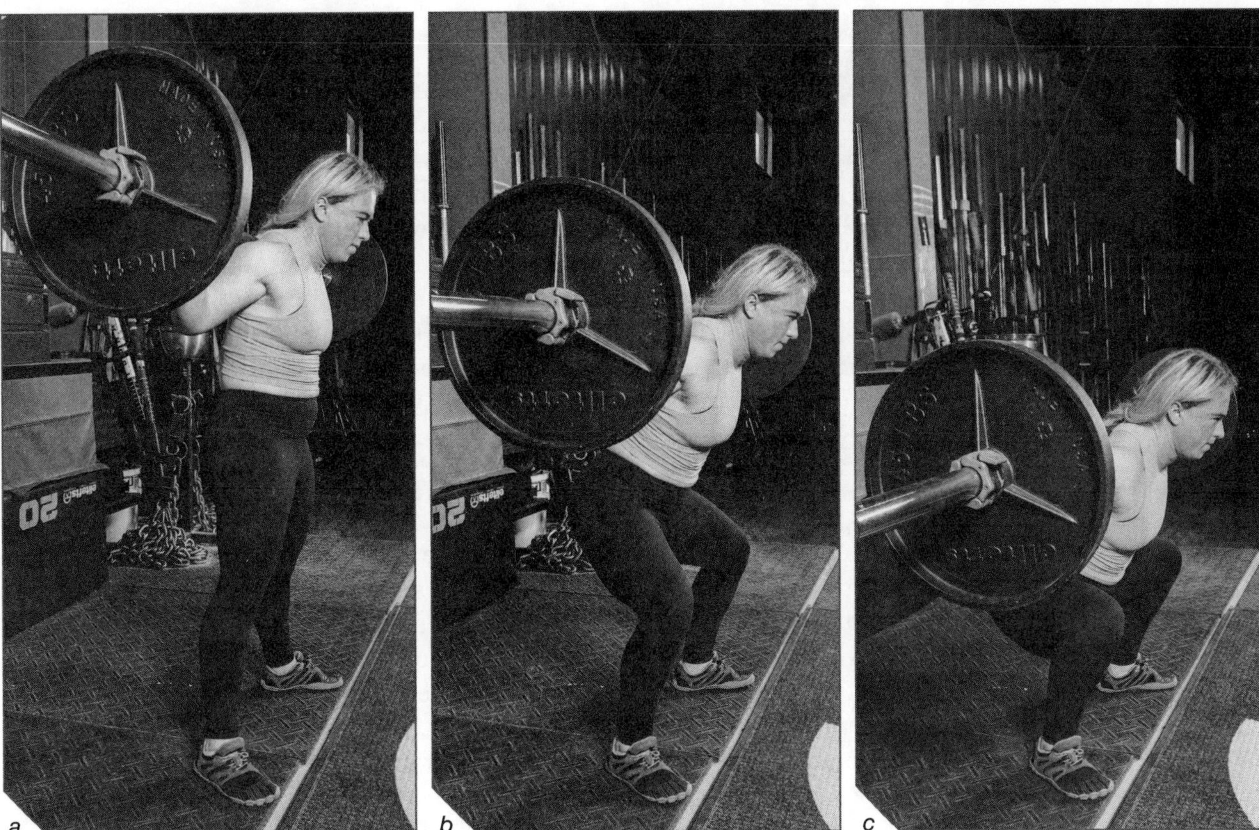

FIGURE 5.4 Stacked ribcage and hip position throughout the squat: *(a)* start, *(b)* midpoint, and *(c)* bottom.

KEY POINT

You will often see lifters using a low bar position who start the movement with the hips already partially flexed. In theory, this isn't a big deal, but you will sacrifice your ability to brace 100 percent maximally if you are trying to set your brace in this position. So, if this is you, either your bar position is too low or you need to grow some bigger rear delts. At the end of the day, if for some reason your squat setup doesn't allow you to stand tall and upright when the bar is on your back, then something is definitely off.

Bar Placement

Since I touched on this previously, I may as well address it now. A huge amount of attention is given to the difference between high bar and low bar positions. Yes, it does change the balance point and the leverages of the lift, but let's be realistic here: The difference in terms of bar position for most people between a high and low bar position is going to be about 1 to 2 inches (2.5 to 5 centimeters). This doesn't change things that much, so they do not need to be treated as two different lifts. Yes, most will be able to move more weight (I will outline why below) with a lower bar position, but in reality, it should come down to whichever one beats you up less and personal preference. Let's take a look.

High Bar Position

The high bar position is when the bar is resting anywhere from the mid to upper traps. This bar position requires less shoulder mobility and allows you to maintain a more upright torso position throughout the lift and leads to more loading through the anterior chain. The higher bar position also means there is a greater workload on the thoracic extensors to stop the chest and shoulders from being "caved in" by the weight. It is generally best suited for lifters with a long torso and short femurs (aka people who are built for squats) because it will shift the load toward what is often their strongest muscle group, the quads, and away from the posterior chain (often a weak point). See figure 5.5*a* for an example of the high bar position for the squat.

Low Bar Position

The low bar position is when the bar is resting on the rear delts. This bar position requires greater shoulder mobility because you have to reach back and down further to get your hands on the bar. As such, a low bar position will usually bring with it a wider grip width, which can make it more difficult to maintain shoulder retraction and back tightness. The lower bar position requires more hip flexion to keep the load centered over the midfoot and therefore leads to more loading through the posterior chain.

By reducing the amount of knee flexion and therefore forward knee travel, you "hit depth" in a higher position in a low bar squat as the knee sits higher relative to the floor in the bottom position—meaning less vertical distance traveled. This along with more recruitment of the posterior chain and a lesser demand on the thoracic extensors (as the load is sitting lower on the thoracic spine) is why most lifters can lift more load with a low bar position. Those with a more deadlift-friendly body structure (short torso, long legs) will generally get a greater benefit from low bar because it will shift the load to their naturally stronger posterior chain. However, some lifters with this build may in turn struggle to hit depth if it requires too high of a degree of hip flexion to keep the bar over the midfoot.

Since the context of this book is about moving maximal weights, I would suggest lifters use a low bar position. Provided you can hit depth while maintaining proper alignment, the low bar position doesn't beat up your elbows and wrists (more on this in a second), and it doesn't feel unnatural for you to do so. See figure 5.5*b* for an example of the low bar position for the squat.

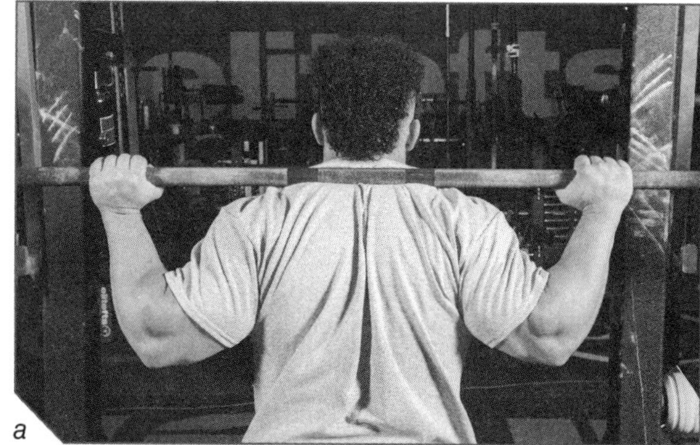
a

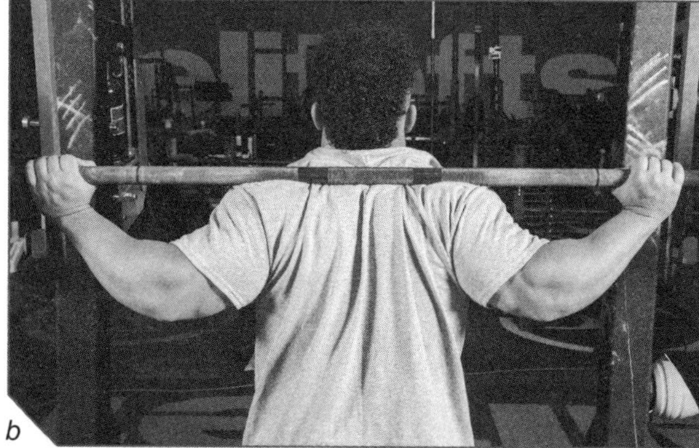
b

FIGURE 5.5 Bar position for the squat: *(a)* high bar and *(b)* low bar.

KEY POINT

Do not make the mistake of thinking there are only two options, high and low bar, when it comes to bar placement. Bar placement is a spectrum. The bar can effectively rest on any part of the upper back between the upper traps and rear delts. So, make sure you experiment with it. Most lifters, in fact, do end up settling on a sort of mid-bar position over time.

Grip Width

Correct grip is key to achieving a stable setup with the bar. It is also very important for keeping your wrist and elbow joints happy since incorrect hand placement can easily lead to tendonitis.

If hand placement for the grip is too narrow, then much of the weight of the bar will rest in your hands rather than on your back, effectively because the height of your hands is higher than the height of your back where the bar is resting. This gives a much worse connection with the bar. It also makes it likely the bar will roll up your back (as your hands are pushing *up* into the bar, due to being wedged in place). Tendonitis will often develop in this circumstance as the weight of the bar is sitting on the wrist and elbow joint rather than on the upper back. Too wide of a grip will simply make it harder to achieve proper back tightness. The wider the hands go relative to the shoulders, the harder it becomes to fully retract the shoulder blades and maximally contract all the muscles associated with that action (which is why using a wider grip on bench requires more upper back stability).

We want the grip width to be as narrow as possible while allowing the wrist to be straight and the weight of the bar to rest fully on the upper back (not in the hand). This will give us the best trade-off between maximal upper back tightness while having the bar resting properly on the back with no undue pressure on the joints. A cocked back wrist position can easily rock back and forth (leading to movement of the bar) and put excessive pressure through the wrist joint. A straight wrist alignment is inherently more stable and will therefore allow you in turn to keep the bar more stable on your back. See figure 5.6 for proper grip position on the bar for the squat compared to a grip that is too wide or too narrow.

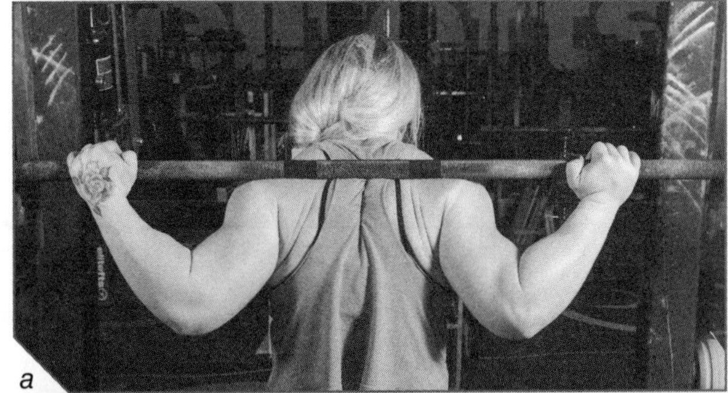
a

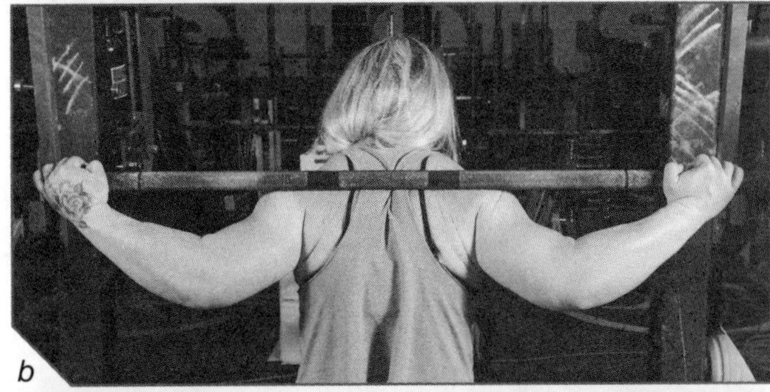
b

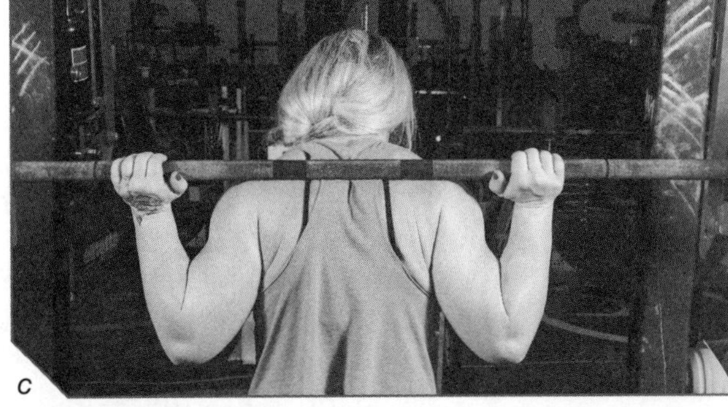
c

FIGURE 5.6 Comparison of grip position on the bar for the squat: *(a)* optimal, *(b)* too wide, and *(c)* too narrow.

As a final note on grip, those who use a low bar position, even with a solid setup, can still develop tendonitis over time, especially if they are squatting and benching frequently. I have found that in many of these cases, using a falcon grip (see figure 5.7), where the little finger is not put over the bar, can almost entirely eradicate this issue. In my experience, it doesn't negatively affect the stability or effectiveness of the setup, and it also sounds really cool. So, it's a win-win all round if this is an issue.

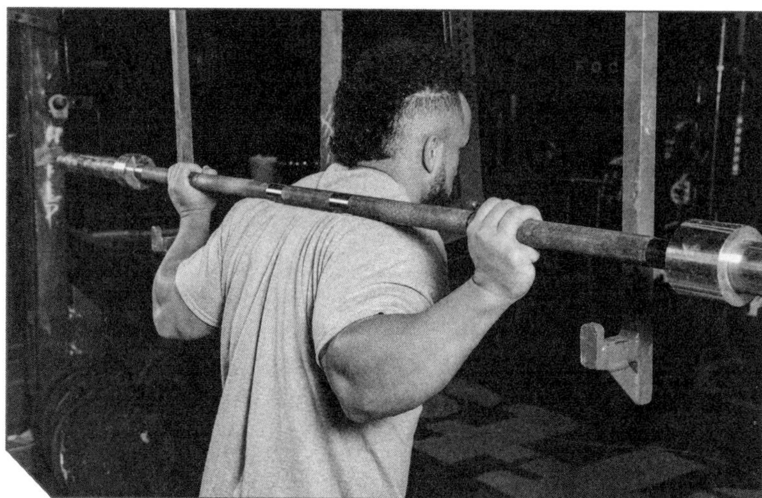

FIGURE 5.7 Falcon grip.

Setting the Upper Back

Once the bar and grip are set, the next step is to give the bar the most stable platform possible to rest on (see figure 5.8). Once the bar is in position, I like to use these three steps to set the upper back (regardless of bar position):

1. Start by squeezing the shoulder blades back and together as hard as possible to get maximal retraction.
2. Drive the elbows even further back and together by squeezing your triceps into your lats. This will further retract the shoulder blades and contract the traps.
3. Pull the bar directly down, into the back through the lats. When done correctly the elbows will only drop slightly as the shoulders depress into the body. If the elbows drop or move forward

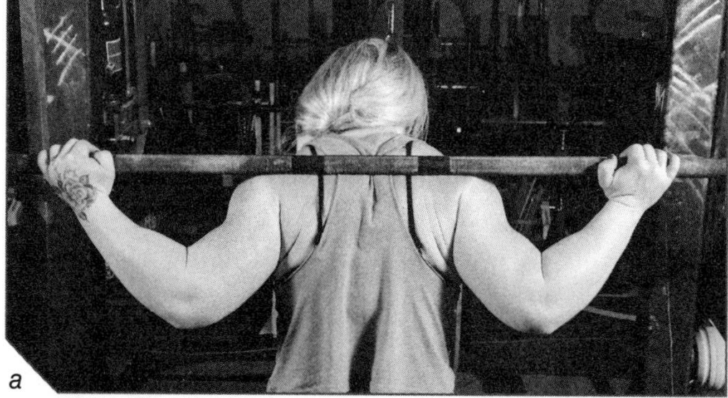

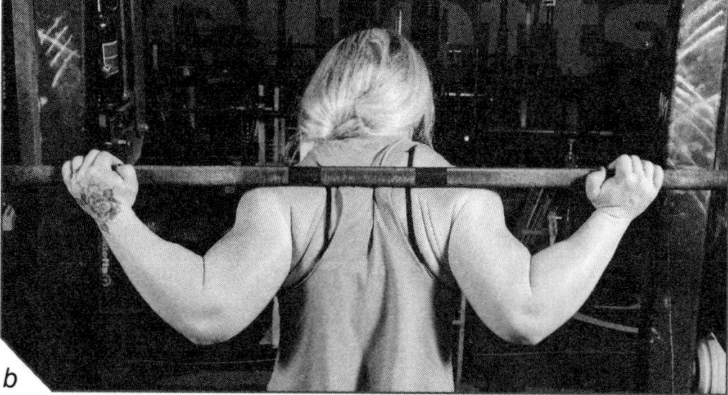

FIGURE 5.8 Comparison of the upper back in the *(a)* neutral and *(b)* set position.

significantly, then all you have done is rotate your shoulder. There is a huge difference between pulling the bar (and shoulders) down into the body through the lats and just rotating the elbows down and forward through the shoulder joint. Setting the lats here is massively important for maintaining torso rigidity and spinal alignment (as discussed with the deadlift).

Elbow Position

Once the upper back is set, there should be no change in elbow position throughout the lift. A change in elbow position shows the shoulders and upper back have changed alignment throughout the lift; it also likely means the bar has rolled in some direction, which is not a recipe for a successful squat. Throughout the squat, simply continue to cue yourself to squeeze your triceps into your lats because this will maintain elbow alignment and upper back tightness.

The elbows rotating down during the descent is often a sign that the lats are being *overused* during the squat. This upper arm movement also then leads to the chest and lumbar spine arching up. This results in a loss of bracing strength and an anterior tilting of the pelvis, which makes it more difficult to hit depth. Remember, once the shoulders have been maximally depressed, the job of the lats is done; they should only be contracting isometrically at that point.

Be aware that bar positioning alters elbow positioning. For example, when squatting high bar, one can get away with having the elbows very low or even directly under the bar (see figure 5.9*a*). This can even be beneficial because it gives a more direct line to pull down on the bar into the traps through the lats. With low bar, however, this is not the case. A higher elbow position is necessary with low bar as it "props up" the rear delts to make them an effective shelf for the bar to rest on (see figure 5.9*b*). If the elbows drop too low, the rear delts will not protrude out far enough from the body for the bar to rest on fully (unless you have enormous rear delts). This is why elbow movement (as addressed in the point above) is even more hazardous when using a low bar position. So, when using a low bar position, the elbows will be pushed up to maintain the shelf; just make sure you don't push them up too high because this will result in the thoracic spine and shoulder girdle rounding forward.

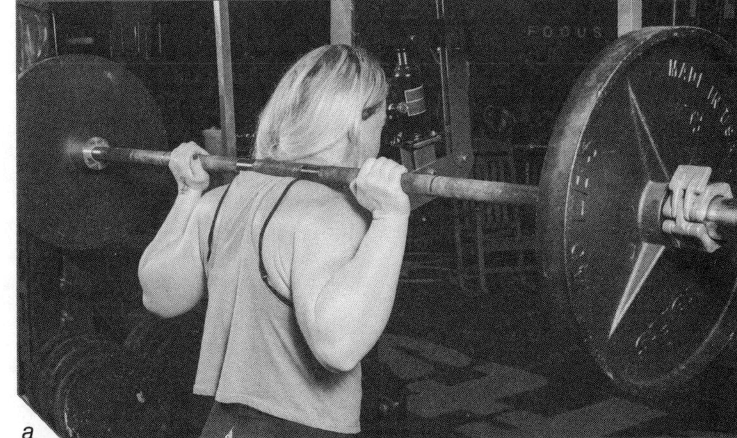

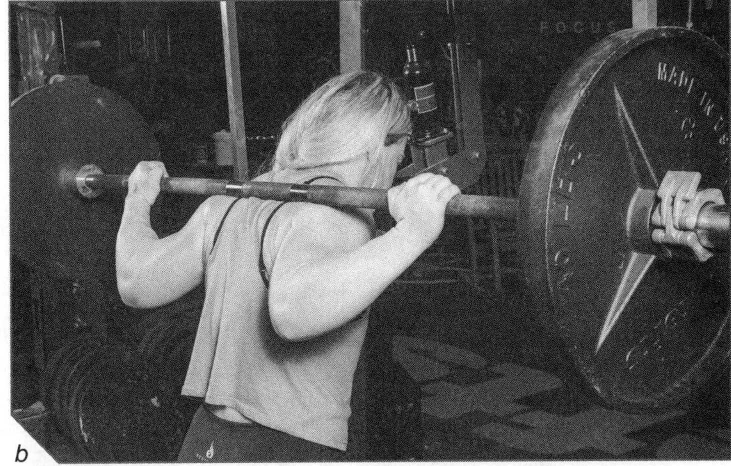

FIGURE 5.9 Elbow position for *(a)* high bar and *(b)* low bar.

Head Position

We want a neutral alignment once again through the entire spine here. So, just as with deadlift, we want the chin slightly tucked and the crown of the head as tall to the sky as possible. We want this alignment to be maintained throughout the lift—so yes, this will mean at the bottom of the squat, your head should be at a downward angle. See figure 5.10 for an example of proper head position during a squat.

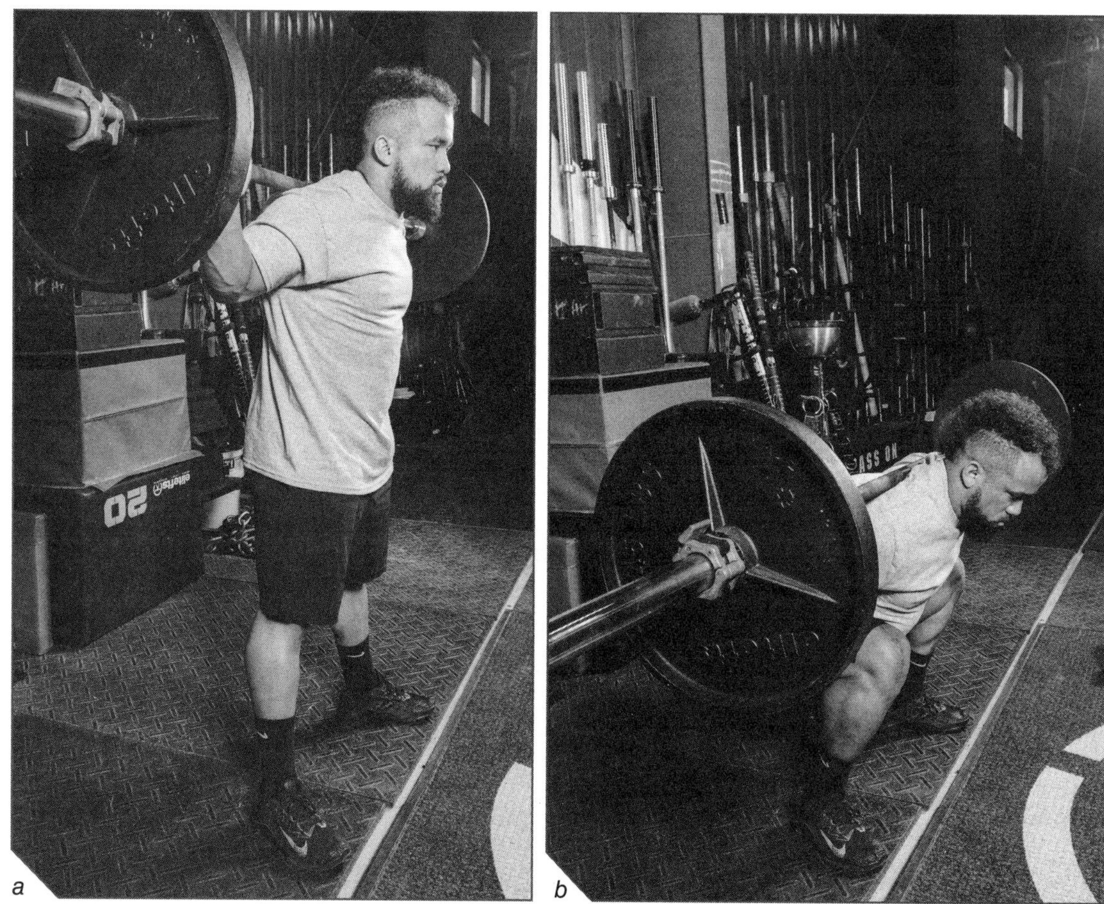

FIGURE 5.10 Correct head position for the squat at the *(a)* start and *(b)* bottom position.

KEY POINT

Many coaches teach lifters to look up and arch the head up during the squat (as well as deadlift), which they justify by saying that it will help you to "keep the chest up" or that "the body goes where the head goes." However, if you have proper functioning of your thoracic and cervical spine, then arching your head up should not bring the chest up with it. Last I checked, the neck is meant to be able to move independently of other segments of the spine. Furthermore, yes, arching the head up can in fact increase neural drive to the traps and thoracic extensors and posterior chain (which could in turn help you keep your chest up, perhaps), but this comes at the expense of reduced neural drive to the abdominals and anterior chain. So that is not a trade-off worth making. As we've said already, spinal alignment is at its strongest when neutral, so let's respect that principle.

Bar Path and Movement Pattern

The desired bar path of the squat is incredibly simple. The bar should stay directly over the midfoot at all times, meaning the bar path should be perfectly vertical during both the eccentric and concentric portions of the exercise. In fact, any deviation from this vertical bar path indicates a technical fault. It could come down to mobility, muscle imbalance, or simply technical skill. Regardless, any deviation that causes the bar to not be directly over the midfoot is inefficient and should be corrected.

Assessing your bar path is easy. Simply film yourself performing a set of squats (from the side) so that you can see your entire body from head to toe (ideally using around 30 to 40 percent of your 1RM). I can't explain why, but often the leverages and balance points just don't seem to work as well with very low loads, or people just don't put the effort in to squat those lower loads correctly. Watch the end of the barbell: Does it stay directly over your midfoot and move vertically? Here are two improper bar paths that we commonly see and how to fix them.

Bar Drifts Forward Over the Toes

If this happens, it is because there is too much hip flexion compared to knee flexion, leading to the torso being pitched too far forward. If this occurs on the descent, it is most often due to poor ankle mobility inhibiting the knees from traveling far enough forward. When the knees hit a brick wall and can't move forward, the body will simply bend from the hip more instead to get lower. However, this often sadly doesn't result in the hip actually moving downward at all, even if the bar is. So, it is not leading to any further depth being achieved; instead, you are being folded in half like a human accordion. If this occurs on the ascent, then this is your typical squat good morning, where the knees extend without the hips, leading to the hips rising up but the shoulders (and therefore the bar along with them) staying still. This is most commonly caused by a weak anterior chain (mainly quads), so the body shifts the weight on to the stronger posterior chain. In theory, this makes sense, but in reality, it puts us in such a weak position that it means the lift will rarely be successful. It also places a much greater amount of shear stress through the spine. Even if you can be successful with this squatting pattern in the short term, it is very inefficient and simply shows you have a weakness that is going to hold you back in the long term.

Bar Drifts Backward Toward the Heels

This is pretty rare, but it happens because there's too much knee flexion relative to hip flexion. On the descent, this is usually caused by people thinking they need to squat perfectly upright; in essence, they are trying to front squat their back squat. You must lean forward in a squat to keep the bar centered over the midfoot; by how much, exactly, will depend on bar position and your leverages. If you are guilty of this, you need to encourage your hips to flex more on the descent. Thinking about pointing your chest toward the floor on the descent and looking down a little more will help. It is particularly rare to see the bar shift back toward the heels on the upward phase of a squat. If you see this, it will be in Olympic-style squatters who are very quad dominant. Here, the knees stay forward for too long to keep the quads loaded while the torso becomes more upright as the hips extend, which is an incredibly difficult position to salvage.

To this point, we have identified the bar path that we want to achieve throughout our lift. Now, let's break down the lift to its constituent segments and see how we achieve that. See figure 5.11 for the full movement of a squat.

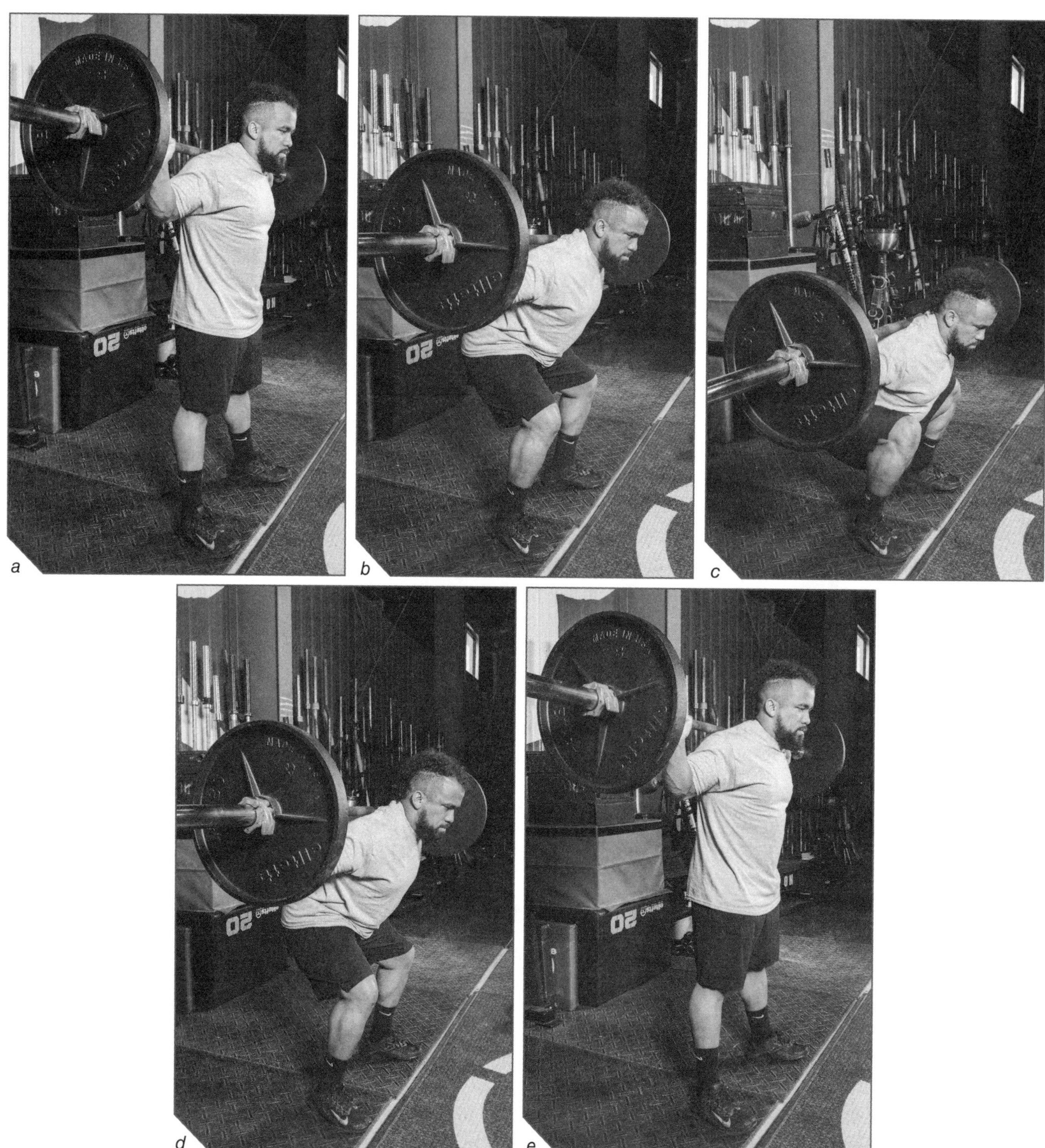

FIGURE 5.11 The segments of the squat: *(a)* start, *(b)* midpoint (end of eccentric phase I), *(c)* bottom (end of eccentric phase II), *(d)* midpoint (end of concentric phase I), and *(e)* finish (end of concentric phase II).

Eccentric Portion

Your goals during the eccentric portion of the squat are as follows:

- Keep the bar directly over the midfoot.
- Maintain bar position and upper back tightness by pulling the bar down into the bar through the lats and squeezing the triceps in toward the lats.
- Maintain hip, knee, and foot alignment by moderately externally rotating the knees. This is best done by gripping the floor through the feet and twisting as if you were trying to rip the floor apart. The kneecap and toes should be oriented in the same direction at all times. Note that so much is made out of "driving the knees out" and "engaging the glutes" that a lot of people actually end up externally rotating the knees out too much, so the knees end up wider than the ankles. This leaves us having further to travel to hit depth (non-vertical shins mean the knee is lower to the ground) as well as placing more pressure on the outside of the foot, leaving the adductors, among other muscles, in a poor position to contribute to the lift. Yes, the glutes are important, and yes, they are a prime mover, but it's not *all* about the glutes here. It's about balance and aligning yourself in a manner that allows all muscle groups to work optimally.
- Stabilize the spine through proper bracing mechanics. This is best represented by the ability to keep the gap between your sternum and belly button (or lowest rib and hip bone) constant throughout the lift. If this gap increases, it means you have extended through the thoracic and lumbar spine. If it decreases, it means you have been "folded in" by the weight through thoracic and lumbar flexion.
- Don't die. This makes the concentric phase very difficult to complete. I struggle with this bit.

KEY POINT

One of the most common issues I see with the squat is an overextension of the spine. We have had "chest up" or "back arched" drilled into us so much that we end up thinking we know we have to be way overextended through the lumbar and thoracic spine to perform a loaded squat. Again, it is about balance here. An overextended spine simply puts your abdominals in a disadvantaged position to create pressure and stability. Likewise, it pre-stretches the glutes, putting them in a worse position to contribute to hip extension. Trust your abs and anterior chain with more of the load, and get your whole body working the way it should.

Just like the deadlift, there are two phases to the movement, which can be distinguished by what happens to the inclination of the torso. In phase I (top half), we have a change in torso angle, relative to the floor, throughout. Whereas in phase II (bottom half), the torso angle stays stable.

Phase I

Once you are set up correctly, the descent should be initiated by breaking from the knee and the hip simultaneously. Doing so will mean you spread the load in a balanced fashion. The knee and the hip have to flex in tandem to keep the load balanced over the midfoot. During the top half of the movement, the knees will be traveling forward over the toes and the hips backward. If you do this correctly, by the time you have reached the midpoint of the descent (give or take), the knees will be as far forward as they are going to be. The torso, too, will be angled as far forward now as it will be at any point in the lift, unless some technical fault occurs. Please note that how far your knees travel forward here is completely determined by leverages, stance width, and bar placement. Those with proportionally longer legs, narrower stances, or a higher bar placement will require more forward knee travel to keep the system in balance. If your knee pass over your toes, that is perfectly fine, provided the bar is maintained in alignment over the midfoot.

KEY POINT

You will often hear that you should break from the knee or hip first to recruit the quad or hip more. While it can work to a degree, it really only works because you are not recruiting those muscles or moving in a manner that loads them correctly in the first place. Also, it can often lead you to squatting in a manner that then favors that joint or muscle group. If you don't let your knees move forward enough (for example) in your squat unless you break from the knee joint first, then this is an issue you need to address. Don't stick a Band-Aid over it. Address the faulty movement pattern.

Phase II

Since the knees are already as far forward as they are going to go, and the torso angle is set, then phase II simply consists of the hips sitting straight down until the bottom position is achieved. During this phase, the shoulders and hips should move in tandem to maintain the torso angle relative to the floor, and the knees should not move further forward.

In the bottom position, you have two options: Relax a little to emphasize the stretch reflex or rebound, or focus on maintaining rigidity and reverse the movement in a more controlled manner. There are several factors, on top of personal preference, that will dictate which will suit you best. Here are the guidelines that generally I go with:

- *Favoring the stretch reflex:* Stable technique (and an experienced lifter); a strong stretch reflex (naturally explosive, good performance in jumping or plyometric-based exercises); proportionally short legs with upright squatting posture; proportionally strong eccentric strength (can control eccentric loads of 110 to 120 percent of 1RM)
- *The "staying tight" approach:* Unreliable technique; naturally slow or a grinding lifting style; proportionally long legs with lots of forward lean; poor eccentric strength; under-developed ligament or tendon strength

Generally, the most important factor I tend to find is the lower body proportions. Those with long legs have longer levers, which always brings with it greater stability demands. So, the idea of partially relaxing and speeding up at the bottom of the squat (the position with the highest stability demands) simply isn't a good one here. The benefit of a stronger muscle contraction out of the bottom position simply doesn't outweigh the negative of reduced stability where the demands are highest. However, a short-legged lifter with short levers to stabilize can likely get away with it and reap the benefits of the stretch reflex.

If you are not choosing to use the stretch reflex in your squat, then your mindset here should be to progressively build up more and more full-body tension as you approach the bottom position. At the bottom of a heavy squat, it should feel like your head is about to explode from the pressure built up. When I coach, I like to say it is as if you were attempting to do a pause squat; you should have enough tension (throughout the whole descent ideally) that you could pause at any time if required. Then, when it comes to reversing the movement, you will be in the best position in terms of stability and muscular tension to do so.

If you are using the stretch reflex, then I still like to coach the descent in the same manner, with one exception: You will relax slightly as you approach the bottom of the lift. If you are efficient with the stretch reflex, then you shouldn't need to free-fall for half of the lift to use it—plus, that leaves too much opportunity for losing positioning. As a general rule, I like to have lifters "relax" just above parallel to allow them enough distance to speed up and catch the bounce without sacrificing control for too long.

Just to be clear, when we say "relax" here, we are talking relatively. There should be a 10 to 20 percent relaxation of the prime movers (quads, hamstrings, glutes) of the lift and nothing else. This is done just enough to allow a stretching of these muscle groups at the bottom without sacrificing positioning (knees stacked directly over ankles, no extra forward movement of the knee). The upper back and abs that are holding your torso position absolutely should not relax at all.

KEY POINT

You will often see the knees move forward at the bottom of the squat when someone is using the stretch reflex or if someone has a very knee dominant or upright squat style. As discussed, the knees should be as far forward as they are going to be by the end of phase I. Forward knee travel at the bottom is usually a subconscious mechanism to work around a weakness: to get a greater stretch reflex (poor strength or stability in the bottom position) or to excessively load the quads (lacking posterior chain strength). It is also likely to cause a forward shift off balance onto the toes in the bottom, which will negatively affect your positioning. The only time this can be beneficial is if you are squatting in knee wraps, which provide a lot of stretch and rebound. In this case, the extra stretching of the wrap at the bottom can exaggerate the effect of the wraps, but even then, you must be careful to make sure it doesn't cause a forward balance shift.

Concentric Portion

Great job. You got to the bottom of the squat—hooray for gravity. Now it's time for the difficult bit. For the upward phase, we go through the same two phases that we did in the downward phase with a few minor differences.

Phase I

During phase I of the concentric portion, the hips and shoulders should rise together (just like in the first phase of the deadlift); that is, the torso angle relative to the floor should stay stable. Unlike on the downward movement, however, the knees do move during this phase. The knees will move back marginally to facilitate a stronger quad drive out of the hole, which means, in turn, that the hips will also shift backward slightly. As this occurs, you should encourage your knees to stay stacked wide, directly over the ankle joint. Allowing them to buckle in out of the hole will reduce your hip and glute strength and more likely lead to a squat good morning–style lift.

It is important during this phase to remember to not only push up into the bar but also back into the bar to avoid the hips moving backward too far. Likewise, you cannot allow the knees to move too far back as it will mean the quads become unloaded and cannot contribute to the next phase of the lift. I like to cue lifters to try to keep their knees over their toes, if they are guilty of letting them shift back too much out of the bottom.

Lifters can fail the lift for a multitude of reasons, but the most common causes are the following:

- Glute strength, if a lifter stays upright. Glutes are recruited most in the bottom position where they are most stretched. So, the lifter is lacking in hip extension strength that could be remedied through the good morning and Romanian deadlift variations, along with some wider-stance squat work.
- Quad strength, if a lifter's hips shift back and up (the typical squat good morning). This occurs as the load is being shifted back onto the posterior chain because the quads cannot produce enough force. This also results in more shear stress through the spine. Strengthening the anterior chain through front-loaded squat variations would be advised here.
- Torso or core stability, if a lifter folds over or collapses. Quite simply, the lifter is unable to maintain enough core rigidity to maintain the spine in alignment under the load, resulting in the bar flexing the spine forward. This can be aided by front-loaded squat variations because of their high demand on core rigidity. But loaded carries would work well here, along with working on your breathing patterning.

How you fail the lift can indicate what you need to work on and improve because it illustrates where your weak point is. In reality, often weaknesses will show up well before you fail a lift, and they will present through bar path or body position changes. This is why it is important to analyze your own lifting regularly.

Phase II

In theory, phase II is the easy bit. The leverages are much more favorable. It is during phase II of the ascent that the torso angle shifts from being forward to being vertical. This is achieved through hip extension, driving the hips forward underneath the bar. While there is knee extension here (and, in fact, top-half-only squats load the quads very effectively), the hip joint goes through a lot more movement in this phase.

During this phase, it is important to remember to keep driving up and back into the bar to encourage knee and hip extension together. Encourage the hips to wedge forward aggressively underneath the bar to lock out the lift as early as possible. The knee and hip joint should lock out simultaneously at the top of the lift. During this phase, the knees will drift inward, inside the knees, as the knee joint extends and the legs straighten. At the top, you should once again be able to stand tall with the bar on your back; if not, then something has shifted in terms of your setup during the rep.

During phase I, lifters will generally fail for one of the following reasons:

- Weak upper back and postural strength, often represented by the chest and shoulders caving forward. Again. Front-loaded squat variations and additional upper back work would be recommended here.
- Weak vastus medialis oblique (VMO), illustrated by poor knee stability and an inability to complete knee extension. Split squat variations are your go-to here if this your issue. I prefer performing them with the front-foot elevated.
- Poor stability. Although this is not generally an issue until weights get truly heavy, it is reasonably common to see truly heavy squats missed at the top because of a loss of balance. Single leg work can often address this situation if the issue is from the hip. Front-sided squat variations can be of use if the issue is torso rigidity. My favorite method, however, is the hanging band technique (HBT).
- Lack of intent. The lifter partially relaxes once they are out of the bottom position, thinking the hard work is done.

Again, these signs can guide you in determining what you need to work on to keep your squat improving by showing you what is the weakest link in the chain.

KEY POINT

The upper back collapsing in the top half of the lift is often preceded by the bar rolling up the back (increasing the workload on the thoracic extensors and changing the balance point). This often occurs because the lifter is subconsciously pushing *up* into the bar through the arms to help lift the weight. You should be pulling down on the bar, through the lats, at all times. Don't try to shoulder-press your 1RM squat!

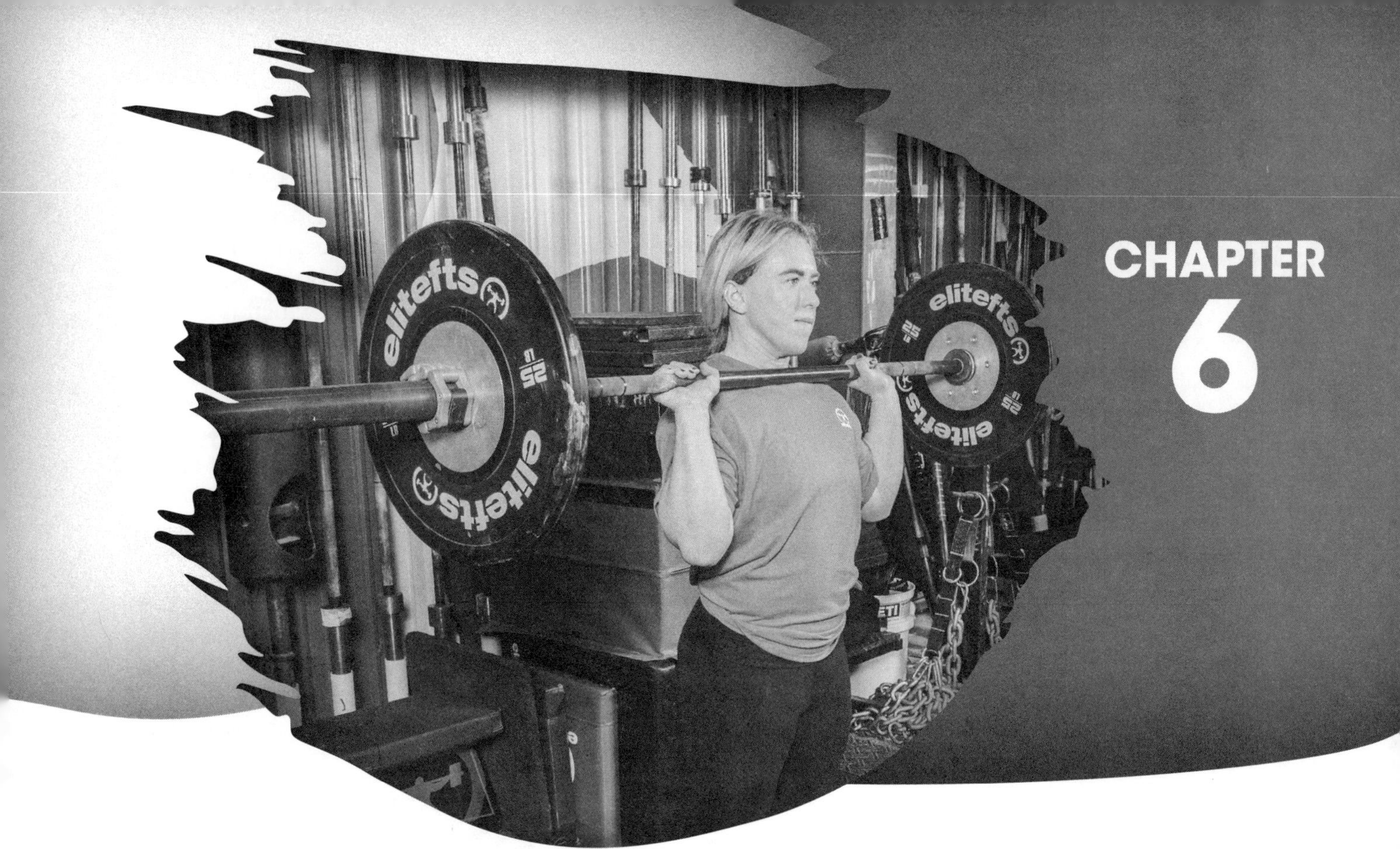

CHAPTER 6

Military Press

For decades, the military press was referred to as "the press" because it was the only press of perceived importance. There were no benches in gyms during these times, and anyway, why would you go to a gym to lie down? The main pressing exercises were overhead presses (press, push press, jerk, etc.), dips, and push-ups. How much weight you could put over your head was seen as a top priority, along with how much weight you could lift from the floor. The best example is Arthur Saxon, who holds the world record in the bent press of 371 pounds (168 kilograms)—look up the bent press to see exactly how impressive that is. Then the world changed, and everyone started bench-pressing, taking selfies in the gym, and posting on TikTok (if that's not devolution, then I don't know what is). It's time to make overhead pressing great again, people.

Just to clarify, we are talking about the military press here, not the arched-back Olympic press. The Olympic clean and press was removed in 1972 because it essentially became a standing incline bench press and a test of which lifter had the most flexible and resilient spine. A military press (hereafter referred to as *press*) is performed with upright (military-like) posture and very little movement through the torso throughout the lift.

So why has the press fallen in popularity? Because it's hard. The press challenges you far beyond the ability of the pressing muscles to produce force. It requires a great deal of stability, coordination, and postural strength (you know, all the stuff most people are terrible at). It also doesn't massage the ego like the bench press can because the loads lifted will be smaller; also, there are fewer ways to cheat a few extra kilos on to the bar (e.g., bouncing off the chest, driving hips up off the bench). Because of the smaller loads lifted, it also requires a lot of patience since progress will seem slow. Adding 5 percent to a lift is great progress; but when that 5 percent only equates to 2 to 3 kilograms (4 to 7 pounds) then it can test even the most determined lifters patience, which is something we seem to be painfully short of as a species now.

Setup

I am going to address setup as if you were performing your presses with the bar in a rack. You could argue a true old-time press would be done without a rack, but then I would have to write a whole extra section on how to power clean it up to position (and by this point, you are likely already half asleep). See figure 6.1 for proper setup for the military press.

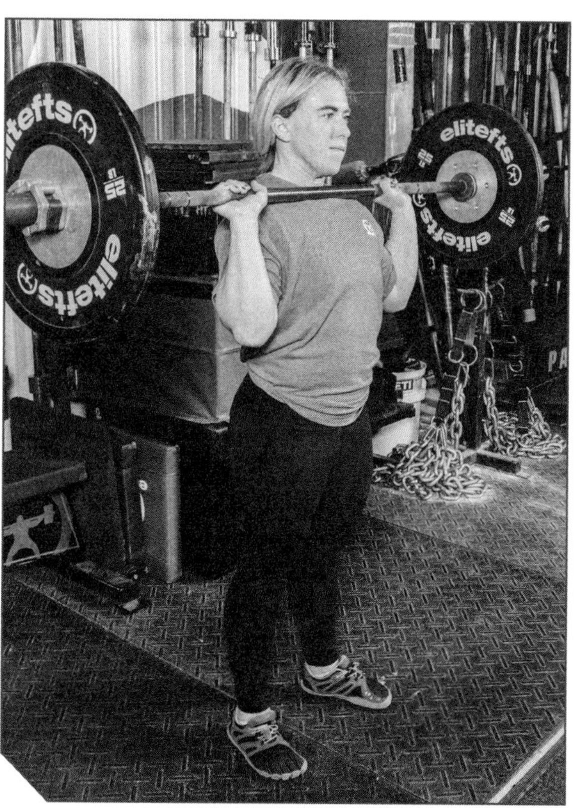

FIGURE 6.1 Setup for the military press.

Stance

Stance width will affect your overall stability throughout the lift. If the stance is too narrow, your base will be too small to provide enough stability. If the stance is too wide, it will almost provide too much stability and allow you to get away with too much back bend.

Between hip width and shoulder width is a very good starting point for most lifters. Personally, I favor a narrower hip-width stance during the press. It emphasizes the core stability element of the lift by being less forgiving when it comes to back bend and leaning back, which, in my opinion, is one of the greatest benefits of the press. Note that you will see some individuals adopt a split stance during the press. This is just a way of cheating to get more support. The back leg can be used to allow a greater degree of backward lean during the lift. This is generally done because of a lack of stability, core strength, or skill. Do it properly or not at all. See figure 6.1 for an example of proper foot position for the military press.

Grip Width

The first step to setting up for a successful press is getting the correct grip width. Most people end up gripping too wide to subconsciously cheat by reducing the range of motion and also recruiting the pecs more once they inevitably lean back.

The grip width should be the widest grip that allows you to achieve the proper alignment in the starting position (addressed below). For 90 percent or more of lifters, this means a grip width just outside your shoulders. This may vary a little depending on your proportions, but setting your grip so that your index fingers are just outside the width of your shoulders in the bottom position will put most people very close to, if not in, the optimal start position. See figure 6.2 for grip position for the military press.

Adopting a grip narrower than this is generally inefficient because it will lead to your arms and shoulders being internally rotated at the bottom position. It will also lead to your hands being partially inhibited by your own shoulders as you press out of the bottom position. Likewise, a wider grip may reduce the range of motion but will lead to the arm and shoulder being too externally rotated in the bottom position. This will stop you from getting your elbow directly under your wrist (more on this shortly) and reduce your starting strength. Also, it's worth noting that the optimal grip for your press will be different from that of your push press or jerk, so don't use your grip on one of these exercises to determine the other.

As well as grip width, you have a few options regarding how to actually grip the bar. Of course, you could just use a regular grip (see figure 6.3*a*), but many lifters struggle to achieve proper alignment with this grip. Over time, this can lead to discomfort or potentially tendonitis. So many lifters benefit from adopting a false grip, where the thumb is pressed into the underside of the bar (see figure 6.3*b*), or a suicide grip, where the thumb is not around the bar (see figure 6.3*c*). You won't drop the bar, and these grips actually allow you to achieve a more neutral wrist position, putting less pressure on the elbow joint. This actually makes it a more joint-friendly option as well as potentially stronger, due to the improved alignment. Note that pressing using fat or axle bars can achieve a similar outcome.

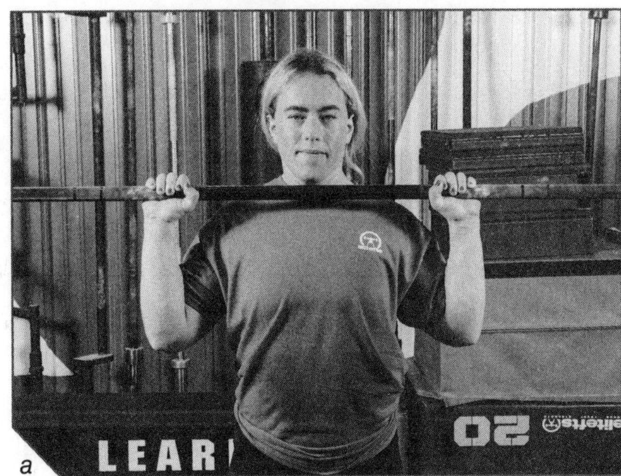

a

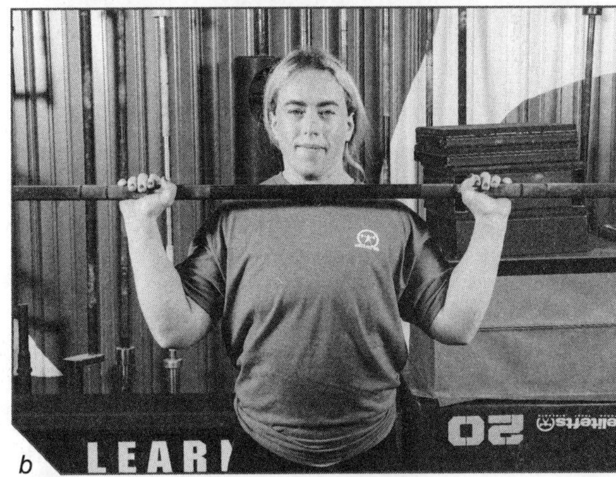

b

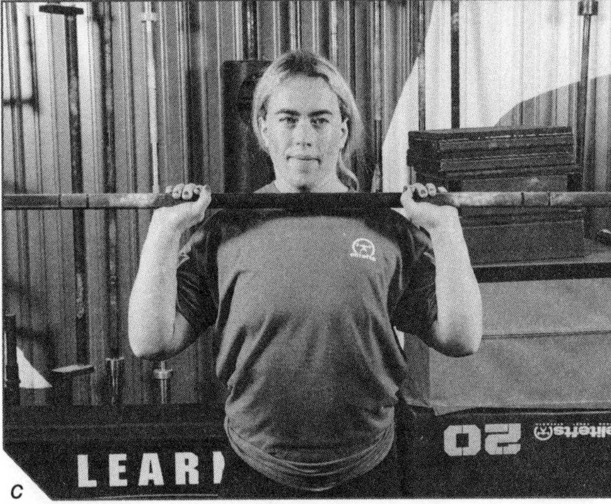

c

FIGURE 6.2 Comparison of grip position on the bar for the military press: *(a)* optimal, *(b)* too wide, and *(c)* too narrow.

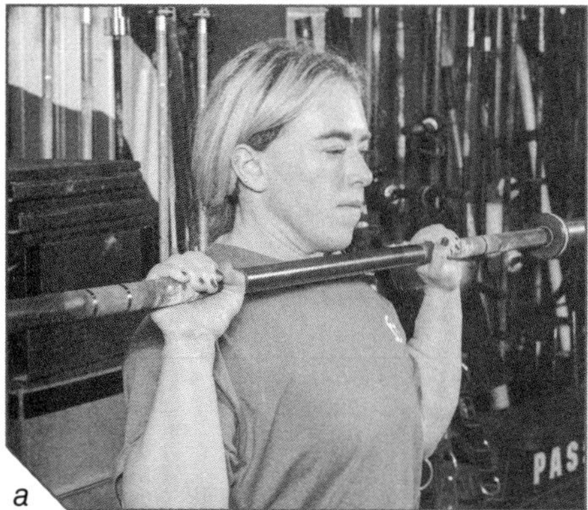

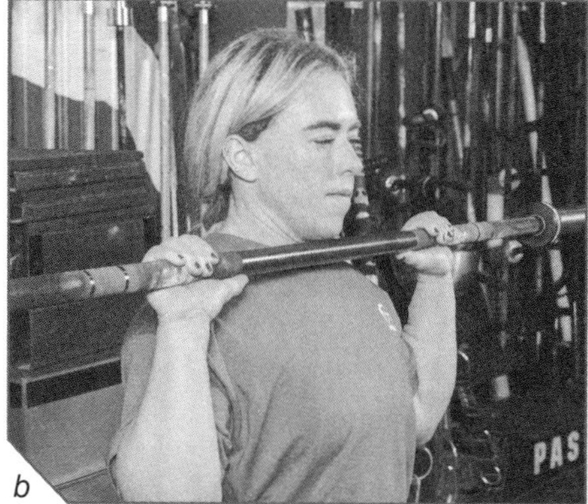

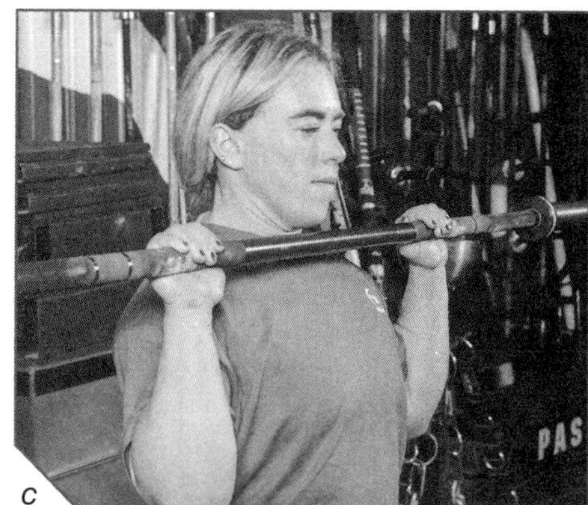

FIGURE 6.3 Types of grips for the military press: *(a)* regular, *(b)* false, and *(c)* suicide.

Wrist and Elbow Position

Once the correct grip width is set, we now need to set up the upper arms and shoulders around it. A common mistake with the press is setting up with the bar too low relative to the body. This results in the elbow joint sitting behind the bar and outside the wrists. Where the bar will start relative to your body is simply a by-product of your arm proportions. If your forearm is considerably longer than your upper arm, then the bar will sit relatively higher compared to your body. The start position of the press, as shown in figure 6.4, is the lowest position in which you can accomplish the following:

- Align the elbow joint directly underneath or, ideally, slightly in front of, the bar.
- Align the elbow joint directly under the wrist joint in terms of lateral space (i.e., when viewed from the front).

This is the most efficient start position and gives us the best alignment to apply force vertically into the bar. In this start position, the bar will be slightly in front of your center of gravity, which will necessitate a very slight backward lean to keep the system in balance.

If you struggle to achieve the start position outlined here, then your mobility needs work. The most likely culprits are going to be the pec minor and lats, so start hammering those areas with soft tissue work and stretching. Yes, it's boring and time-consuming, but not as boring and time-consuming as being injured (or weak).

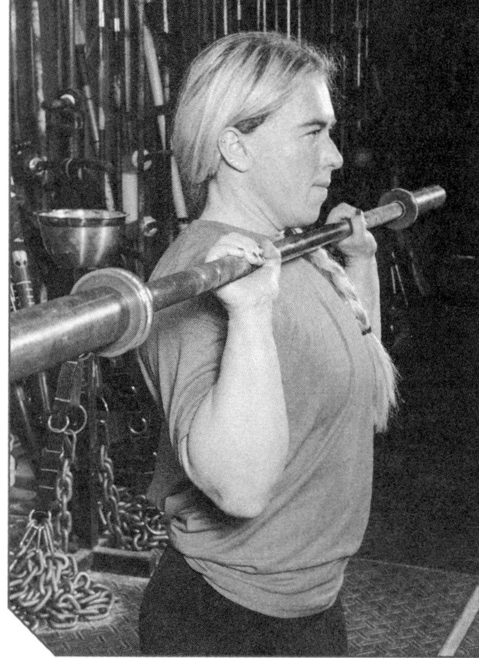

FIGURE 6.4 Correct alignment for the start of the military press.

KEY POINT

While the start position outlined for the military press is optimal for this exercise, note that it is not the best start position for the push press or the jerk. The push press and jerk rely heavily on the transfer of force from the legs into the bar and so benefit from starting in the front rack position, in contact with the delts. This allows a much greater transfer of force from the legs into the bar. The push press can be done reasonably well from the same starting position as the press (and is employed often by lifters who lack the mobility to achieve proper front rack positioning—just look at World's Strongest Man competitors), but it does result in less efficient force transfer. The press can be done from a front rack position, but it doesn't really carry any benefit. Likewise, achieving a proper front rack position requires a lot more mobility, which many lifters lack.

Upper Back Position

As in many lifts, it is common to see lifters overextended through the lumbar spine and over-retracted through the shoulder blades when performing the press. Because the average person now has the upper back posture of a Neanderthal, we are constantly drilled to "pull your shoulders back!"—to the point where those with half-decent posture end up performing their lifts with overly retracted shoulders.

The upper back should be set in slight retraction while maintaining a neutral thoracic spine and centrated shoulders. What this means in plain language is to slightly retract your shoulders while keeping your shoulders as wide as possible (imagine trying to keep your collarbone as wide as possible). This positioning allows the shoulders to be centrated properly and the scapulae to be in the best position to stabilize them throughout the movement (see figure 6.5). Having the shoulders overly retracted impinges on the scapulae's ability to glide properly, therefore reducing shoulder stability.

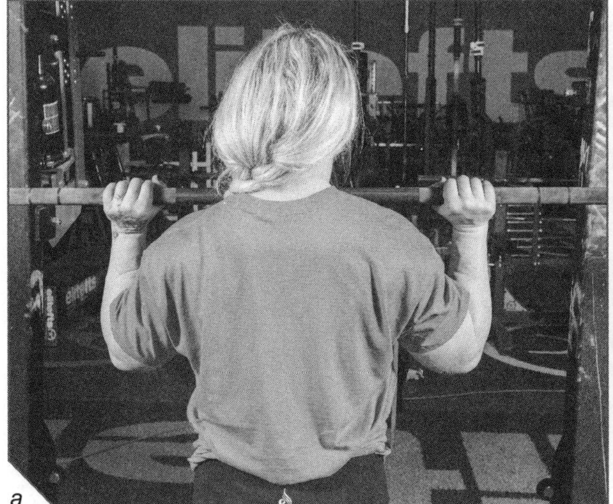

a

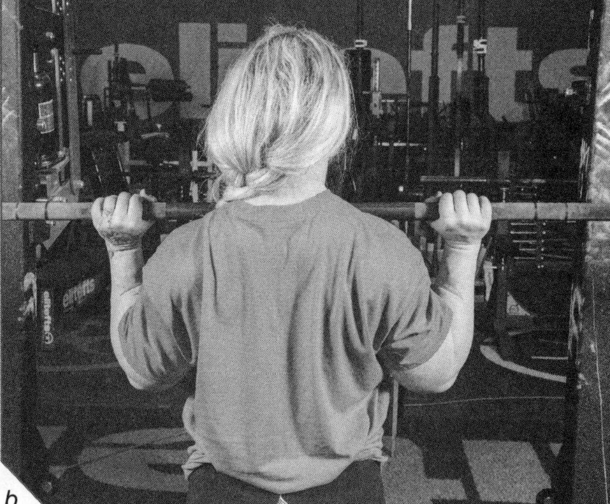

b

FIGURE 6.5 Comparison of the upper back in a *(a)* relaxed and *(b)* retracted position.

KEY POINT

Overhead pressing is a brilliant tool for teaching correct scapular control and movement, which is massively important for performing well in the press (and bench press). Unlike the bench press, however, the press allows the scapulae to glide uninhibited during the movement, which in turn allows a more natural relationship with the upper arm. Also, since the arm moves through a greater range of motion compared to a horizontal press, so do the scapulae. This fact, combined with the greater stability demands required by overhead pressing, make it far more demanding when it comes to glenohumeral control. An overhead press performed standing is also a fantastic way of improving core strength and stability because of the high demands of stabilizing a load that is so far away from your center of gravity.

Torso and Hip Position

One of the many reasons the press is such a great exercise is because it challenges your torso rigidity probably better than any other exercise. As the arms extend overhead, the lats lengthen and begin to pull upward on the rib cage. This upward pull needs to be counteracted by a downward pull by the abdominals. The further the arm extends, the harder it is to resist this upward pull. Add to that the fact that you have a (hopefully, for your sake) heavy barbell moving overhead, progressively further from your center of gravity, which makes it even more challenging. That the barbell goes from starting slightly in front of your center of gravity to being in line with it also compounds this effect.

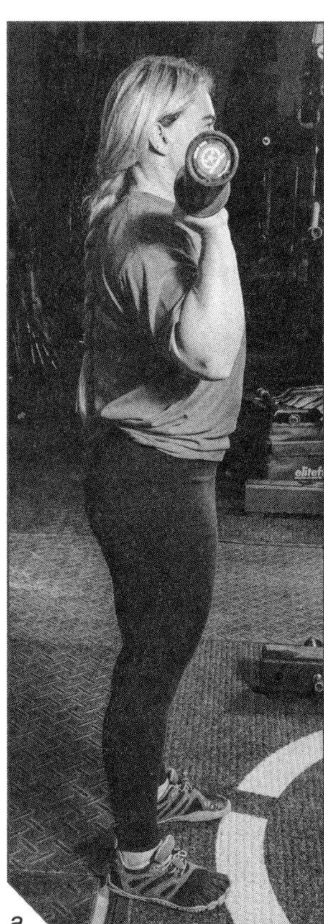

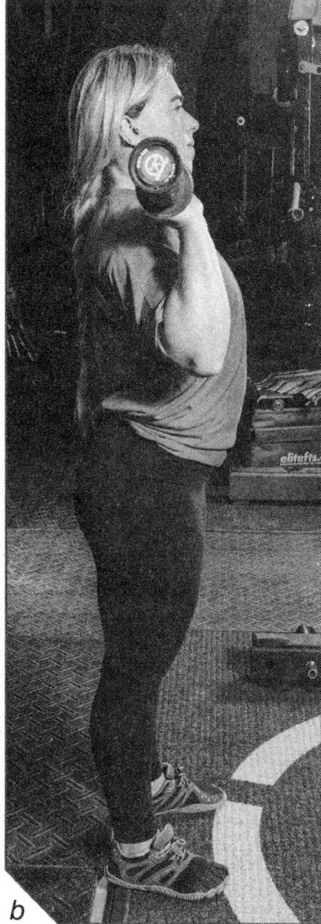

FIGURE 6.6 Comparison of a *(a)* neutral alignment of the spine for the military press and *(b)* an over-arched posture.

Just like in the squat and deadlift, we are looking for neutral spinal alignment throughout (see figure 6.6 for an example of neutral alignment for the military press compared to the commonly-seen over-arched position). This means chin slightly tucked, ribs pulled down, and pelvis directly underneath them, with one slight difference: a small degree of backward lean in the start position. In the start position, the torso will have a slight backward lean to account for the load being in front of you or your center of gravity. This is necessary to keep the system in balance. This backward lean will remain until the bar can move back over the head and realign with your center of gravity. In the top position, the bar and arm should be in a vertical alignment over your center of gravity.

Note that at the start of the lift, it is very common to see individuals lean back and arch through the lumbar spine to initiate the lift. This happens for several reasons:

- To gain leverage to recruit the upper pecs more (more pressing power)—not necessarily a bad thing
- Pressing the bar forward away from the body—wrong
- Losing spinal alignment because of improper bracing or start position—even more wrong

A small amount of backward lean and lumbar extension during the press isn't a bad thing. In fact, it is required for moving maximal weights overhead. However, the point is that it cannot be achieved at the cost of losing your brace and alignment. When we talk about neutral spinal alignment, we are not talking about one very specific position; there is a degree of leeway in both directions. And that is what we want to focus on—staying within neutral range. I would define neutral range as the range in which you can keep your rib cage and diaphragm stacked directly over your hips and pelvic floor muscles. So, basically, if the gap between your sternum and your belly button increases (in the case of lumbar extension) or decreases (in the case of lumbar flexion), then you are now outside the neutral range, and I am very disappointed in you. This can be easy to tell if you are wearing a belt because you will feel that you lose contact with the belt somewhere around your midsection, depending on whether you have fallen into extension or flexion.

In summary, yes, a small amount of extension or backward lean is fine at the beginning of the lift, but this must be corrected after phase I is complete (see the next section on Bar Path and Movement Pattern), and it cannot be done at the expense of losing neutral alignment and bracing. In my experience, most people will always tend to lean back too far, so you are better off focusing on minimizing the backward lean as much as possible; in turn, you will generally keep it to a reasonable degree, unless you are attempting a weight you have no right lifting.

Bar Path and Movement Pattern

As mentioned previously, the press represents an extra challenge in terms of stability and balance, and unlike the squat and deadlift, it doesn't follow a vertical bar path. Because most humans tend to have a head, the bar has to start out in front of the body and then finish directly over the center of gravity in the top position. So, the bar path of the press will curve backward to achieve this. And again, unlike the squat and deadlift, we spend some of this movement with the bar *not* over our center of gravity. Our goal is to navigate the bar back in line with that point as efficiently as possible. See figure 6.7 for the full movement of a military press.

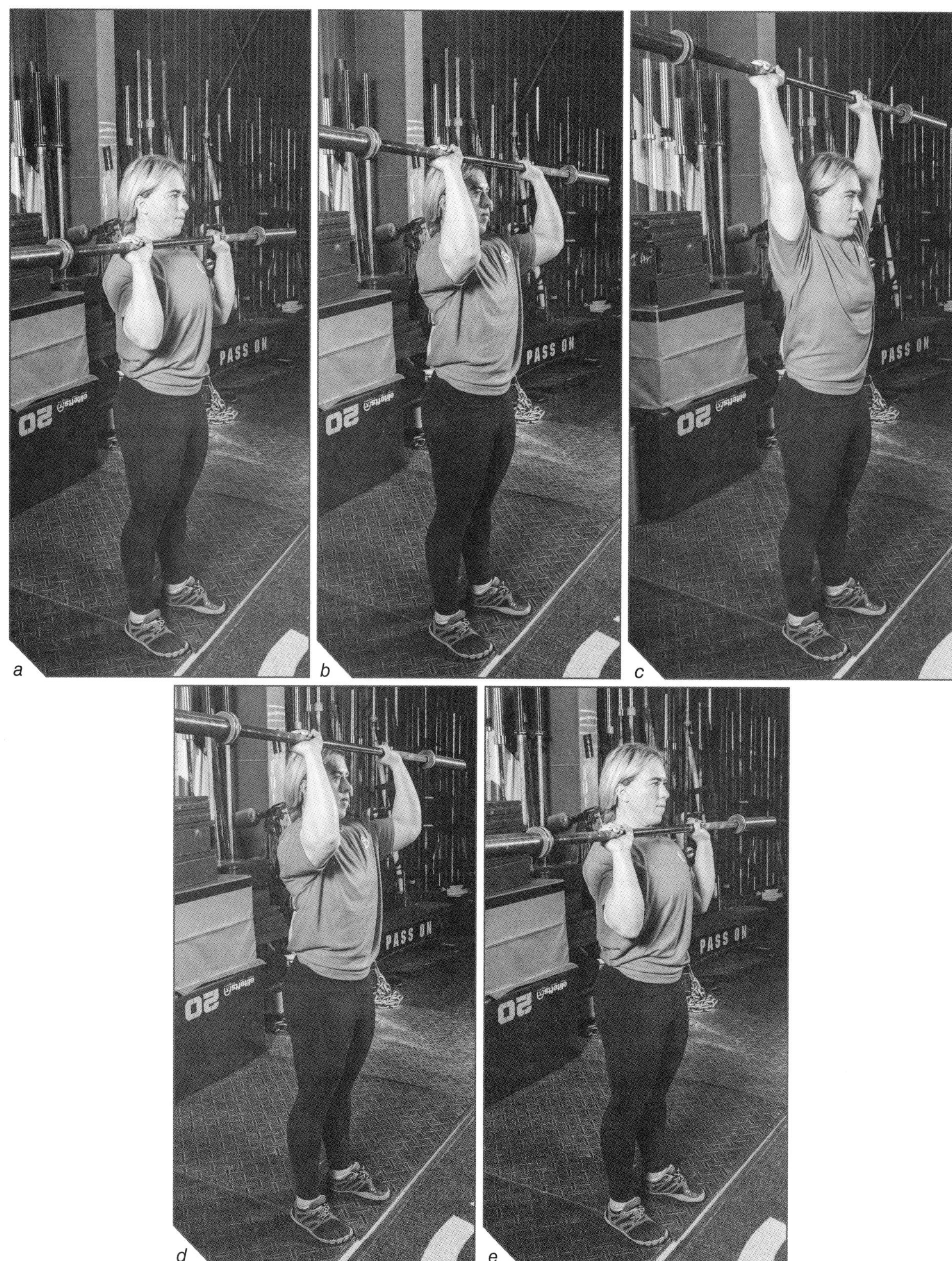

FIGURE 6.7 The segments of a military press: *(a)* start, *(b)* midpoint (end of concentric phase I), *(c)* top (end of concentric phase II), *(d)* midpoint (end of eccentric phase I), and *(e)* finish (end of eccentric phase II).

Concentric Portion

Once again, our movement is split into two phases. First, we have a phase where we must press the bar while it is in front of our center of gravity (due to our head being in the way). Then we have a second phase where the bar moves backward over our head to be aligned with our center of gravity, and the lift can be completed.

Phase I

Phase I of the press starts in the bottom position and finishes once the bar is just above forehead height. During phase I, the bar is in front of the body (unless you want to try pressing the bar through your face), and the elbows and forearms stay in the same alignment, stacked vertically under the bar, in front of you. The bar path for this phase should be vertical or with an extremely slight backward curve. As mentioned previously, there will usually be a slight backward lean during this phase to gain leverage and to allow the bar to stay as close to the center of gravity as possible without hitting the face.

Initiating, phase I is done by actively rotating the scapulae upward. In fact, you can essentially "steal" the first inch or two of movement just from this action if you are wired in well to your scapulae without any real active pressing, as it were. If you are not, the press is the perfect tool to teach you to feel out the natural glide of your scapulae and learn to control it. So, the scapulae initiate the movement by rotating upward, and then the front delts and the clavicular portion of the pecs (to a smaller degree) take over the main pressing work. During this phase, the shoulders stay in position; any rising or shrugging of the shoulders at this point will take the front delt and pecs out of optimal alignment, meaning they can contribute less.

KEY POINT

Shrugging the shoulders during phase I is not optimal for force production, so why do we so commonly see it? Generally speaking, it comes down to the compounding effect of several factors:

- *Poor postural awareness or control*: The lifter doesn't know how to keep the shoulders depressed while the arms move overhead. Temporarily swapping to less demanding variations of the press (such as the landmine press) can allow this to be improved on.
- *Strong or overactive upper traps*: Generally, this occurs in lifters with poor posture or poor programming. When the bar is being pressed overhead, we need even pull on the scapulae from above (upper traps) and below (lower traps, lats), but the upper traps end up dominating, resulting in the scapulae elevating. Strengthening the lats and lower traps can correct this imbalance.
- *Poor starting strength*: The lifter struggles during the early phase of the lift and shrugs up to create extra momentum. This works to a degree, but then because of suboptimal shoulder alignment, it ends up moving the sticking point to further on in the lift (often around forehead height). This is commonly seen in lifters who like to use the stretch reflex out of the bottom position (not performing reps from a dead-stop), leaving them short of practice at creating force from a dead-stop at that point. Pin presses can be your friend here.

Phase II

Phase II begins around or just above forehead level and finishes with the bar locked out directly overhead. During phase II, the bar drifts backward to align with the center of gravity, and the elbows will externally rotate to stay under the wrists. As the bar passes the forehead, it should start to drift backward in a gradual manner. The bar should end up aligned over the midfoot about halfway through this phase. At this point, the elbows will also be fully externally rotated so that they are pointing directly sideways out from the body. Any earlier will take the delts out of the equation too early and leave you doing a really terrible triceps extension with a bar that is floating a couple of inches over your head.

Once the bar is roughly halfway through phase II, the triceps are in a mechanically advantageous enough position to finish the lift. If this backward movement is done too late, then you leave yourself with the bar out in front of the body (usually accompanied with an exaggerated lumbar arch) and with no leverage to finish the lift. At the finish point of the lift, the arm should be locked and completely vertical, with the wrist, elbow, and shoulder joint stacked directly under the bar. There should be a vertical line down from the bar, through the arm, all the way to the midfoot. The simplest test for this is to see whether you can hold a heavy press over your head at the top of the lift for at least a few seconds. If not, then your finish position probably needs to improve. If you are in a properly stacked position, this shouldn't be an issue, even with a near maximal load.

KEY POINT

A loss of positioning at the top of the press is most often caused by tight lats or by poor bracing ability (often they go hand in hand). As the arm extends overhead, the lat muscle stretches, due to the attachment point being on the upper arm. If the lat is too tight, then it won't allow the arm to fully extend overhead. To compensate, the ribs will flare up and the lumbar spine will extend, shortening the lat from the origin end, in turn allowing enough room for the arm to fully extend.

Even with ample mobility, poor bracing strength can still cause a loss of positioning. As the arm extends overhead, the upward pull on the rib cage from the lat increases in magnitude. If this upward pull cannot be matched by a downward pull on the ribs by the abdominals, then the result will also be that the rib cage flares up. Now, the tighter the lat is, the stronger that upward pull is, which explains why these issues are often interlinked. You then have the compounding factor of the further the bar moves overhead, the harder you must work to stabilize it (due to longer levers).

In these cases, practicing movements such as the Savickas press and including more core dominant work in your training would be a good call. Plus stretching your lats couldn't hurt, either.

Eccentric Portion

Simply speaking, the downward phase of the lift should be a mirror image of the upward phase. So, the descent will begin with a short (vertical) downward phase before the elbows begin internally rotating and bringing the bar forward. Once the bar is roughly at forehead level (depending on lever length), the elbows will be directly under the wrists and also either directly under, or slightly in front of, the barbell. The bar then travels directly down in front of the head to return to the original start position.

The most common fault seen on the descent generally is keeping the elbows flared out for too long so that they end up being outside the wrists (see figure 6.8). This is done because it keeps the bar directly over the center of gravity for longer. To be blunt, this is purely the result of laziness. On the descent, lifters can't be bothered to keep their bracing and alignment up, so instead of bringing the bar down properly by tucking through the elbows (which puts the bar in front of the center of gravity, which equals more core work), they keep them flared. Then they get the bar to just above their skull with their elbows all over the place and have to tuck them in really fast to get the bar in front of their head. This descent path is bad for your elbows and for your shoulders, and it also means you're lazy—don't do it.

If you struggle with this, then do all your presses with slow eccentrics until you can nail it every time. Or keep the same bar path until you get it wrong and end up with an impinged shoulder or the bar crushes your skull. But don't say I didn't tell you so.

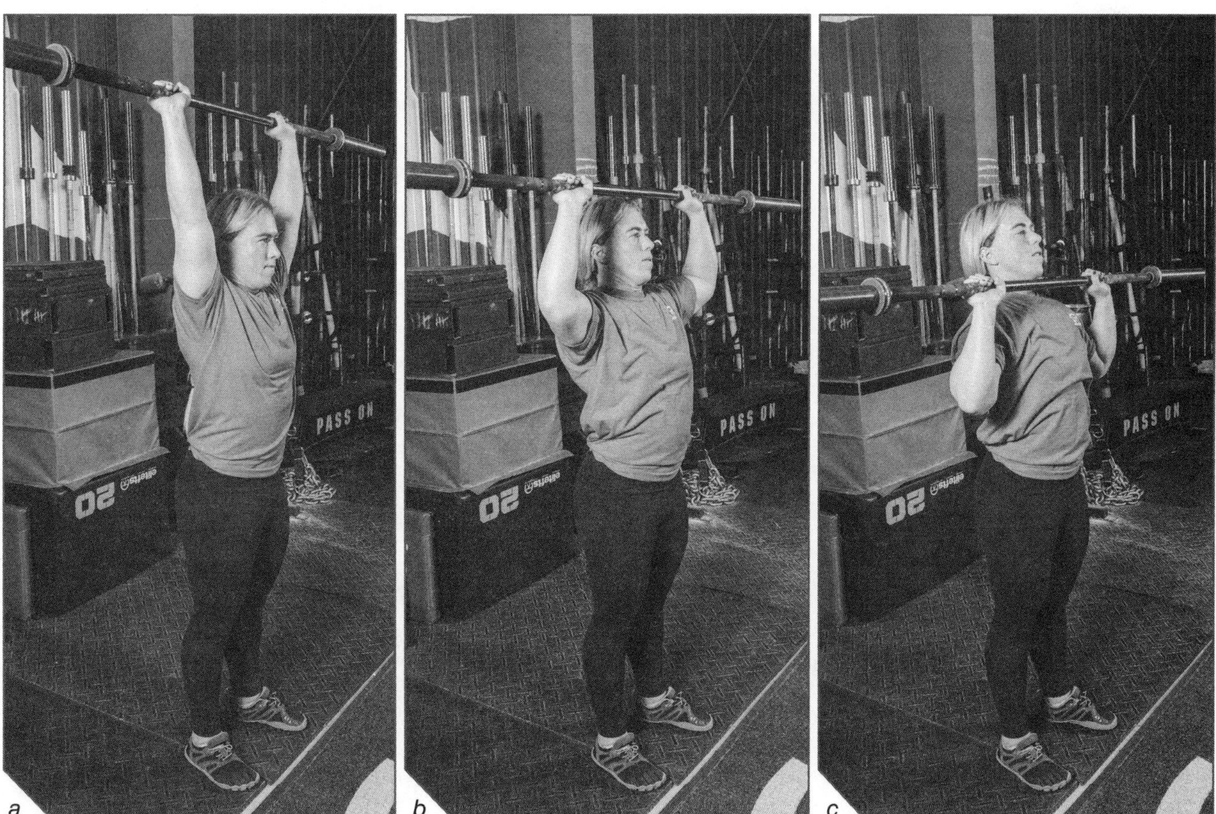

FIGURE 6.8 Incorrect technique on the eccentric portion of the military press: *(a)* start, *(b)* midpoint, and *(c)* finish.

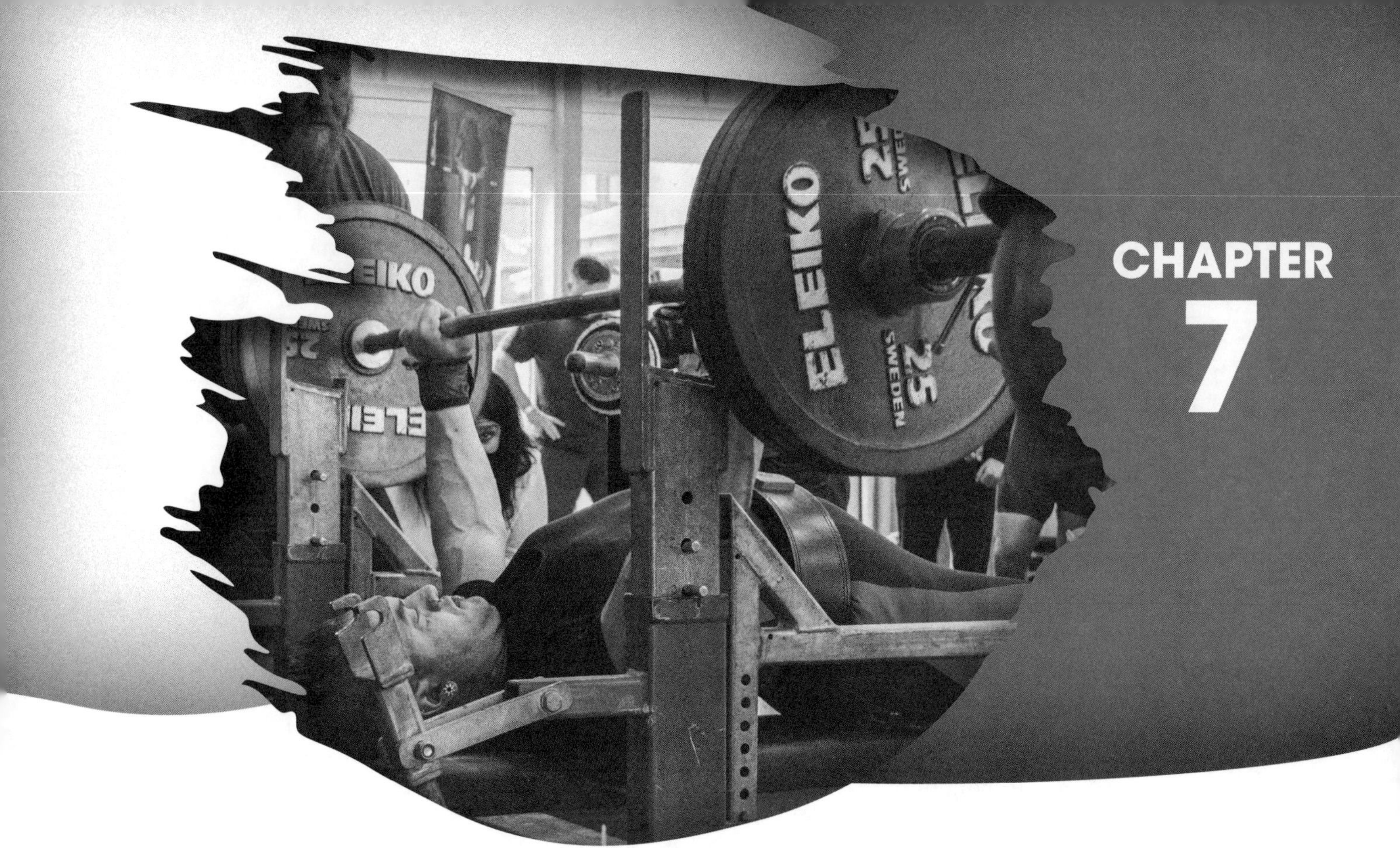

CHAPTER 7

Bench Press

I (Tom) often get very bemused looks when I tell people, including coaches, that I think the bench press is the most technical of the big lifts. I mean, how complicated can it be to lie down and push something away from you? As a result, I find that lifters tend to be overly confident in the quality of their bench press. The reality is that your bench press probably needs just as much work as your other lifts; you just aren't consciously aware of your incompetence.

Where the bench press differs from the other lifts is that there are a lot more individual nuances and preferences that come in to play. With the other lifts, you can give pretty solid guidelines for 80 to 90 percent of the mechanics based purely on physics and levers, for instance. But with the bench press, not so much. Many people can end up strongest using setups (e.g., grip width, foot position) that are in theory suboptimal, and then there is the difference between what is optimal for men and women. Owing to that variation, this chapter is a bit of a beast, but it is purely about the complexity of the lift.

When performed correctly, the bench press is just as much of a full body lift as any of the others that we have covered so far. Louie Simmons, the founder of Westside Barbell, used to talk about all the lifters he had observed over the years who blew out their quads while benching. Similarly, when I was competing at the European Championships in 2017, I tore my quad while squatting (as if I needed another reason to hate squats). Nothing major, but it was enough to make walking around a bit of a pain. I lost about 15 to 20 percent off my bench press purely from not being able to use my right leg properly during the lift. A solid bench press setup requires tension through the entire body, from the hands on the bar down to the feet. Any weak link in that chain is going to cost you power and stability.

Setup

In this section, I want to address a setup with flat feet and on the tiptoes. My preferred setup is with flat feet, so I'll spend the most time covering this setup in the same order that I teach it and have people set up in person.

Setting Up with Flat Feet

This is the setup process for those who want to bench with their feet flat on the floor (see figure 7.1 for an example of the proper flat feet setup for the bench press). This setup is covered first because it is what I find works best for the majority of people (who aren't competitive powerlifters, at least), but also because some lifting federations will only allow you to set up this way. If you want to bench on your tiptoes, don't worry, we have you covered. But the process is different.

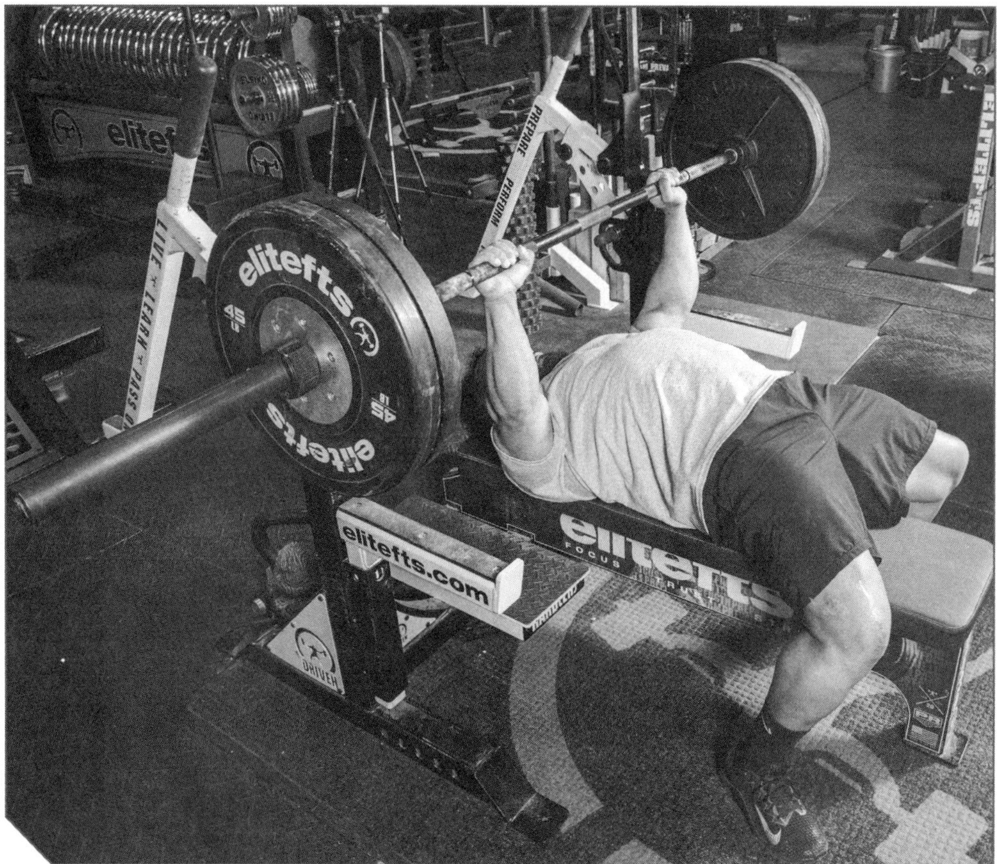

FIGURE 7.1 Setup for the bench press: flat feet.

Grip Width

Where you grip the bar is going to be determined by your wingspan to a large degree. So, when finding your optimal grip placement, you can't really depend on arbitrary measures such as "little fingers on the rings," as an example. It is common to see 1.5 times shoulder width suggested as your grip width, and to be honest, this isn't a bad suggestion. But we are here to move maximal poundage, so we need to find what is optimal rather than settle for OK.

For beginner and intermediate lifters, you want to start with the widest possible grip width that allows you to keep the elbow stacked directly under the wrist in the bottom position of the lift (see figure 7.2). This is going to depend on your upper and lower arm length as well as the size of your arch. To test this, film your bench press looking up your body and then look specifically at your forearm positioning when the bar is on your chest, and simply keep working the grip out until you can no longer achieve a vertical forearm. This gives us the best mix of a shortened range of motion, stacked joints, and a lower demand on upper back stability (compared to a wider grip). Essentially, this gives us a pretty safe setup in which injury risk is low (the pecs aren't in an overly stretched position, the upper back stability is reasonably easy to maintain) and achieving correct alignment isn't too difficult because the elbow can stay directly under the wrist throughout the entire lift.

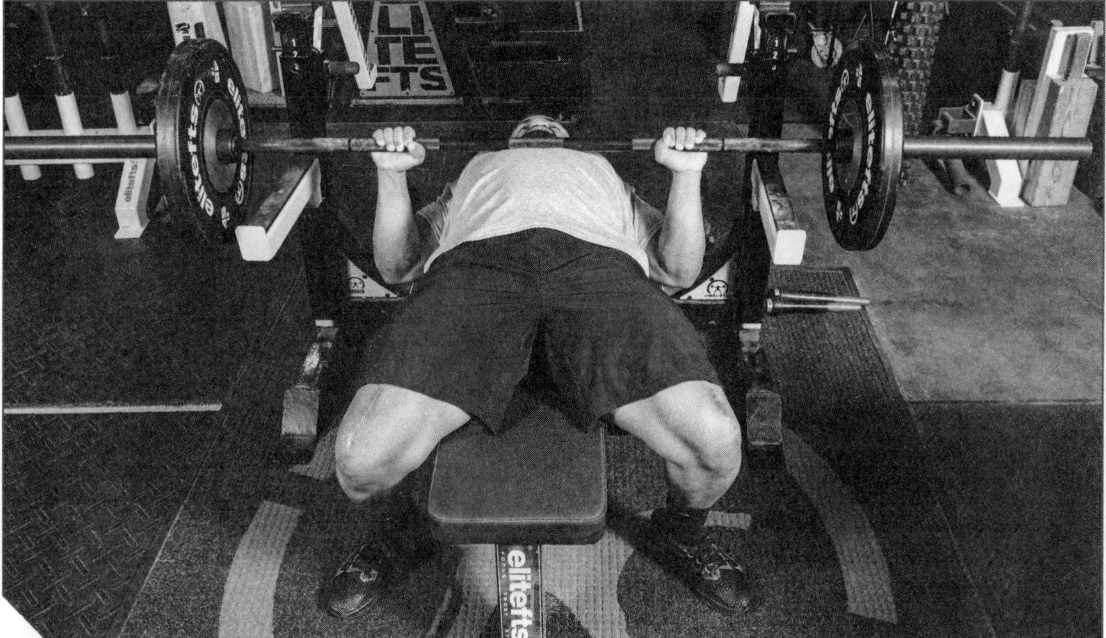

FIGURE 7.2 The widest grip that allows the lifter to maintain a stacked forearm during the bench press is the best starting point.

As you become more proficient at the bench press, you can move your grip wider (see figure 7.3), although that doesn't mean everyone should. This comes with the benefits of a reduced range of motion and increased pec recruitment (not universally a good thing), but it has the downsides of increased upper back and stability demands, because keeping your shoulders pinned back is harder with a wider grip. It will also mean that you do not have a vertically stacked forearm throughout the lift (inherently less stable). Generally, you are going to benefit from a wider grip if you fall into one of these categories:

- *Have long arms or a wingspan that is an inch (3cm or more) greater than your height*. You will be a pec dominant presser, so emphasizing the pecs will benefit you. Plus, since you will have a large range of motion, you have more to gain from shortening it.
- *Have good leg drive*. A wider grip places the pecs under a greater stretch at the bottom of the lift, meaning your sticking point is more likely to be toward the bottom end of the lift compared to a narrow grip. Leg drive can help you navigate around this mechanical disadvantage.
- *Are female*. If you are female, then you will generally benefit from a wider grip because you will have less potential for upper body muscle relative to a male. So, you have more to gain from improving leverages and shortening range of motion as you have less raw pressing power to rely on. If you can't produce as much force, reduce the amount of force you must create to complete the lift—simple. Also, women will have more lumbar spine flexibility (to help accommodate for the postural shift during pregnancy), which means they can achieve a larger arch generally than men.

It's important to remember that when using a wider grip, you will not achieve a stacked or vertical forearm throughout the lift, but what is important is that the outward angle of the forearm should be constant throughout the lift. So, for example, if your forearms are angled out at 15 degrees when the bar is on the chest, then the forearms should be at this 15-degree angle throughout the whole lift.

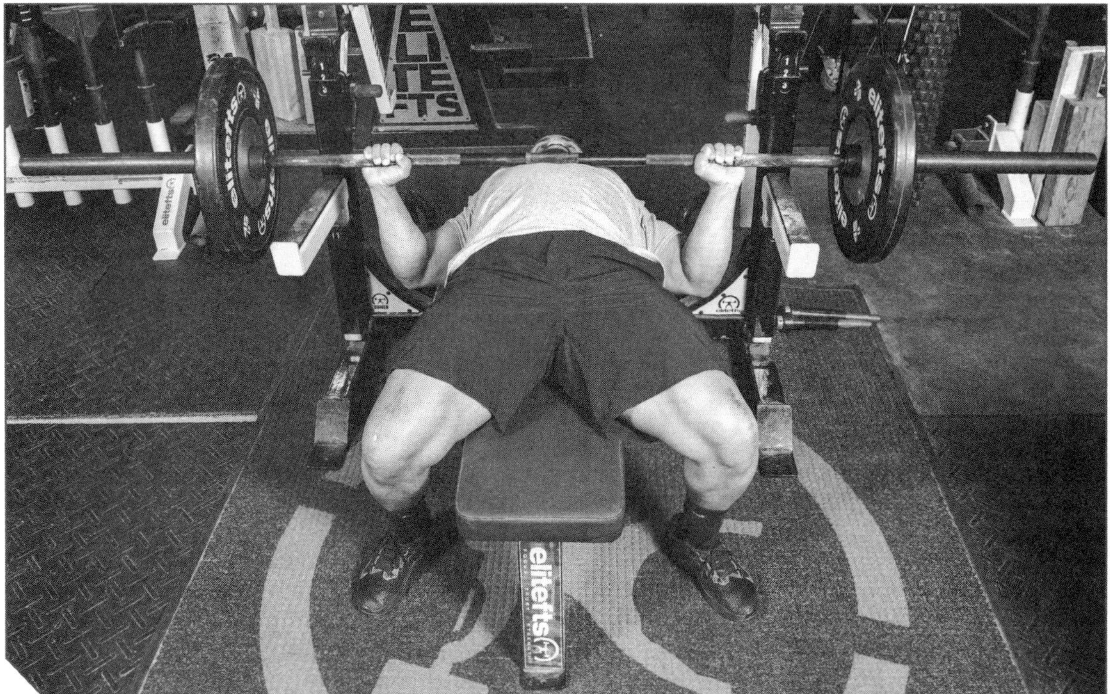

FIGURE 7.3 A wider grip means that the wrist joint will be outside the elbow at the bottom of the lift, resulting in a non-vertical forearm.

Finally, is there such a thing as too wide? Yes. At some point, the advantage of shortening the range of motion is outweighed by putting the shoulders and triceps in a disadvantageous position (so they can contribute less), upper back or stability demands being too high, and the upper arm being in such a flared-out position that it aggravates the shoulder joint because it cannot track properly. As a general rule, I don't like to see the forearm angled out at more than 30 degrees. Any more than this and one ends up running into the disadvantages listed above and increasing the risk of injury.

KEY POINT

It is important to remember that once you find your optimal grip width, that doesn't mean that it is going to be your optimal grip forever. For example, if you improve your flexibility and get a bigger arch, then you may benefit from going wider to take advantage of a higher touch point. Likewise, if you strengthen your upper back significantly, you may now have enough stability to use a wider grip. Bodyweight fluctuations also affect optimal grip width because weight gain brings with it more passive joint stability and maybe a higher chest position, which may facilitate a wider grip. The reverse would be true for weight loss. My optimal grip is about an inch (3 centimeters) narrower (per side) when I weigh around 200 pounds (91 kilograms) compared to 220 pounds (100 kilograms).

Wrist Position

A cocked back wrist position is likely the most common fault seen in bench press. This wrist position places the bar back behind the wrist joint so that the bar is no longer stacked directly over the elbow joint (see figure 7.4). This is not only inefficient but also makes it more likely the bar will be driven too far back over the shoulders and head on the concentric portion, leading to a failed lift. Think of it like a punch. You wouldn't punch with a cocked back wrist because it would lead to poor force transfer.

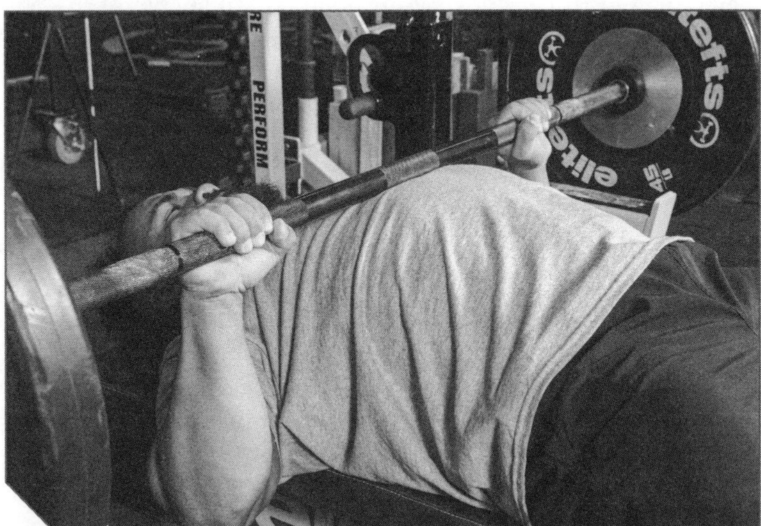

FIGURE 7.4 Correct wrist alignment for the bench press.

The most common reason for this fault is in fact elbow positioning. When the elbows are flared out too much, they will end up behind the bar (as in closer to the head) during the lift. To correct this, the wrists will then cock back to allow the bar to move back over the elbows. If this is a fault of yours, then no, you don't need to tie your wrist wraps tighter; instead, you likely need to fix your elbow positioning. It may also be that you are trying to hold the bar too high in your hand. You want the bar to sink as low into your palm as possible. Note, however, that there are few high-level bench pressers who use what is an extremely advanced technique with a maximum legal (super-wide) grip and a purposely heavily cocked back wrist position. This allows them to limit the range of motion massively, and the wrist position actually allows them to over-tuck the elbows while touching a higher point on the torso. This is an extremely intricate and stressful technique used by a very small number of benchers; this is likely not for you.

Setting the Upper Back

The upper back forms the foundation from which we can apply force to the bar. As such, a loose upper back is the biggest power leak that you can have in a bench press. In fact, you could probably argue that no bench press has really been missed because of an inability to create enough force to move the bar (unless attempting something way too heavy); rather, it was the inability to provide enough stability to channel that force into the bar that caused the lift to fail.

The biggest benefit of a correct thoracic arch during a proper bench press setup is in fact the ability to provide more stability for the upper back and shoulder joint. Yes, it also has other benefits, such as reducing the range of motion (by raising the chest up off the bench) and facilitating a greater use of the pecs in the lift (by turning it into a kind of semi-decline bench), but the main benefit is from the upper back stability that is gained, which is often overlooked. The injury risk of the lift is also reduced by the enhanced stability and by limiting the range of motion (once the elbow starts traveling below the level of the shoulder during a bench, the shoulder stress increases markedly). A proper thoracic arch also facilitates a better transfer of leg drive into the bar (this will be discussed later).

When setting up, begin by lying flat on the bench with your feet on the end of the bench (see figure 7.5*a*). Push yourself back along the bench until the bar is roughly level with your upper chest (your head will likely be off the bench at this point; see figure 7.5*b*). From this position, perform a glute bridge by pushing your feet into the bench and driving your hips as high as possible (see figure 7.5*c*). Once the hips are set, it is important to keep them as high as possible while we set the upper back because it will allow us to get the weight sitting higher up on the traps.

With the hips elevated, pull your upper body up off the bench using the bar (think inverted row); at this point, only your feet will be on the bench (see figure 7.5*d*). While the upper body is elevated off the bench, you are going to set your shoulders by rolling them down and back into your body as far as possible (you should feel your lats contract when you do so). You are looking to set the shoulders as low into the body as possible (think about making your neck as long as possible) and rotating them so that the chest is pulled up.

Once you have done this, you are going to retract the shoulder blades (squeeze your shoulder blades together), which will further arch the chest up, before laying your upper body back down on the bench (see figure 7.5*e*). When you do this, it is important to have the contact point of your upper body with the bench as high up on your traps as possible. You want it to feel as if your weight is resting almost on the base of your neck as opposed to down on your mid-back. Otherwise, you haven't really set up with an arch.

Once you have done this, you should now be in a position where your grip is on the bar, your upper back is arched and on the bench with your weight resting high up on your traps, and your hips are elevated. With your upper back set, now we need to set the hips and feet.

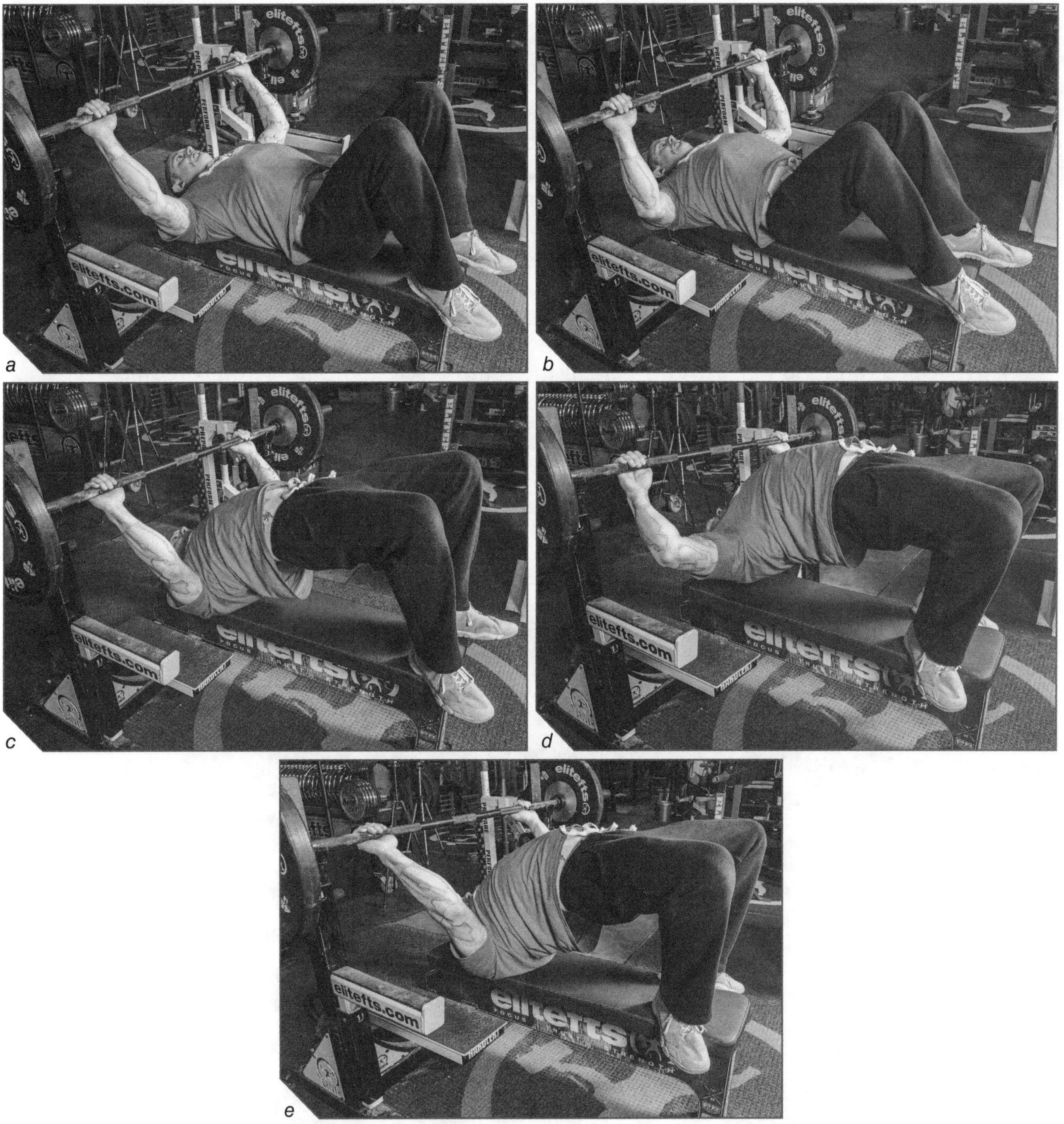

FIGURE 7.5 Setting the arch for the bench press.

KEY POINT

Many coaches teach you to retract as much as possible during this part of the setup. In theory, it makes perfect sense to have bigger arch, more upper back tension, and so on. However, this isn't strictly true. During the lowering phase of the bench press, the shoulder joint goes through extension. As this extension occurs, there needs to be some degree of shoulder retraction to keep the shoulder joint centrated. If the shoulders start in a maximally retracted position, then you have removed their ability to retract further during the eccentric. This will lead to poor joint alignment in the bottom position and a higher amount of stress on the shoulder joint and the pecs. During the setup, use 80 to 90 percent of your possible shoulder retraction and your shoulder will be able to move more efficiently. A good test for this is simply that you should be able to feel your shoulder blades pull back and together slightly during the descent, which will also result in a very small rise of the sternum, which is a good visual cue.

Position on the Bench

Once you have reached this part of the setup, you should have your eye line directly under the bar if handing off to yourself (see figure 7.6). This gives the best mix of being under the bar enough to make unracking the bar doable but also being far enough down the bench that you are not going to be smashing into the J-hook uprights on every rep. If you are getting a handout, then you can be slightly further down the bench because you will be getting help out of the rack.

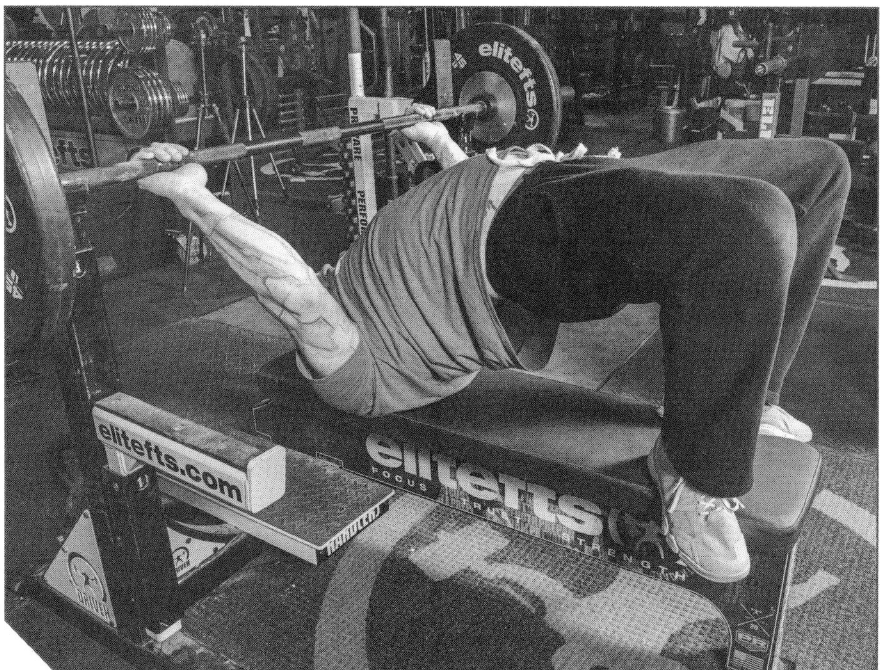

FIGURE 7.6 Correct body position on the bench relative to the bar.

KEY POINT

More flexible lifters can run into the issue of being able to arch too much in their setup. As advantageous as an arch can be in the bench press, it is not the be-all and end-all. Remember, the main benefit of the arch is to improve stability, so an excessive thoracic arch will actually mean that not all of the shoulder blade is resting on the bench. If a large part of the shoulder blade is not supported by the bench, then your upper back and shoulder stability is going to decrease dramatically. It is very similar to using a bench that is too narrow, if you have ever had that displeasure. If this occurs, then we are detracting from the main purpose of the arch. So, as a general rule, you should set up using the biggest thoracic arch you can (following the guidelines presented in this section) as long as your shoulder blades mostly remain supported on the bench. If you are very flexible, then you may have to purposely tone down how much you arch.

Hip and Foot Position

Our grip is now set on the bar and our upper back is set on the bench. From this position, we now need to set the hips and feet. This can make or break your setup because it will determine whether you are able to maintain your upper back setup and how much leg drive you can get. If you get this wrong, you will also end up with your butt coming off the bench when you drive through the legs.

We start the process by placing the feet down on the floor one at a time. If you are placing your left leg down first, then you would continue to push hard down into the bench through the right leg, as the hip needs to stay as elevated as possible while you do this. As the right leg is pushing into the bench, the left leg will be lowered down and the left foot will be placed on the floor on tiptoes as far back toward the head and as close to the bench (without touching it) as possible (see figure 7.7*a*). Once the left foot is planted on tiptoes, push through it as hard as possible to provide stability, and keep the hip elevated while the right leg is now lowered and the right foot is planted in the exact same manner as the left (see figure 7.7*b*). With both feet on tiptoes, you will now push the hips as far up the bench toward your shoulders as you can get it (see figure 7.7*c*). Make sure your butt is firmly planted on the bench in this position and not just hovering in contact, or else it will rise off when you drive through the legs.

Now to adjust the feet. Currently, your feet should be on tiptoes as far back toward our head as possible and close to the bench. The goal is to get them flat on the floor starting from a position in which you can only keep the heels on the floor through downward pressure from the legs. To achieve this, the feet are shuffled forward (down the bench) until you get to a position where you can just get your heels down on the floor; it should take at least a 70 to 80 percent effort from your legs to keep the heels down on the floor if you get this right (see figure 7.7*d*). A good test for this is simply to relax after you have set up; when you relax, the heels should instantly pop up off the floor and consequently the chest should drop (due to the arch partially collapsing).

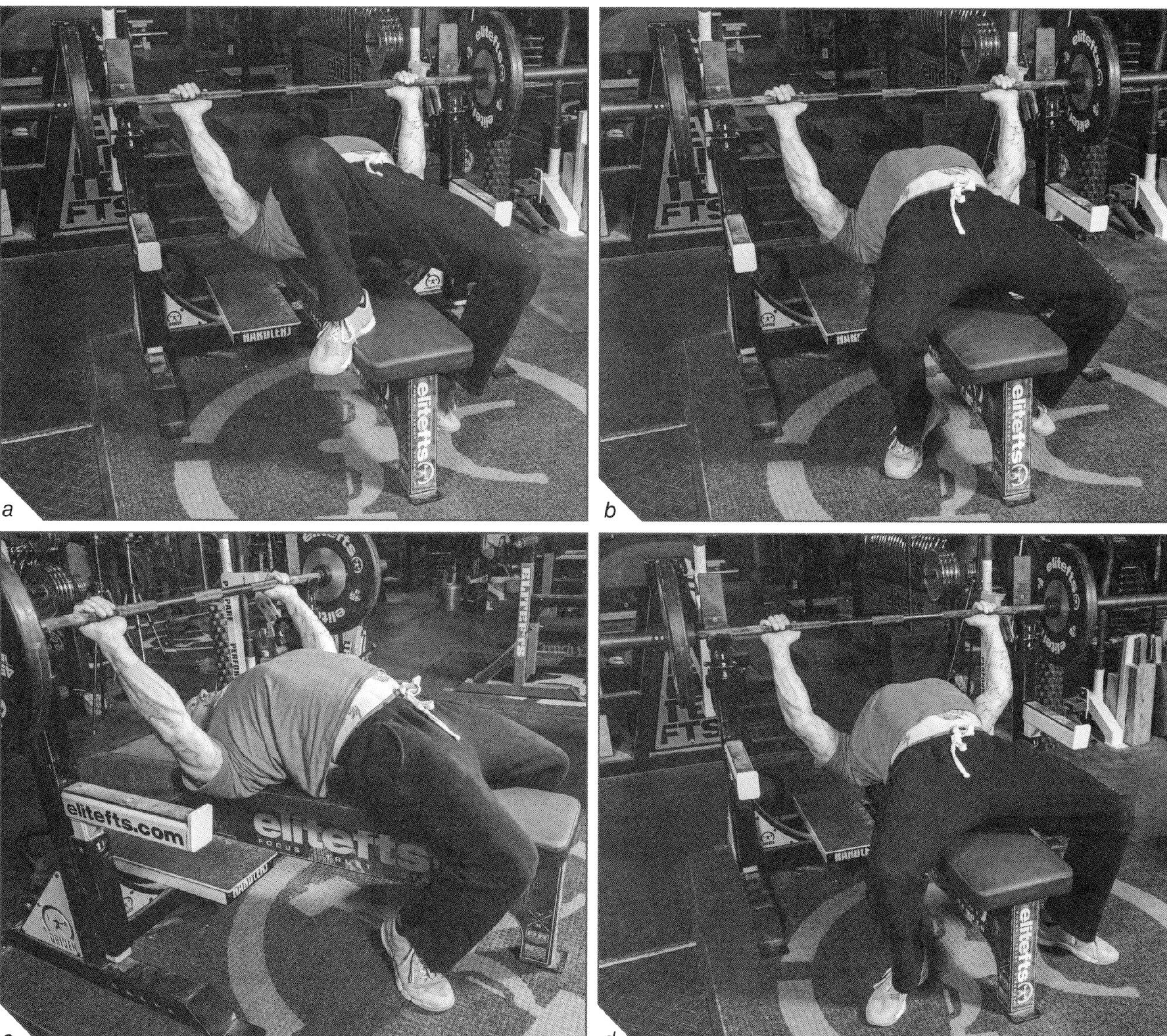

FIGURE 7.7 Setting the hips and feet.

Foot Angle

How you have your feet angled (as in pointing forward down the bench or angled out to the side) can be quite personal. I generally like to have lifters angle their feet out as much as possible without being uncomfortable. Why? Angling the feet out rotates the femur out also, which can help to create and maintain tension in the glutes and allows the knee to be lower relative to the hip while staying tucked further under the body (see figure 7.8). The level of the knee relative to the hip is a key determinant of whether the butt will come off the bench, so getting the knee lower without sacrificing stability (the more tucked under the body the foot is, the more stability it provides) is a big plus. Also, having the feet angled further outward provides more grip against the floor when pushing through the legs (think about turning skis sideways while skiing to slow down).

If you are benching with your feet angled out (which I would advise that you at least try) as opposed to straight forward, follow the steps above, but stop shuf-

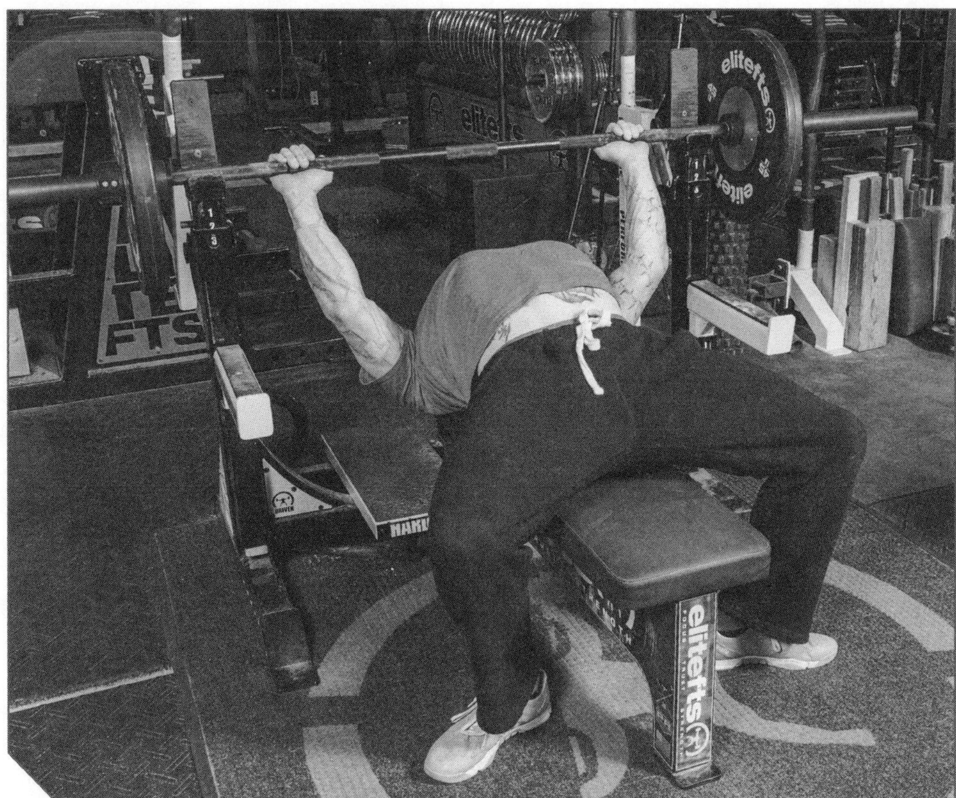

FIGURE 7.8 Foot setup for the bench press with additional external rotation.

fling your feet forward just short of being able to get your heels down. From this position, you then "screw" your feet into the floor as you angle them out until you can just get your heels on the floor. Job done.

KEY POINT

Note that the height of the bench you are using will make a difference to your setup. A lower bench will mean your knee sits higher relative to your hip, giving you more leg drive but also making it more likely that your butt will come off the bench. On a higher bench, you may struggle to reach the floor if you are vertically challenged, and at a minimum, a high bench will likely reduce leg drive and the size of your arch. When using a different height bench, the goal is to achieve the same alignment of hip and knee in terms of vertical distance. As a simple guide, if using a bench that is higher than your normal bench, have your feet narrower and more tucked underneath you. This effectively makes your legs longer in terms of vertical distance. The opposite would then be true if the bench is lower (feet wider or further away from your head).

If you have gone through this whole setup procedure correctly, then there shouldn't be a relaxed muscle in your body. The bench should not be a place where you are comfortable. Yes, you will get used to it over time, but it will simply be less uncomfortable as opposed to comfortable. If your bench press setup is a position you don't mind spending a lot of time in, then you are not doing it well enough.

Unracking the Bar

It is very common to see people set up reasonably well and then ruin half their work by unracking the bar atrociously. By this I mean that while unracking the bar, they allow their shoulders to protract and elevate while allowing the chest to drop. A proper unrack shouldn't compromise any of these things. Usually, this is a sign that someone is trying to make the unrack feel easier (i.e., by being lazy). A proper unrack should consist of two different motions:

- *Extension of the elbow:* You should be setting the rack height so that the bar sits 1 to 2 inches (2.5 to 5 cm) lower than your outstretched arm.
- *Shoulder extension:* Think straight arm pulldown.

The tricep extends the elbow joint just enough to get the bar over the pin, and the lats pull the bar (horizontally relative to the floor) to get the bar directly over the shoulder joint to the start position of the press (see figure 7.9). When done properly, neither of these actions should cause a deterioration of your setup. If you can't get your head around it, then try doing straight arm pulldowns and some bench lockouts (last few inches of the press) in your warm-up for bench, as these are the constituent parts of the unrack.

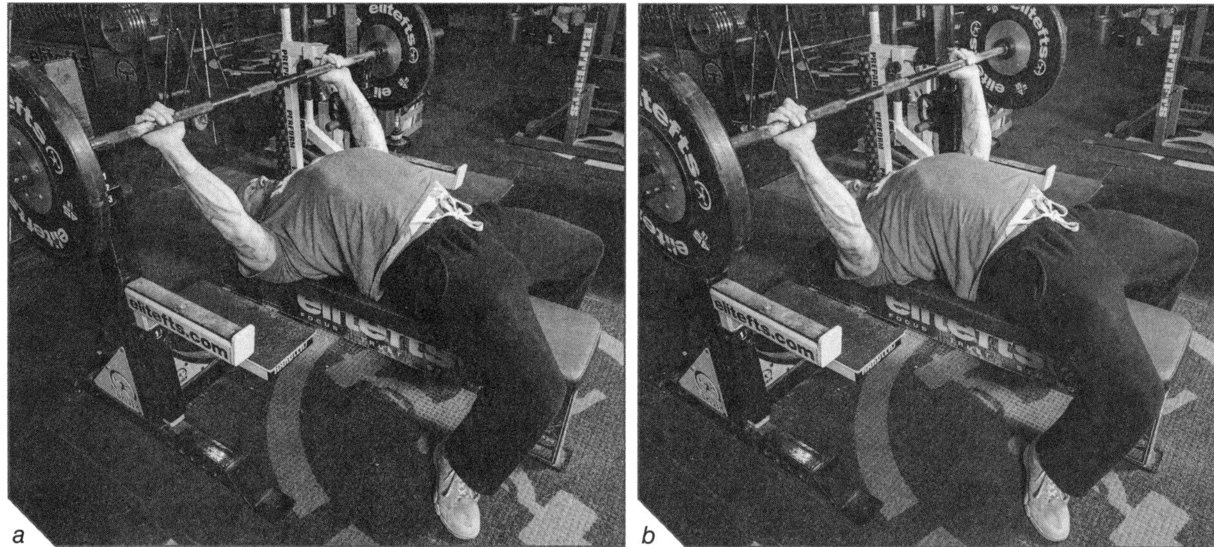

FIGURE 7.9 A correctly executed unrack should not compromise the setup: *(a)* before the unrack and *(b)* after the unrack.

Setting Up on Tiptoes

Now we will address the differences when setting up on tiptoes as opposed to flat feet. The benefit of benching on tiptoes is an increased arch, which means reduced ROM. The downside is less stability and less leg drive, since less of the foot is in contact with the floor. As a result, this tends to be more beneficial for women than men because usually women benefit more from improving leverages (discussed above). They also tend to be more flexible, so they gain more "arch" from moving to tiptoes.

When setting up on tiptoes, the feet are set on the floor first and then you set the rest of the body around them. It can be tricky to know exactly where to put your feet to set up, but the easiest way to at least get very close is to sit on the bench where your butt would normally be when you are benching. In this position, then set your feet on tiptoes as far under your body and as close to the bench as possible (see figure 7.10). Make sure, however, that the balls of your feet are on the ground. When I say tiptoes here, I don't literally mean just the ends of your toes touching the floor. That is way too unstable.

To set up with the feet tip-toed, you pretty much do the same process as described above, only with your feet already on the floor. Drive the toes into the floor and pull your hips up and your upper back off the bench (inverted row) to set the upper back with your weight as high up on the traps as possible. Then place the hips down on the bench as close to your shoulders as possible while ensuring there is solid contact. If you have set your feet in the right position, then at this point your setup should be done.

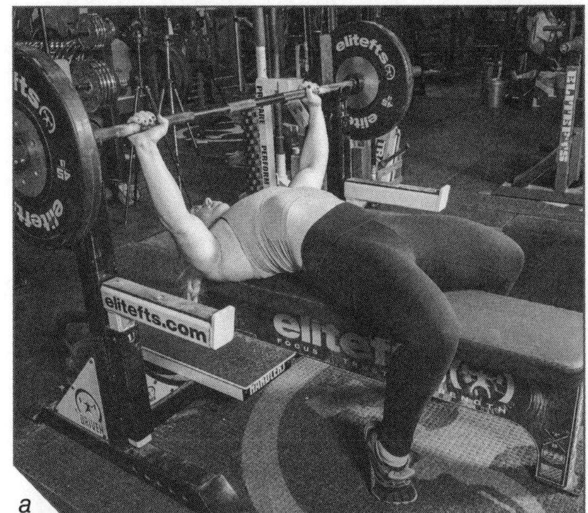

a

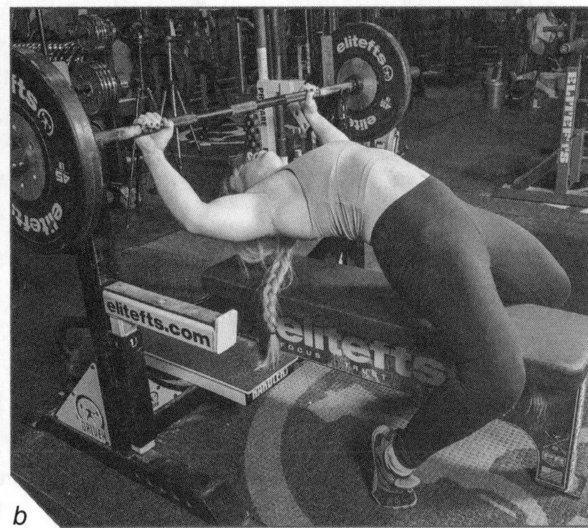

b

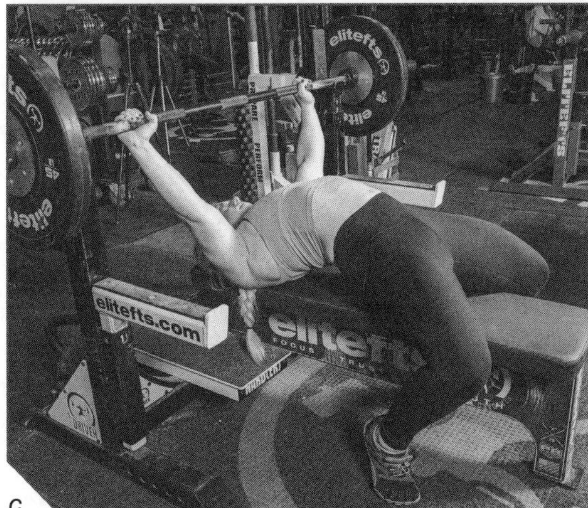

c

FIGURE 7.10 The tip-toe setup: *(a)* initial foot position, *(b)* performing the inverted row to set the upper back, and *(c)* the final setup.

KEY POINT

If your butt is rising off the bench when you have set up on tiptoes, then it means your knee is too high relative to your hip (provided you are doing the leg drive correctly). The simplest way to solve this is to set up with your feet in the same position down the bench but simply wider, because this will drop the knee down. Keep setting up with your feet a little wider until you can maximally drive through the legs without your butt coming up.

Bar Path and Movement Pattern

We've nailed our setup and managed to unrack the empty bar. At this point, the bar should be starting directly over the shoulder joint so that the arm is perfectly vertical and the shoulder, elbow, and wrist joint are stacked directly under the bar (when viewed from the side). This is where things start to get complicated.

Bar path, in fact, varies somewhat based on a few factors, including limb length, grip width, and even experience or skill level (on the upward phase). One thing that I want to emphasize is that most of the time the bar path is not vertical. Many coaches, especially those coaching equipped bench press, try to teach that the bar path for a bench press is a straight line. It is not, for 95 percent (or more) of lifters. The only way you can get a vertical bar path is if you can get the contact point of the bar with the chest directly over the shoulder joint. This is a wonderful set of leverages to have in the bench press, if you can achieve it, but the sad reality is that very few lifters can. Achieving a vertical bar path generally involves using a very wide grip (usually max the legal grip width), having a very big arch, or having a large rib cage and barrel chest. If you can get a vertical bar path then great—you'll likely hit some huge benches. For the other 99 percent of us, we will have a horizontal component to our bar path, meaning it will be a curve, to at least some degree. See figure 7.11 for the full movement of a bench press.

Eccentric Portion

The best way to characterize the downward phase is an inverted J shape. Unless you are one of the few who can achieve a vertical bar path, then the bar path is going to be curved in nature. How curved the bar path is will simply depend on how far down the torso your touch point is (the horizontal component of the bar path). The size of the horizontal component will depend on these factors:

- *Size of your arch*: bigger arch = less horizontal travel
- *Size of chest and rib cage*: bigger = less horizontal travel
- *Grip width*: wider grip = less horizontal travel

It is important to realize that unlike the squat and deadlift, where the desired bar path is always vertical, the bench press bar path will vary, but there are still some hard-and-fast rules.

Phase I

The length of phase I will depend on how curved the bar path is. The more horizontal distance you must cover, the longer phase I will last. The vast majority (but not quite all) of the horizontal travel is covered during phase I. This is achieved by shoulder extension through the lats (think straight arm pulldown, just like the unrack) while the elbows flex and tuck inward toward the rib cage. The elbow and shoulder joint must bend in unison to keep the forearm stacked under the bar as it travels over the body. The longer phase I lasts, the more the elbows will have to tuck in toward the body to cover the horizontal distance required.

During this phase, the upper back and shoulder blades will stay pinned in place as the shoulder flexes. However, almost all of the downward rotation of the scapulae will occur here because of the inward rotation of the upper arm and elbow (adduction). Controlling this scapular rotation is absolutely key to maintaining upper back stability during the descent. If you can't feel your scapulae while you

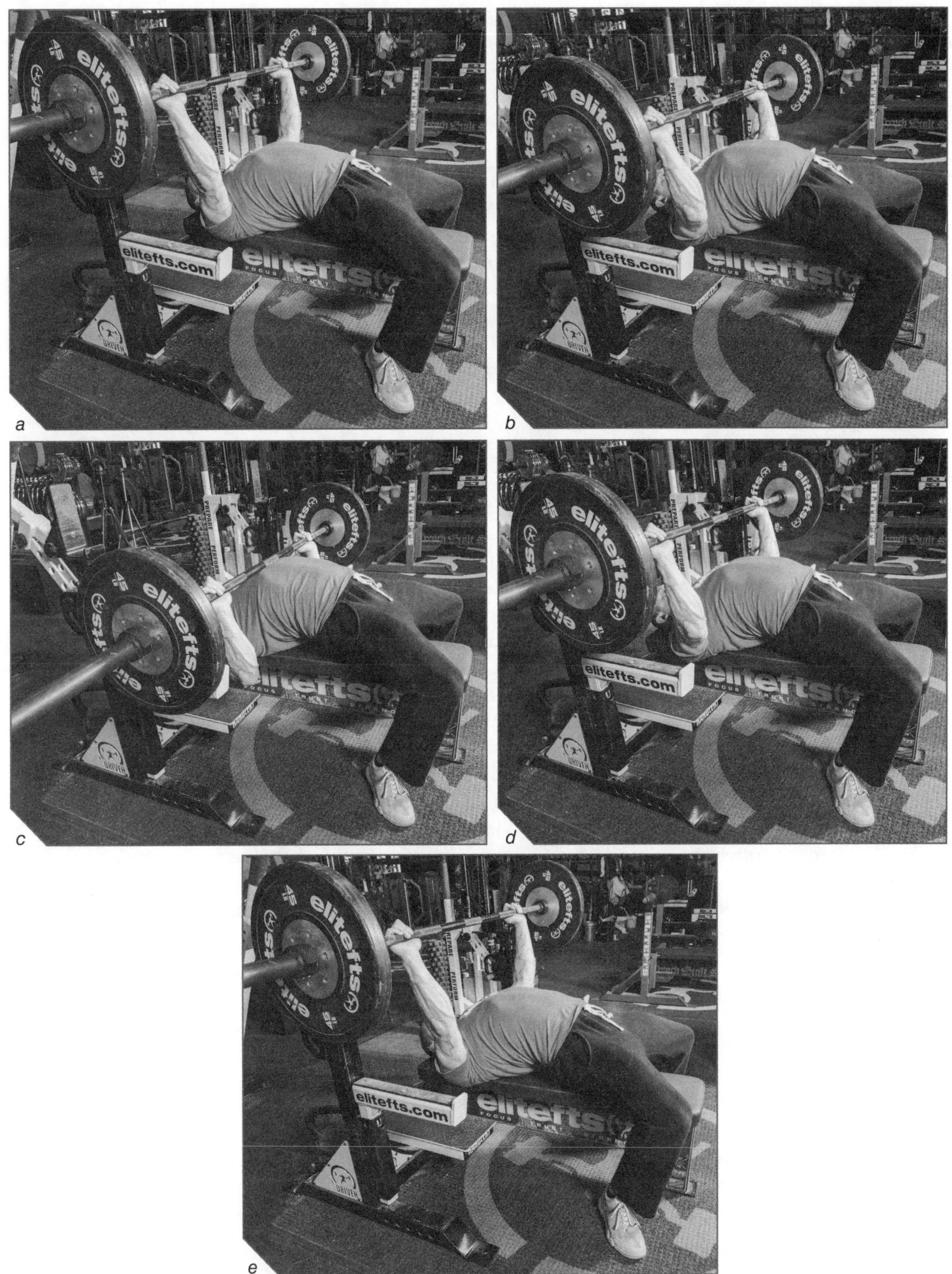

FIGURE 7.11 Segments of a bench press: *(a)* start, *(b)* midpoint (end of eccentric phase I), *(c)* bottom (end of eccentric phase II), *(d)* midpoint (end of concentric phase I), and *(e)* finish (end of concentric phase II).

bench, then this is something you need to address. It is especially important to keep the rear delts contracted during this phase (as with the entire descent) to help anchor and centrate the shoulder joint while the upper arm adducts.

By the time phase I is complete, the bar will be directly over (or very close to) the touch point on the torso, and the elbows will be directly under the bar when both viewed from the side and when looking up the bench. That is, unless you use a wide grip width, the elbow remains inside the wrist joint. In this case, by the time phase I is complete, the elbow joint will be as close to being under the wrist as it is going to be in the lift.

During phase I, the hamstrings also have a key role to play. The hamstrings actively pull the body down and into the bench (imagine doing a leg curl but with your body moving instead of your feet). If the setup is done well, this can be seen as a movement of the body down the bench slightly. This essentially sets you up for a greater degree of leg drive on the concentric. The pulling-down action into the bench can also help plant the body into the bench more, providing more stability.

Phase II

Again, the length of phase II will depend on the factors listed at the start of phase I. This phase is characterized by a vertical (or near vertical) downward movement of the bar while the elbow joint stays stacked vertical (or as close to vertical as it will be) under the bar. During this phase, there is no further tucking of the elbow, and the movement is akin to a seated row done with a bench press grip. As a result, there is little to no rotation of the scapulae at this point, and the main pulling muscles are the rhomboids, traps, and rear delts (as opposed to the lats during phase I). At this point, the main role of the lats is to anchor the shoulder joint, which is still hugely important because the demands on shoulder stability increase the lower the bar is in the movement.

It is during phase II that not setting up with full retraction becomes key. During the row-like motion to get the bar to the chest, the shoulders need to be able to retract a small amount to keep the shoulder joint centrated and to reduce stress on the joint and the pecs. This shoulder retraction during the lower part of the descent if often viewable as a small upward movement of the sternum toward the bar, which can be a great cue to encourage this movement.

Obviously, during this phase, we are going to bring the bar into contact with the chest. The manner in which the bar makes contact with the chest can be a very personal thing. There are three different strategies in terms of making contact with the chest: light touch, slight sink, and large sink.

Light Touch

The bar is brought down until it is just in contact with the chest (see figure 7.12). Here, the focus is on maintaining upper back tightness at all costs. The benefit to this method is that you are minimizing the range of motion and limiting the likelihood of losing back tightness or alignment as the bar sinks into the chest. The downside is that it greatly reduces the amount of leg drive you can get off the chest due to the minimal contact with the bar. This tends to work best under these conditions:

- You have poor leg drive on the bench (especially if you bench on tiptoes).
- Your bar path is vertical or near vertical (i.e., wide grip, big arch, short arms). This is because leg drive only really contributes to the horizontal

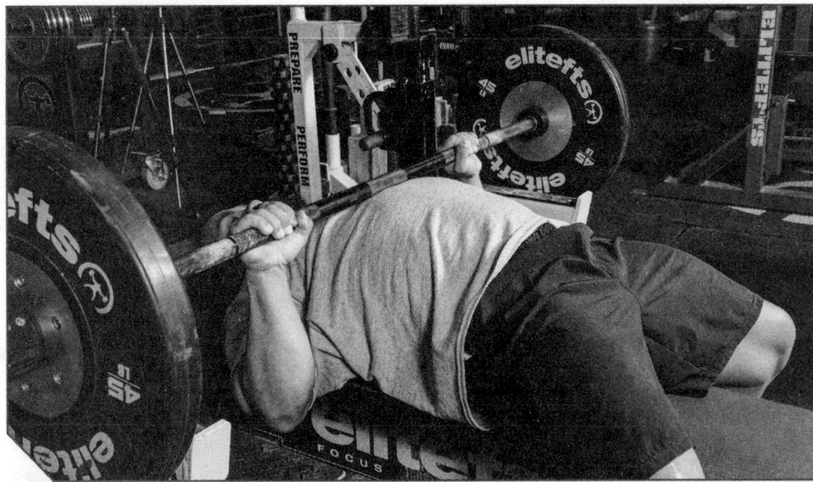

FIGURE 7.12 With a light touch technique, the bar is brought down until it barely makes contact with the chest.

component of the press. So, if your bar path has little to no horizontal component, then it isn't of much use.

- Your upper back strength is a weakness. In this case, you won't be able to get away with losing any tightness when you sink it into your chest.

Slight Sink

This is likely the most common technique. The bar should sink slightly down into the chest while keeping the forearms vertically stacked under the bar (see figure 7.13). During this sinking movement, it is important to focus on pulling the elbows directly down and trying to further retract the shoulder blades to keep the upper back and forearm as set as we would like. This ends up being the best option for most lifters because it gives a great middle ground of not adding too much range of motion to the lift (meaning joint alignment isn't compromised) but allowing a greater use of leg drive owing to the more solid contact between the bar and the body. The important thing to remember here is that the sinking motion of the bar into the chest is a controlled "pull" into the chest. It's a continuation of the seated row-like movement in phase II. It is not an excuse to relax and be lazy.

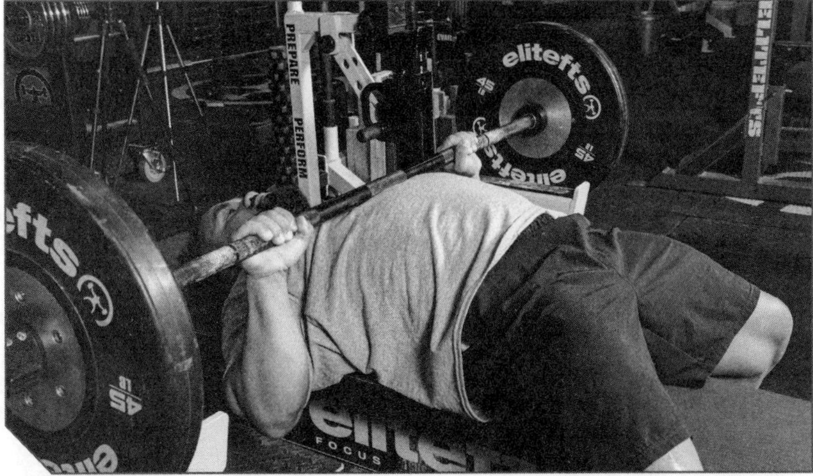

FIGURE 7.13 With a slight sink technique, the bar is allowed to slightly sink into the ribcage at the bottom of the lift.

Large Sink

This last option is almost like performing a horizontal push press and isn't that commonly seen. Dan Green has used this method very successfully to bench-press some seriously impressive numbers: 237.5 kilograms (523.6 pounds) while competing in the under 110kg/242lb weight category. This method involves an exaggerated sinking of the bar into the chest (see figure 7.14). This movement will mean the elbows will end up behind the bar in the bottom position due to the bar sinking further down the body and the shoulder extending further. This is also accompanied by a movement of the whole body down the bench, facilitated mainly by the leg curl movement (discussed earlier) but also the weight of the bar pushing the body down into the bench.

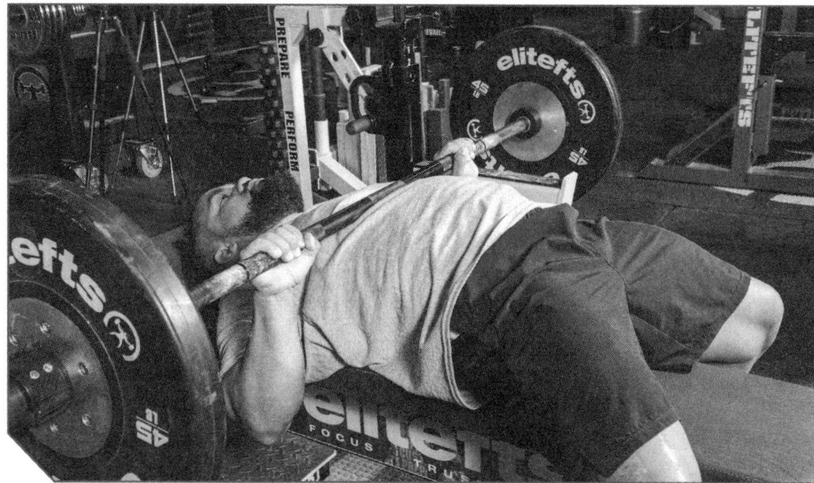

FIGURE 7.14 With a large sink technique ,the bar is allowed to sink a considerable amount into the chest to the point where the forearm angle is altered.

This is essentially like pulling back on a rubber band. The hamstrings and back (along with the weight of the bar) have pulled the body down and into the bench. The body can now be driven up the bench through the quads, which will be visible as a clear movement of the body up the bench. This means the leg drive can contribute a huge amount of force into the bar (horizontally) and make the first third to half of the movement much easier due to momentum.

Sounds great, right? The downside here is that you must have an incredibly good setup and technique to not have your butt come off the bench during the leg drive. Not only that, but the movement of the body up and down the bench can make it very easy to lose your upper back setup. Furthermore, you have to get the timing of the leg drive and bar path on the concentric perfect (especially if you are pausing), or else you will lose control and power (just like a push press).

This is an advanced technique that should only be used by lifters who already have a very solid technique on the bench press. The people who have the most to gain from this technique are lifters who are naturally explosive (relying on speed to get through sticking points) or have long arms (meaning they have a lot of horizontal distance to travel, which the enhanced leg drive will help with).

KEY POINT

You will either see lifters keep their head back against the bench throughout the descent or bring their head up to watch or follow the bar down to the chest. Unless you compete in a federation that doesn't allow you to move your head, then neither of these is inherently bad.

Keeping the head down during the descent makes it easier to keep the upper back set and easier to pull the shoulder blades back and together during phase II, since the upward head movement will lengthen the cervical spine (and therefore, to a lesser degree, the upper thoracic spine). On the other hand, allowing the head to raise during the descent allows you to watch the bar on the way down and can increase motor control and proprioception. This one is pretty much going to be entirely down to personal preference. The only time I would say that either option is an issue is when lifters *must* raise their head up off the bench because of restricted mobility (mainly around the pec minor and front delts). If this is you, I would strongly suggest working on your mobility because you're a pec tear waiting to happen. Likewise, if raising the head off the bench is accompanied with a loss of shoulder retraction and a drop in sternum position, then this also needs to be remedied.

Concentric Portion

So, we have successfully negotiated our way into the precarious position of having a very heavy barbell on our chest. Now what? The first thing we need to address here is the leg drive. The upward phase of the bench press is initiated by the leg drive. It is what breaks the inertia and begins the reversal of the bar. The best way I can describe it is that the upward phase of the bench press is performed like a wave up the body, starting in the feet and legs and working up the body to the arms and shoulders. Visualizing it as a lying-down push press also works.

So how do you use leg drive? This will actually vary depending on your foot position. If you set up using flat feet, then leg drive is primarily a horizontal drive up the bench through the quads and, to a lesser degree, the glutes. Here there are two components to the leg drive:

- *A push through the quads up the bench:* Imagine trying to push your body up the bench toward the uprights. If you have your feet reasonably straightforward, you can also think about trying to push your toes out through the front of your shoes.
- *A contraction of glutes:* Squeeze your glutes, hard. If you need me to explain how to do it, then you have bigger issues than a weak bench press.

These two actions need to be done simultaneously and with 100 percent effort to make the leg drive as effective as possible. Once the leg drive has been initiated, the lower body should not relax at any point throughout the whole upward phase, and the legs should be continuing to drive up the bench. Otherwise, you risk losing your setup as the legs relax while you are still pressing the bar. Once the leg drive has been performed, it's time to actually press the bar.

If you bench using a tiptoe setup, then things are slightly different. Because of the foot position, you have no ability to drive the toes forward into the floor through the quads (which is why you get less leg drive). Instead, to get some momentum from the quads and glutes, we attempt to stamp the heels down toward the floor as hard as possible.

If you have set up correctly, the heels should barely move, no matter how hard you push. However, this violent driving down of the heels will cause the glutes and quads to contract intensely and allow us to impart some momentum into the bar.

KEY POINT

If the setup is correct, then your butt should stay on the bench during the leg drive; in fact, it shouldn't physically be able to move enough to come off the bench. If it does, then you have relaxed your lower body during the descent, allowing the hips to sit in a different position and the arch to collapse (relaxing your coiled spring, as it were). The other option is that you are performing the leg drive incorrectly and pushing your feet down into the floor (which pushes the hips up) as opposed to pushing the feet forward horizontally. It's pretty common to see this creep in as weights get close to maximal loads. People may subconsciously think they can't press it, and so they end up driving excessively through the legs and hips to get it off the chest.

As we have already mentioned, the bar path will vary based on several factors. On the concentric portion of the lift, there are also different styles of bar path, usually based on an individual's proportions and natural strengths and weaknesses. Most lifters will use what is called a curved bar path, but a very few advanced lifters may use what is called the double-curved bar path. These lifters are quite a small minority. Yet, for the sake of clarity, we will address both styles.

Curved Bar Path

The vast majority of lifters will use a curved bar path, essentially matching the bar path of the eccentric portion of the lift.

Phase I We obviously begin phase I of the concentric portion where we left off in phase II of the eccentric portion, with the bar in contact with the chest. For the vast majority of lifters, the upward bar path will closely mimic the downward path. So, in the same way that the amount of curvature on the downward path depends on various factors, the same is true on the upward phase (see figure 7.15).

Phase I on the concentric is primarily driven by the pecs as well as the leg drive (unless you use a light touch). During this phase, the bar path is again near vertical, and the elbows only rotate externally very slightly, meaning there is little to no rotation of the scapulae. As well as driving through the pecs, it is important to flex the lats hard during this phase to keep the shoulders packed and provide stability for the upper arm while the shoulder is in its most extended position.

It is important during this phase to keep the elbow from flaring too much because this will take the pecs out of the equation. Remember, the pec is generally in the best position to apply force through the upper arm when it is roughly 45 degrees from the body due to muscle fiber alignment. Flaring early will lead to the bar drifting back over the body too early, before the delts and triceps are in a good position to finish the lift. This is most commonly seen in lifters who either have weak pecs (they subconsciously try to take the load away from the

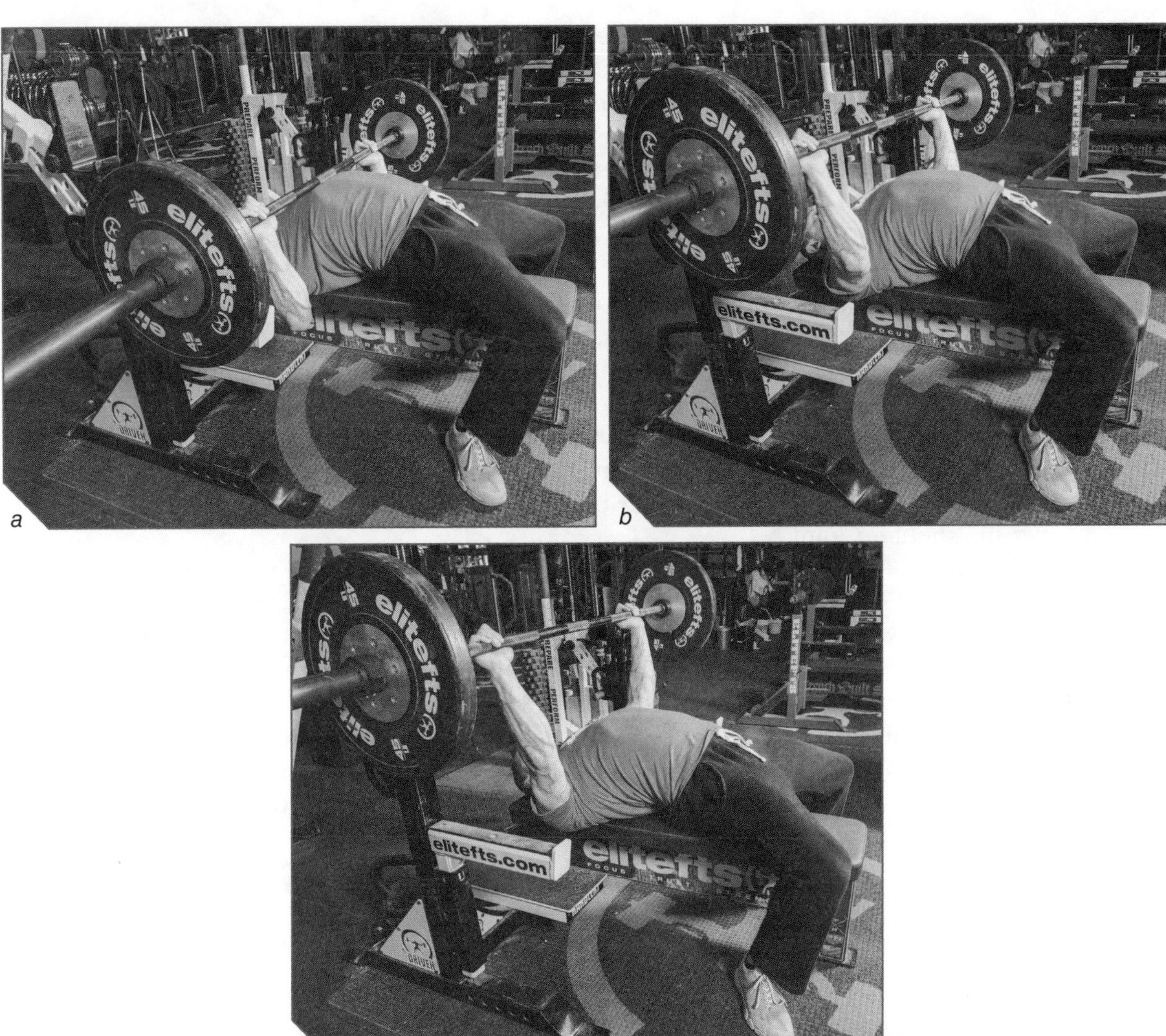

FIGURE 7.15 Concentric phases of the bench press: *(a)* start of phase I, *(b)* end of phase I and start of phase II, and *(c)* end of phase II.

pecs) or those who have weak lats (the lats actively internally rotate the upper arm to stop the elbow from flaring).

KEY POINT

If you are someone who tends to under- or over-tuck the elbows during the bench, then focusing on your hand pressure can help solve this. If you tend to over-tuck your elbows, imagine that you are trying to pull the bar apart (think band pull apart) and snap the bar in half in the direction of down the body (snap the bar between your hands in a manner that places more pressure on the inside index finger side of the palm compared to outside the palm). If you under-tuck your elbows, then you need to think about snapping the bar in the opposite direction, up the body (imagine snapping the bar in a manner that places more pressure on the outside of the palm compared to the inside).

Phase II As we transition from phase I to phase II, the loading will shift from the pecs over to the shoulders and triceps. The pecs are still playing a role during phase II, but they are simply doing less of the work proportionally. This is why the most common sticking point for the bench press is at 2 to 3 inches (5 to 8 centimeters) off the chest, where the loading begins to transition to the delts and triceps. This is also generally where the momentum from the leg drive begins to die out. So, mastering this transition is key to working through that sticking point.

As we begin phase II, the bar is going to start to drift back over the body toward the shoulders. To facilitate this, the elbows are going to need to flare out to the side to keep the elbows directly under the wrist joint. This means that the scapulae also have to rotate upward to allow the upper arm to rotate. This scapular rotation needs to be allowed without sacrificing the upper back setup (i.e., not allowing your shoulders to shrug up). The elbows will continue to flare out as the arm extends and the bar drifts back to its final position, stacked directly over the shoulder joint.

Note that a very common fault seen during phase II of the bench press is "overpressing." This is where the shoulders protract as the arms extend, leaving the upper back in a weakened position and the thoracic arch reduced. The best way to test this is to see the position at which the bar becomes locked out while you are performing a set of multiple reps. If you are guilty of the heinous crime of overpressing, then as the reps go on the shoulders will gradually protract, leaving the arm effectively longer (and the chest lower). The result will be that the bar finishes in a progressively higher position, further away from the body.

If this is the case, then you need to focus on your upper back strength and the ability to keep the shoulders retracted while your arms extend. Slow eccentric pulling work is great here. Also, you may need to switch your thinking from "press the bar away" to "straighten the arms" in order to encourage the shoulders to stay back.

Double-Curved Bar Path

This bar path is much more technical and difficult to execute, but this style is used by some advanced lifters with great success. It is important to note, though, that many lifters will never use this bar path, and it is not always the best option. This bar path tends to favor those who are very triceps dominant or have short arms, because it shifts the loads over to the triceps considerably earlier in the lift.

During the first phase of this bar path, the bar is pressed up in the same manner as in phase I. However, once the bar has moved a few inches, essentially to where phase II of the upward phase begins, the elbows are then flared out aggressively. This exaggerated outward rotation drifts the bar back over the shoulder joint much earlier in the lift. With this bar path, the bar will be over the shoulder joint for a large proportion of the concentric, as opposed to right at the end of the lift with the regular curved bar path. This then leaves the remainder of the lift to be completed as an almost pure triceps extension movement.

The result of this technique is a double-curved bar path in which the bar travels vertically off the chest a very small amount before curving back over the shoulder joint and finally being pressed in an almost vertical line over the shoulder to lock out. As I said, this is an advanced method, which isn't even necessarily stronger for all lifters. But if you are an advanced bench presser with strong triceps, then it may worth giving it a go.

KEY POINT

It's very important to remember that the bench press is a whole-body movement, and dismounting the bench is part of that. When dismounting the bench, perform a sit-up-like motion before standing up. This sit-up motion means you have performed your ab training for the week and now no longer need to lie on a mat pretending to enjoy crunches and planks. Train smart, not hard, folks.

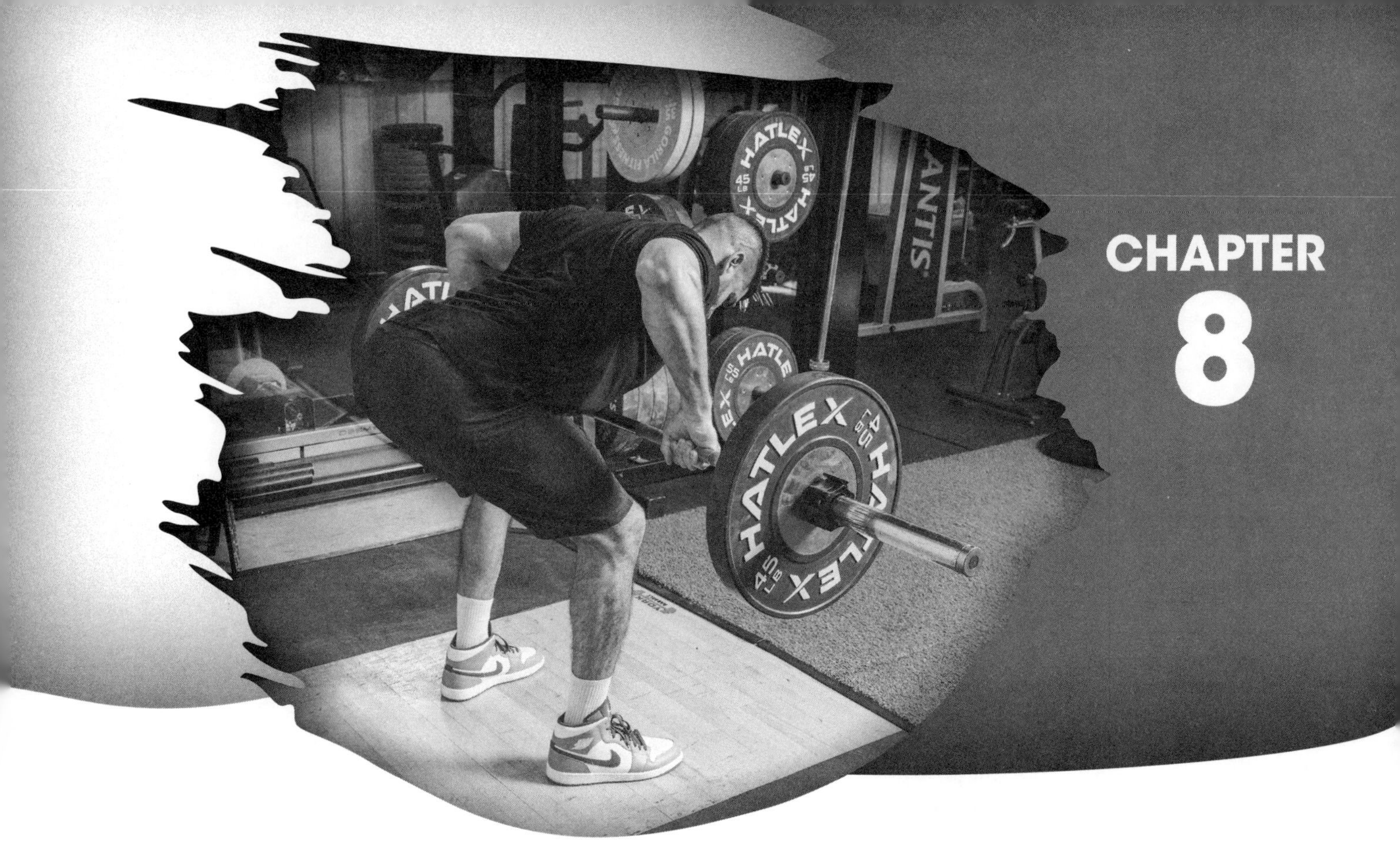

CHAPTER 8

Pendlay Row

Made popular by American weightlifting coach Glenn Pendlay, the Pendlay row is in essence a strict barbell row done with the torso parallel to the ground. This is possibly the single best pulling exercise for improving back strength in the big lifts. In fact, it probably deserves to be classed as a big lift in and of itself, at least if you value balance (which you should if you value long-term strength). The Pendlay row has these advantages when it comes to improving the "big lifts":

- *Posterior chain loading:* The torso being held perpendicular to the floor throughout the lift greatly increases the amount of full-body tension required to perform the lift. The hamstrings and glutes have to contract isometrically to a high degree to hold the hip angle (relative to the floor) stable throughout the lift. This is one of the main reasons the Pendlay row improves deadlift "starting strength" so well.
- *Bracing or core stability:* Maintaining spinal alignment while rowing a heavy load with a torso perpendicular to the floor requires tremendous core stability. The abs and spinal erectors need to work very hard to prevent lumbar flexion. Yet another reason this is great for improving your deadlift bottom-end strength.
- *Angle of pull:* The bar path and torso position combined give this variation a different angle of pull to other rowing variations. This bar path mimics the

line of pull on the downward phase of the bench press pretty well, which means it tends to carry over well to the bench press also. This angle also means the Pendlay row is great at stimulating the rhomboids, traps, and rear delts, which play a huge role in upper back stability in all the big lifts.

- *Full-body tension:* The Pendlay row teaches you how to use the upper back maximally while locking the torso into position against a load, which is conveniently how we use the upper back in all the big lifts.
- *Difficult to cheat:* A lot of "bent over" rows just end up becoming a poorly executed shrug. The perpendicular torso position makes cheating in this manner much more difficult. In fact, if you cheat by dropping the hips down to get the torso more vertical (improving your pulling leverages), you will simply end up pulling the bar straight into your knees (that'll teach you). We will discuss some approved cheating methods on this lift later, however.

Setup

Setting up for a Pendlay row is very similar to setting up for a deadlift, provided you use the moral and upstanding conventional stance, of course. The stance width, foot angle, and all the associated cues are going to be the exact same here as for the deadlift. How you set your upper back (e.g., retracting, twisting the elbows back) and brace is also pretty much the same. The differences in setting up for a Pendlay row will be covered in this section. See figure 8.1 for proper setup for a Pendlay row.

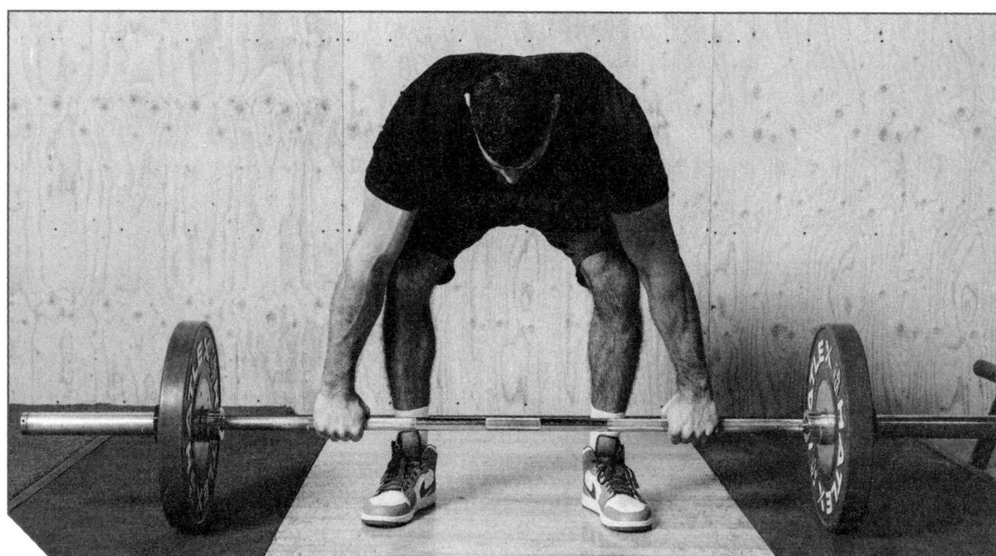

FIGURE 8.1 Setup for the Pendlay row.

Grip Width

Your grip width will be wider than the one you use to deadlift. A narrow grip would result in a bar path that pulls back toward the hip and targets the lats more, which is not the aim here. We want a grip width that allows us to keep the elbow and upper arm reasonably flared out and allows the bar to be pulled to the lower chest or the upper stomach (depending on your proportions). If you have some Olympic lifting experience, then your clean grip is a good place to start (see figure 8.2). If not, then going one hand width wider than your regular deadlift grip will put the majority of lifters in the right place (see figure 8.3).

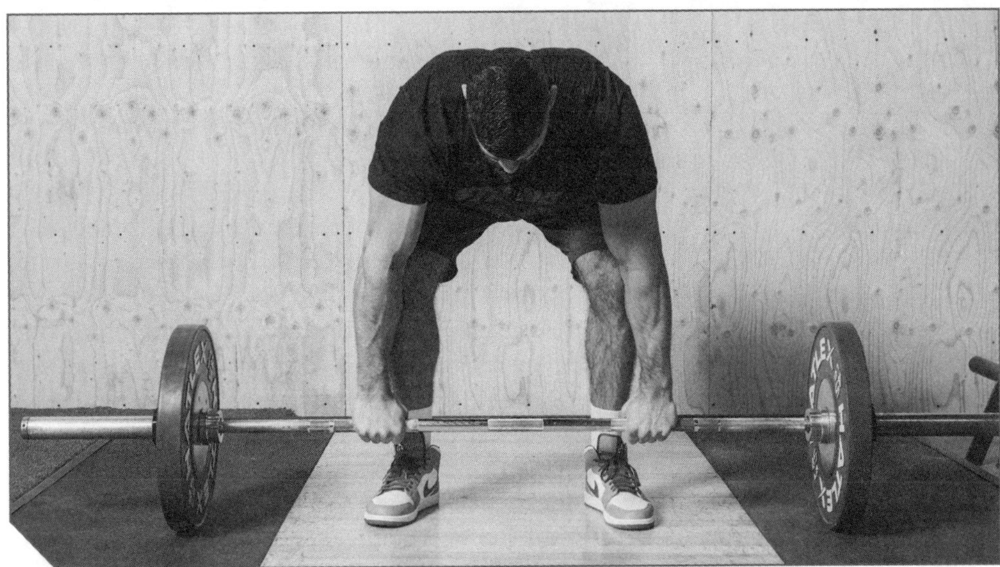

FIGURE 8.2 Clean grip for the Pendlay row.

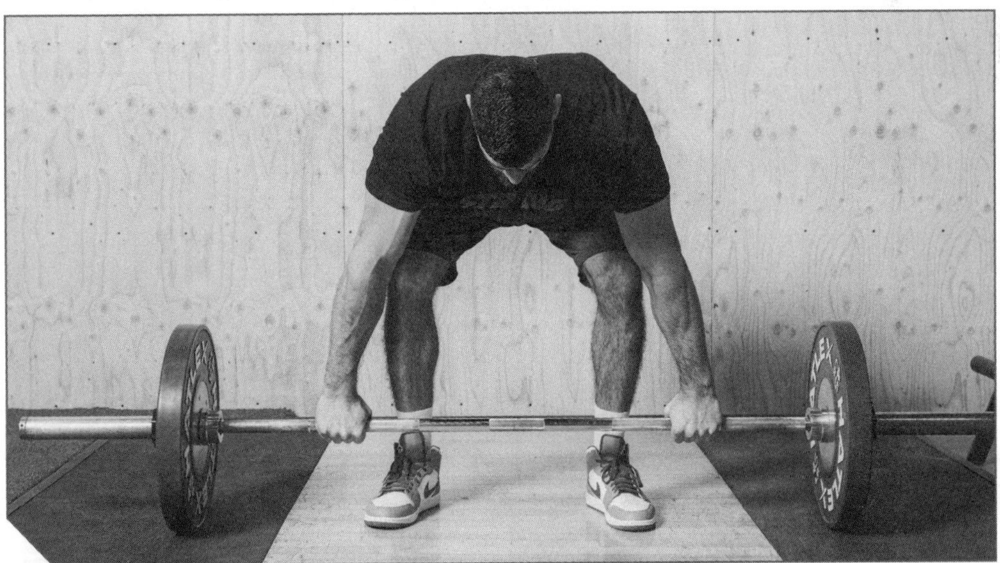

FIGURE 8.3 Grip for the Pendlay row with one hand width wider than a regular deadlift grip.

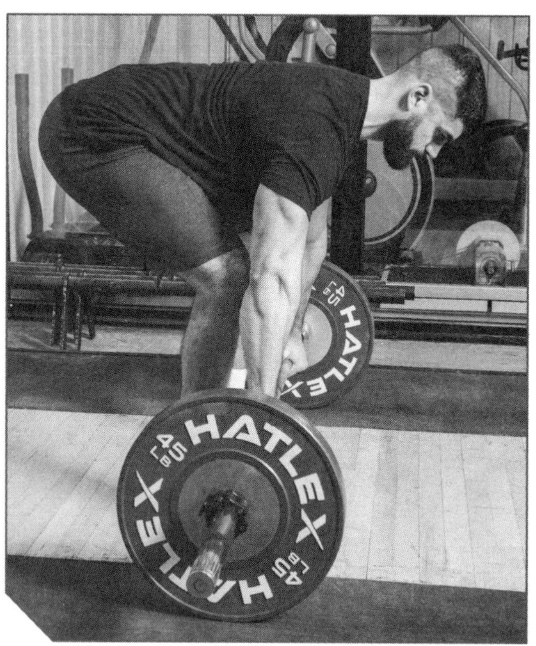

FIGURE 8.4 Proper hip height for the Pendlay row.

Hip Height

When setting up for a deadlift, the knees are over the bar. This position makes it quite difficult to row the bar directly up, if you value your kneecaps, that is. So, we get around this issue in two ways. First, we are going to set the hips slightly higher. This will give us an almost vertical shin angle, which will help clear the path for the bar during the row. Remember that the hips must still be lower than the shoulders. See figure 8.4 for an example of proper hip height for a Pendlay row.

Bar Placement

The second way we get around the "I can't row a barbell through my kneecaps" issue is by altering the bar position. Here, we are going to set the bar in front of the midfoot. The bar should be set directly underneath the scapulae. Remember, the shoulders will be set slightly further forward since we are setting the hips higher (see figure 8.5).

After all, the scapulae are the anchor for all the muscles that are responsible for rowing the bar, so setting up underneath them gives us a very stable starting point from which to set tension in all the right places. How far in front of the midfoot you need the bar to be will vary depending on your proportions (heck, those with very long torsos may still end up with the bar over the midfoot). What we are looking for is the armpits being directly over the bar and a slight backward angle of the arm.

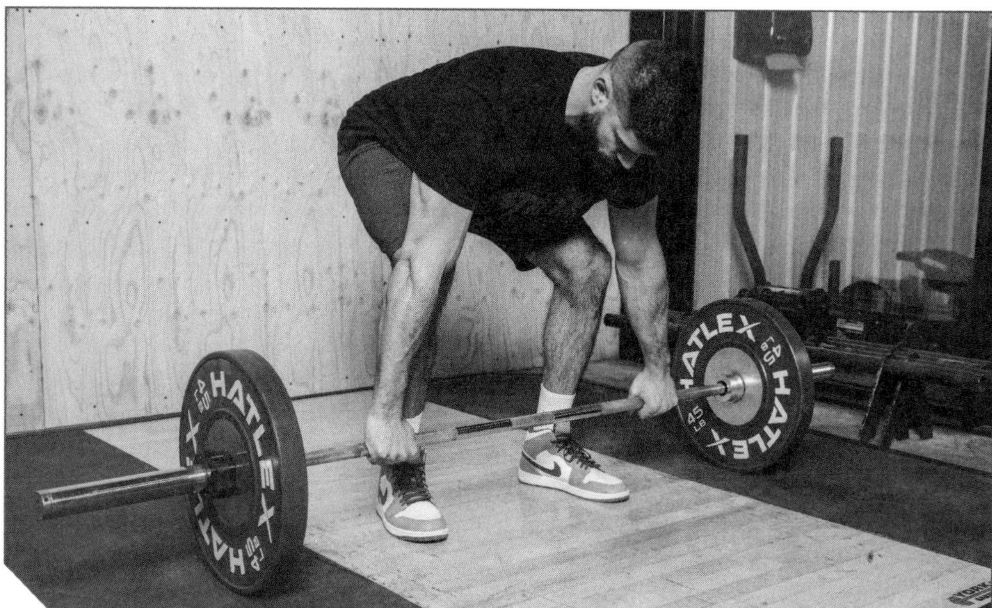

FIGURE 8.5 Bar placement for the Pendlay row.

Upper Back and Elbow Position

In a deadlift, we externally rotate the upper arm and elbow maximally to get as much lat tension as possible. With a Pendlay row, we want to target the rhomboids, traps, and rear delts more, so we need to have less external rotation. In their natural position, the elbows will be pointing directly out to the side, 90 degrees to the body. During our setup, we want to use a small amount of external rotation to pack the shoulders and give us some lat tension, so we are aiming for the elbows and upper arms to be rotated roughly 45 to 60 degrees relative to the body (see figure 8.6). Think of it as setting the upper arm at a similar angle to your body as it would be at the bottom of your bench press.

Then, unlike the deadlift, we are going to aim for maximal shoulder retraction, since we are going to be doing a row, after all. When we perform this retraction, imagine that you are going to try to get the bar off the floor purely from the motion of shrugging back. When you do this correctly, you should be feeling a lot of tension throughout your upper back and around your scapulae.

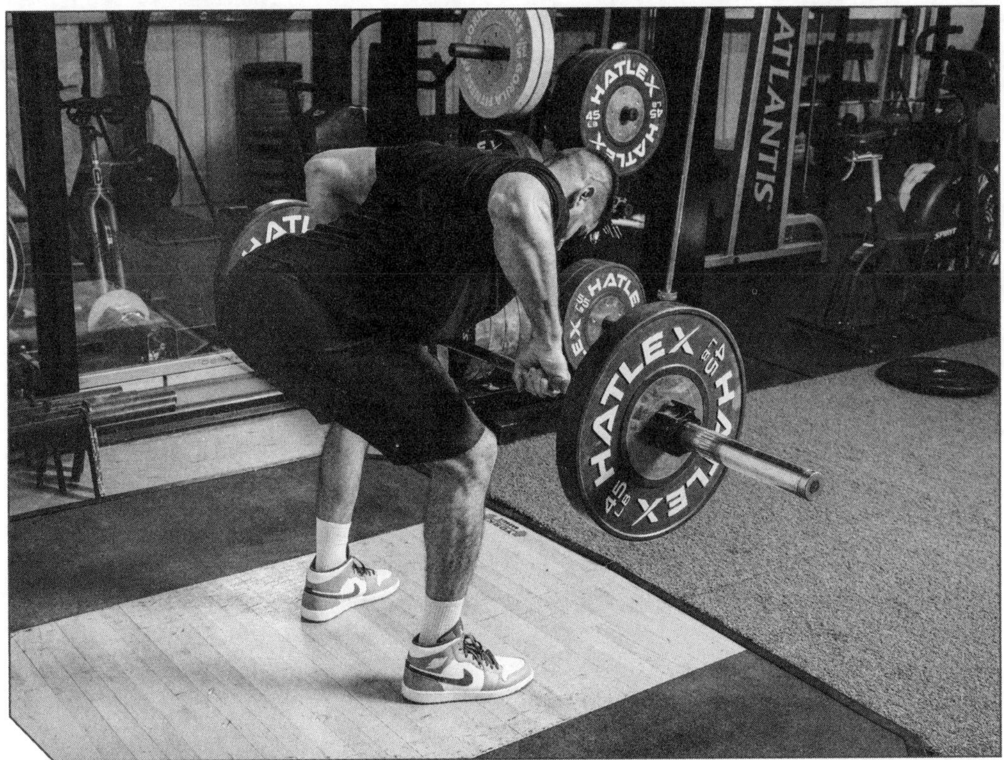

FIGURE 8.6 External rotation of the elbows and upper arms to create lat tension during the setup for the Pendlay row.

Bar Path and Movement Pattern

If you have set up correctly, then it should almost feel like the bar is about to start floating off the floor just from the tension you have created through your whole body, especially the upper back, during the setup. This is the perfect scenario for us to initiate the concentric portion of the lift since the bar is already on the verge of moving, just from the body tension alone that we have created. See figure 8.7 for the full movement for a Pendlay row.

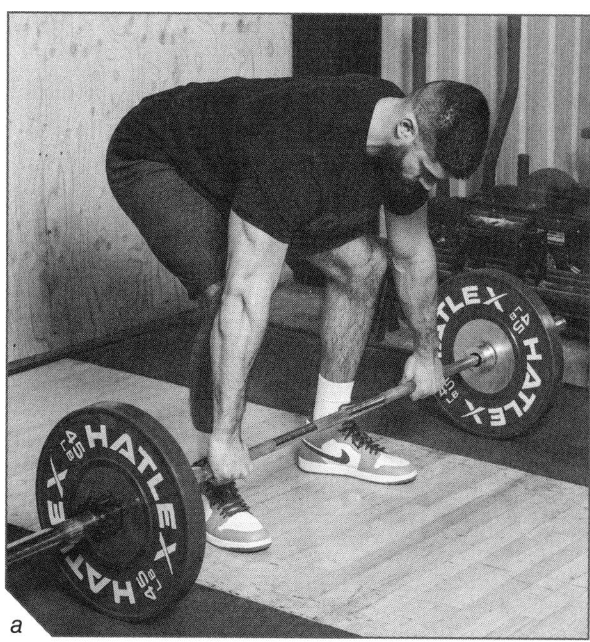

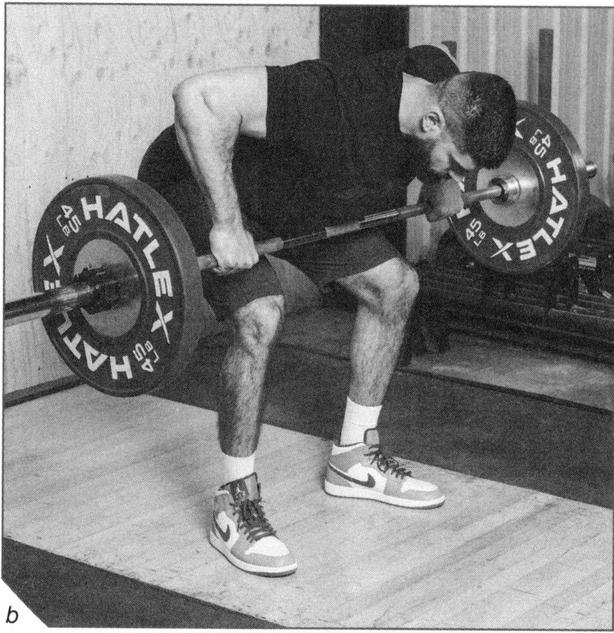

FIGURE 8.7 Pendlay row.

Concentric Portion

The actual rowing movement here is very simple, in theory; the difficult part of the lift is maintaining the body alignment throughout the lift. As you initiate the pull, the most common mistake you can make is to drive through the legs to help break the bar off the floor, even if it's subconscious. The best way to get around this is to isometrically contract the hamstrings and hip flexors as you begin the pull, as if you were trying to pull yourself down toward the floor or the bar. Likewise, it's important to think about keeping your chest and shoulders over the bar to discourage the hips from extending and changing the torso angle.

The pull needs to be initiated aggressively and powerfully through the upper back, especially the rear delts, rhomboids, and traps. The Pendlay row is heavily dependent on the momentum created during the first half of the pull. This is because the pulling muscles are in such a mechanically weak position toward the top of the lift (especially with gravity pulling directly against us, unlike during a regular bent-over row) that a certain amount of momentum needs to be created earlier on in the lift to achieve the finish position. Throughout the pull, the elbow angle, relative to the body, should stay the same. It is the job of the lats to fix the upper arms at this angle during the lift, which is why it is important to keep them contracted, even if they are not the prime mover of the lift.

KEY POINT

Lifters may cock their wrists in a vain attempt to help achieve the top position, the idea being that cocking the wrists will elevate the bar slightly to help get contact with the torso. Again, this is usually done because the weight is too heavy or simply because of poor pulling mechanics (it is something the lifter does during other pulling movements). Keep the wrists stacked throughout the whole lift.

The bar should be pulled until it makes contact with the torso, where possible. Not all lifters will be able to achieve contact with the torso, depending on their proportions. Those with long arms (especially long forearms) or a small rib cage may have to compromise their pulling mechanics to achieve contact between the bar and torso. In this scenario, the goal is simply to pull the bar as close to the body as possible without sacrificing alignment and to make sure that the range of motion stays consistent, especially as the loads increase.

For those who can achieve contact between the bar and the torso, the bar will make contact somewhere between the lower chest and upper stomach, depending on your grip width and proportions. At the top of the lift, the forearm should be vertical (wrist directly under the elbow joint). If this is not the case, then your grip width needs to be adjusted. For instance, if the wrist is inside the elbow joint at the top of the lift, then your grip needs to be wider.

KEY POINT

It is common to see lifters bend their knees during the top half of the pulling phase. This is done primarily to get the torso lower to the floor to make the top position easier to achieve. This is either done because the weight is too heavy to lift to the top position or because the set up didn't create enough full-body tension to maintain positioning, causing a power leak. Set up with more full-body tension, and make sure you are using appropriate loading.

Eccentric Portion

When training for strength, the Pendlay row is going to be performed with loads that make it almost impossible to slow down the eccentric portion of the lift to a significant degree—at least during the top half of the lift, due to the poor leverages. While you may not be able to significantly slow down the downward phase (with maximal loads at least), you should make as much effort as possible to control the bar back to the floor. The downside to just letting the bar drop back to the floor, except for the lack of any eccentric stimulus, is that it also encourages the rest of the body to relax, which can result in poor spinal alignment. And that is never a great idea while there is a heavy barbell in your hands. I see this as a similar situation to what we see in most lifters when it comes to lowering their deadlifts. They pay no attention to the lowering phase and, as a result, have terrible eccentric strength; more often than not, they end up getting injured on the lowering phase rather than the actual lifting phase. The goal during the eccentric phase is to maintain spinal alignment and torso rigidity along with the elbow angle relative to the torso. Your positioning during the downward phase should be the exact same as during the upward phase, the only difference being that the bar is likely moving quicker on the decent.

On the downward phase, you should be contracting the spinal erectors and abdominals maximally to maintain your spinal alignment to avoid being pulled into lumbar flexion by the bar. The lats also need to remain tense to hold the elbow angle stable while the bar is lowered. Likewise, the traps need to stay maximally contracted as the arms extend to stop the shoulders from being pulled into protraction by the bar. So, as you can see, just because you can't control the downward movement of the bar fully, that doesn't mean this phase of the lift doesn't require a lot of effort.

Once the bar is returned to the floor the setup process is then repeated. There is no such thing as a touch-and-go Pendlay row. With the nature of the downward phase of the lift, there is simply no way you can have the prerequisite positioning and muscular tension to pull the bar in the same manner without resetting properly. I would fully expect there to be a short break in between reps, as there would be with a heavy set of deadlifts, while the correct setup is attained.

KEY POINT

Just like the upward phase, it is also common to see lifters bend the knee on the downward phase. Why? Because maintaining a torso position parallel to the floor is difficult, and bending the knee allows the torso to be more upright. This is straight up a bad idea because it leaves you very likely to have the bar smash into your kneecap during the descent. Not only that, but one of the biggest benefits of this exercise, aside from getting a jacked upper back, is the whole-body postural strength stimulus. By moving away from that horizontal torso position, you are short-changing yourself on one of the biggest benefits of the lift.

Variations of the Pendlay Row

There are two key variations of the Pendlay row that you are going to also need to know. Both variations are essentially specific ways of "cheating" to further overload the back. However, just to be clear, these variations are not an excuse to get sloppy and not pay attention. They involve using momentum in a very specific way to maximize the loading of the back muscles as well as the carryover to the other lifts (especially deadlift).

Cheat Pendlay Row

In this variation, a degree of leg drive is used to create extra momentum in the bottom half of the lift. The setup for this variation can mimic your deadlift setup, except with the wider grip. The bar is started over the midfoot, and the hip height is the same as when setting up for a deadlift. The reason for this is that since we are using a leg drive off the floor, the shin and knee will move backward during the start of the lift (just like during a deadlift)—meaning we no longer have the issue of the bar hitting the knee.

In your deadlift setup, with the exception of a slightly wider grip and a slightly different upper back setup (as addressed previously), you will this time initiate the lift through a strong quad drive (again, just like a deadlift). As a result, the hips and shoulders will rise together, meaning the torso angle remains the same as the bar leaves the floor. Once the bar is around mid-shin level, the knee should be back far enough to clear a path for the bar to be pulled up. At this point, the upper body pull can then be initiated. This upper body pull is exactly the same as the strict Pendlay row. See figure 8.8 for a cheat Pendlay row.

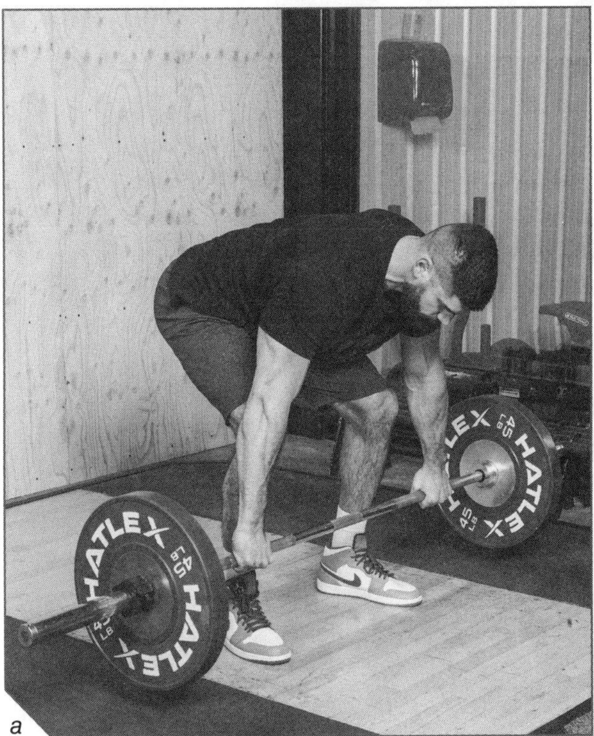

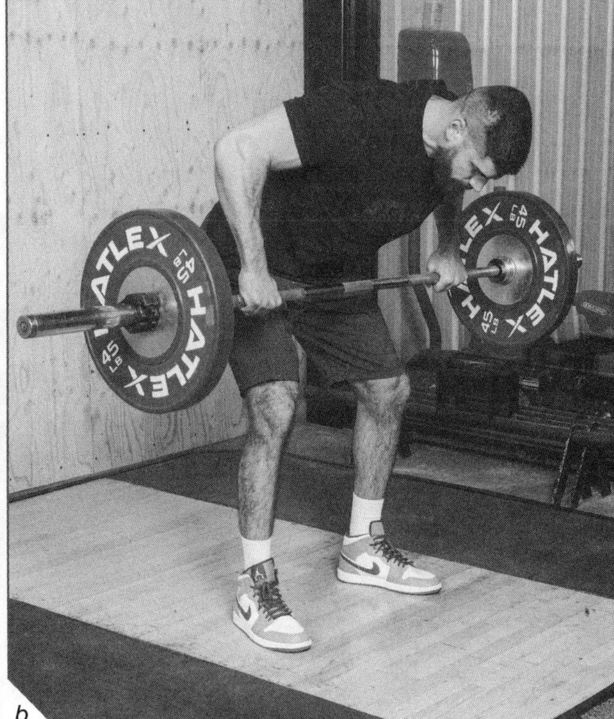

FIGURE 8.8 Cheat Pendlay row.

Deadlift Row

The difference here is that the leg drive portion of the lift is continued for longer. The setup is the exact same as the cheat Pendlay row variation, but instead the bar is deadlifted until it gets to just above knee level. Once the bar is deadlifted to knee level, it is instead rowed to the stomach with the elbows and upper arms in a less flared position (closer to the sides). More leg drive coupled with the slightly more upright torso position and shorter range of pull means that this variation can be loaded up considerably heavier than the regular Pendlay row, making it fantastic for overloading the upper back.

Since both of these variations allow more load to be used, the points I made about the downward phase of the strict Pendlay row are even more important. Maintaining good spinal alignment and bracing during the downward phase are absolutely paramount here to keep the injury risk low and get the most out of these variations. See figure 8.9 for a deadlift row.

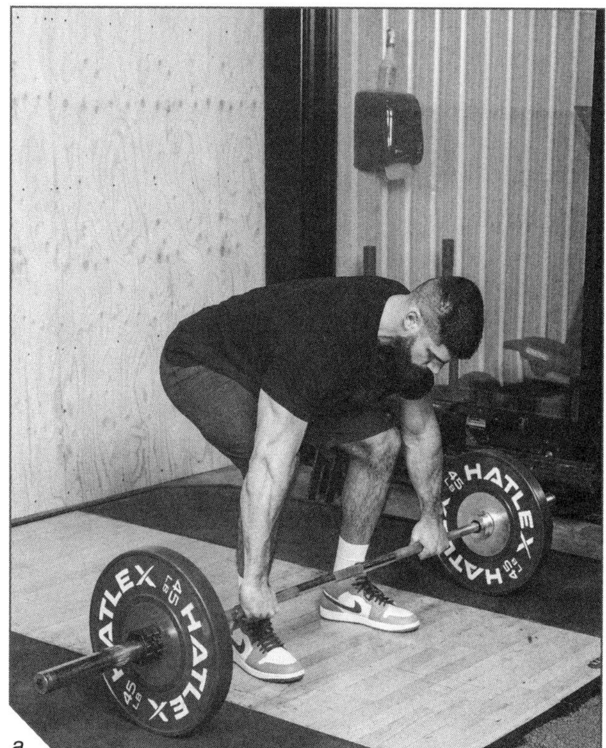

a

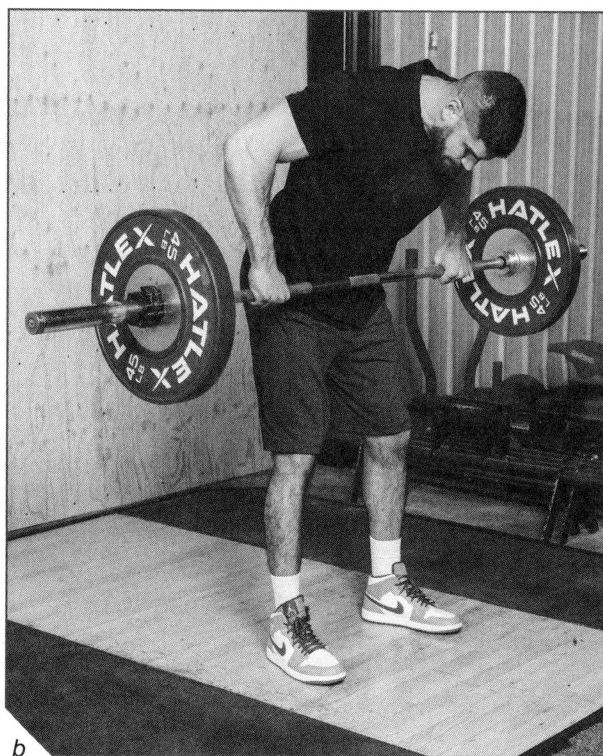

b

FIGURE 8.9 Deadlift row.

KEY POINT

With the higher load and higher dependency on leg drive in the first half of the lift in a deadlift row, it is even more common to see lifters try to gain leverage in the top half of the lift by bending the knee and rounding through the back. Once again, if this is you, stop cheating. You are either using too much weight, lacking in full-body tension, or not creating enough momentum with the leg drive at the start of the lift.

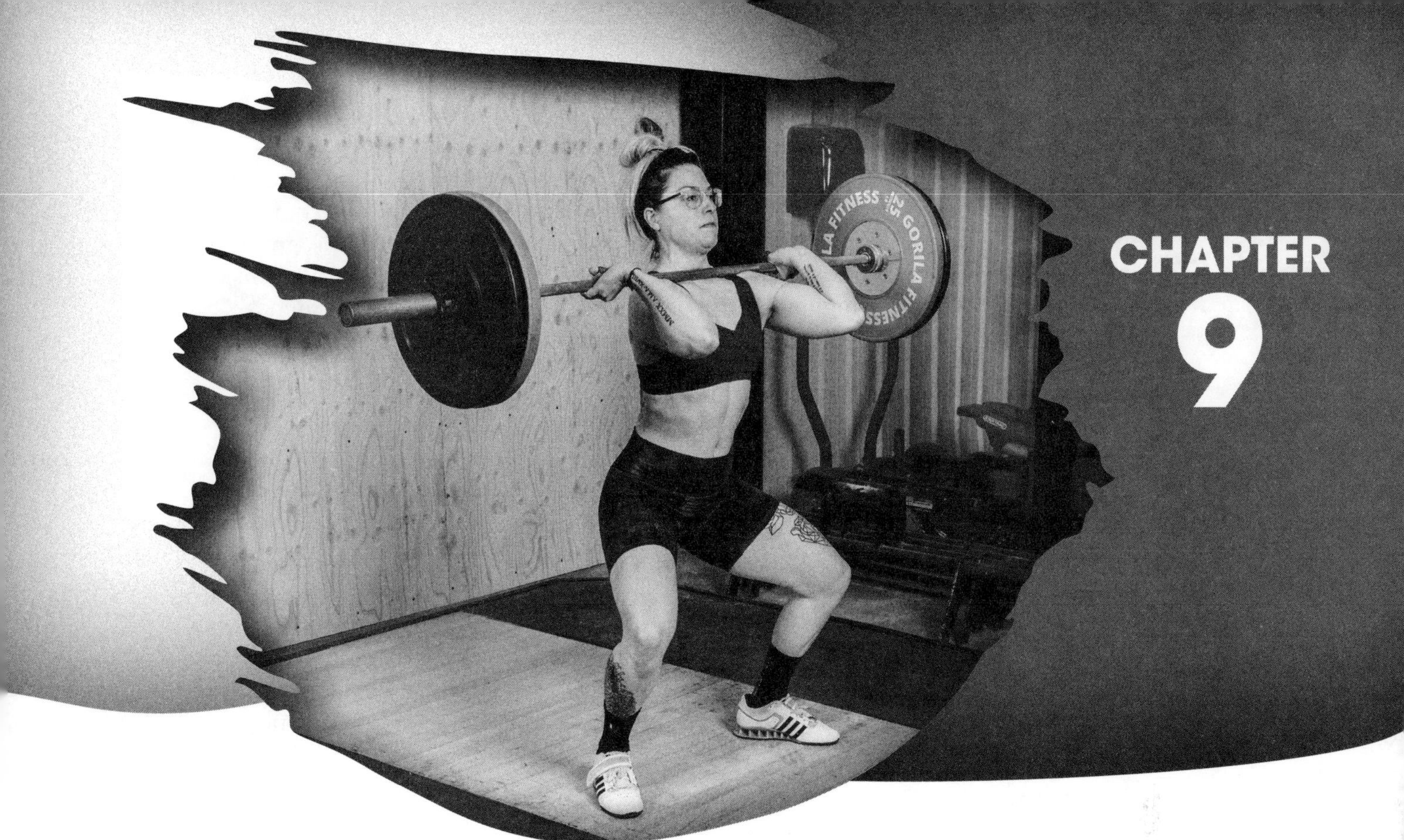

CHAPTER 9

Explosive Pulls

Up until the mid-1950s, explosive pulling was a huge part of the training of most strong lifters. Back then, weightlifting (Olympic lifting) dominated among lifting sports (there was no powerlifting yet, and bodybuilding competitions were in their infancy), and the original strongmen and lifting contests pretty much always included explosive movements. They were known as "the quick lifts," and they normally included lifts such as the one- or two-hand snatch or the one- or two-hand clean and jerk. In fact, the first official weightlifting competitions (that would go on to become Olympic lifting) included five contested lifts:

- One-hand snatch
- One-hand clean and jerk
- Two-hands clean and press
- Two-hands snatch
- Two-hands clean and jerk

When the one-hand lifts were dropped from competition in 1928 (contests were way too long), only three competition lifts remained: the clean and press, the snatch, and the clean and jerk.

These competitions were maintained from 1928 through the 1972 Olympic Games, after which the clean and press was dropped from competition, mostly because the judging had become too permissive. Lifters turned the traditional strict military press into a form of overhead lift with a huge degree of back bend to get under the bar and press much heavier loads. I mention all this only to point out that in the 1950s and before, the quick lifts were part of most serious training programs. Even the courses sold with barbell sets (e.g., the York barbell courses or the Milo course) usually included high pulls and power cleans, sometimes even snatches.

I (Christian) am a big believer in explosive lifting. Of course, I am biased because my origins lie in weightlifting. But I started doing them even before that. I started doing them at around 14 years of age, and as a strength coach, I've pretty much always included explosive pulls in the training of the athletes I work with. Personally, I find that no other exercises are as effective as the high pull to build the traps. For that reason alone, they have their place in this system. While working up to accomplish a power clean is a cool target to shoot for, it is not necessary if your main goal is simply to look jacked and become strong and powerful. The scaled versions of explosive pulling—such as the power shrug, low pulls, and high pulls—are enough for those goals. Usually, I like to have someone progress from power shrugs to low pulls and finally high pulls, and if they have the mobility, coordination, and desire to learn, we can move on to power cleans or even power snatches.

Explosive pulls come in a great many variations. The three main differentiating factors are:

- *Pulling height*: This refers to how high you pull the barbell. For example, in a power shrug, the bar will normally reach a position close to the navel. In a low pull, you reach a height between your navel and the high part of the abdomen. In a high pull, you should reach your chest or even collarbone. In a clean, you actually bring the bar to the shoulders, and in the snatch, straight to the overhead position. I find that the longer the pull is (except for the snatch), the more the natural tendency will be to overuse the arms, which can make the exercise less effective and more dangerous. That's why I like to start with shorter-range pulls to really program the bias toward producing power through the hips, traps, and calves and not early arm pull. Of course, the shorter-range pulls also allow you to use more weight, which makes them worth utilizing even if you are technically solid with the longer-range variations.
- *Starting position*: You can start your exercise from the floor, from blocks (above or below knees), or from the hang (above or below knees). Lifts from above the knees (block or hang) are much easier to learn, and if all you want is strength, power, and size, they are your best choice. "From the hang" lends itself better to hypertrophy, and I prefer to use lifts from the blocks or pins for maximum strength and power development.
- *Grip width*: There are three main grip widths you can use: clean grip (slightly wider than shoulders), snatch grip (wide grip), and hybrid (between clean and snatch grip). The width of the grip influences how likely you are to rely more on your arms. A narrower grip will favor using the arms to pull, whereas wider makes it more mechanically efficient to hit the traps.

Setup

The most important position to master, whether you perform your explosive pulls from the floor, hang, or blocks (which we will cover next in this section), is what I call "the power position." Essentially, when the bar is just above the knees (lower third of the thigh), this is when you violently stand up to impart momentum to the bar. Unsurprisingly, this position mimics the optimal jumping position. To set up in the power position, the feet are about hip-width apart (some will be better with a tad wider or narrower stance, as discussed in chapter 4, on the deadlift). The hips are set back, and the knees are bent at around a 100-degree angle, roughly level with the midfoot. The shoulders are in line with the toes (so forward of the knees). The elbows are turned out, and the lats are engaged (again, see chapter 4 on the deadlift for more detail on how to do this) to keep the bar close. Because the lats are engaged, the bar will be inside the shoulders. Even when you explode, the longer the bar can stay inside the shoulders, the better leverage you'll have at the end of the explosion.

Your choice of start position will alter how much work you need to do to get to the power position. But remember, regardless of where you choose to start your lift, the end goal is the same. Get your body and the bar aligned in the power position so that you can properly explode upward and impart momentum into the bar.

- *If you start from the floor*, the first pull (from the floor to above the knees) is only there to get you into that power position properly, not to create momentum. A big mistake people make with explosive pulls from the floor is accelerating from the floor. See figure 9.1 for an example for a power clean and figure 9.2 for an example for a power snatch.
- *If you start from the hang* (standing up as in the finish position of a deadlift), you get to the power position by lowering the bar down to above the knees, as if you were doing a Romanian deadlift. See figure 9.3 for an example for a power clean and figure 9.4 for an example for a power snatch.
- *If you start from blocks*, you can simply set yourself up in the proper position right way. See figure 9.5 for an example for a power clean.

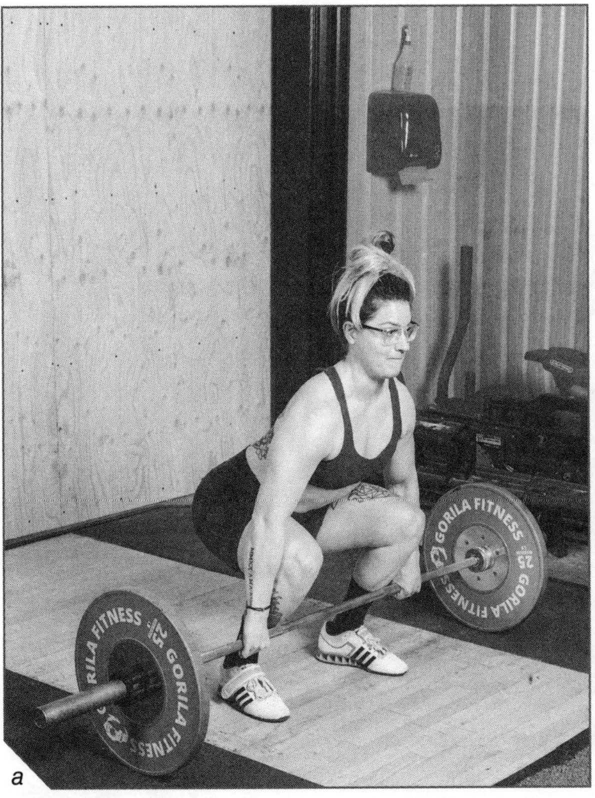

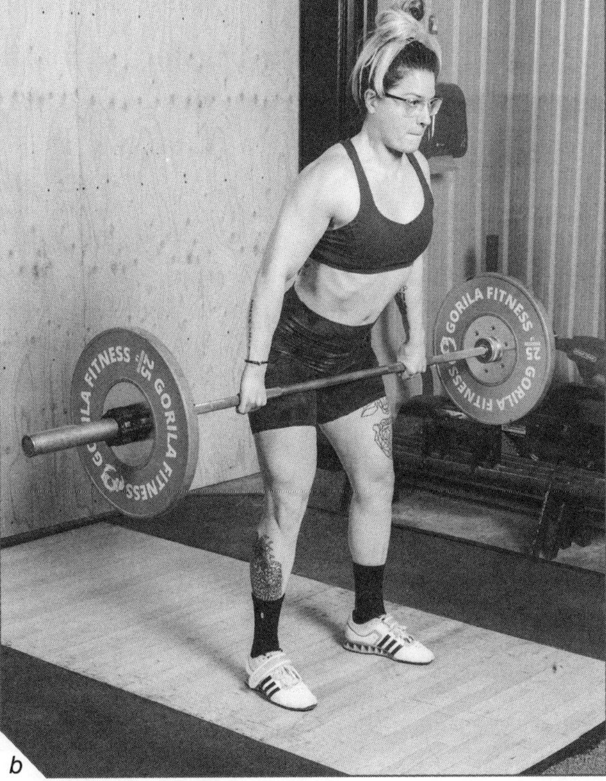

FIGURE 9.1 Getting into the power position from the floor for a power clean.

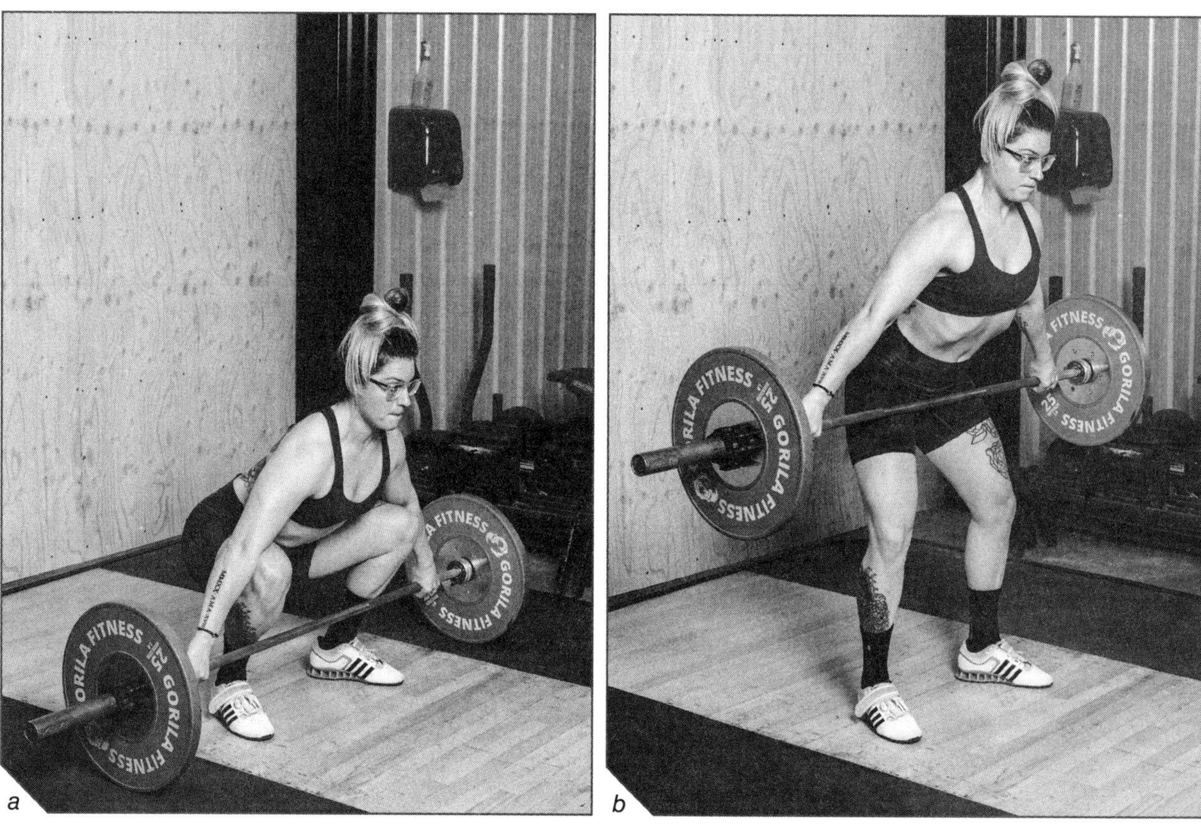

FIGURE 9.2 Getting into the power position from the floor for a power snatch.

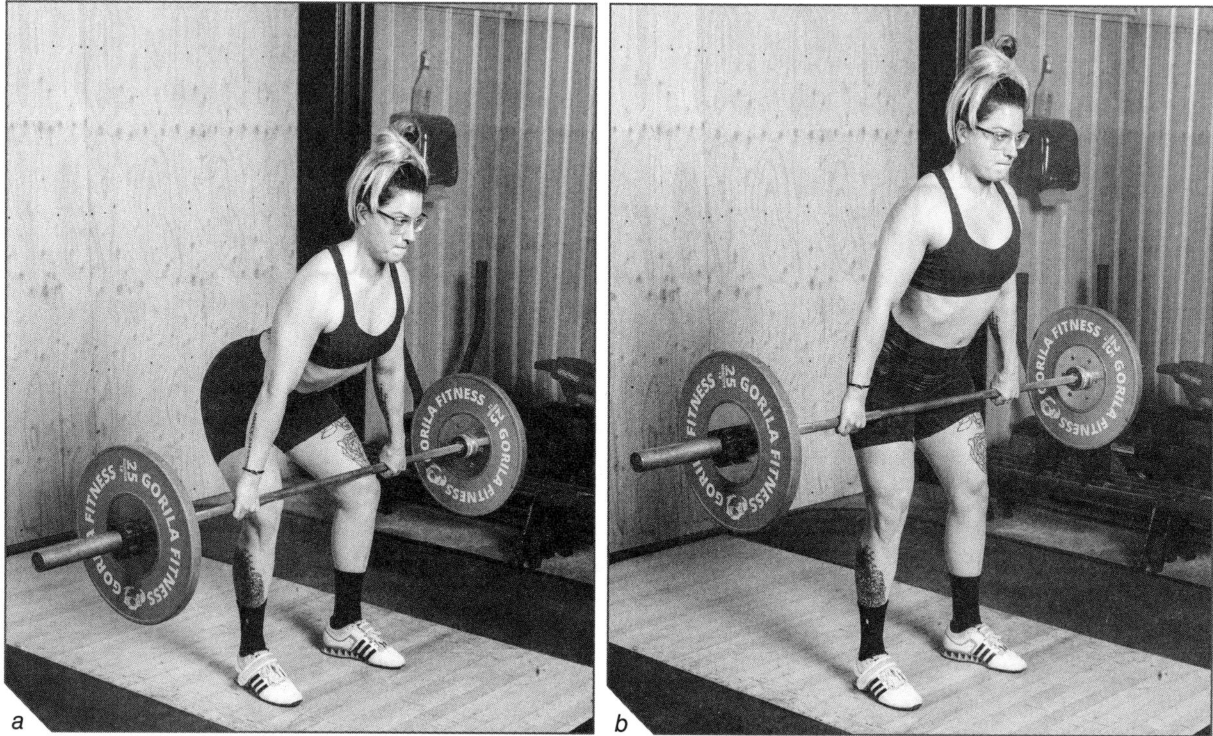

FIGURE 9.3 Getting into the power position from the hang for a power clean.

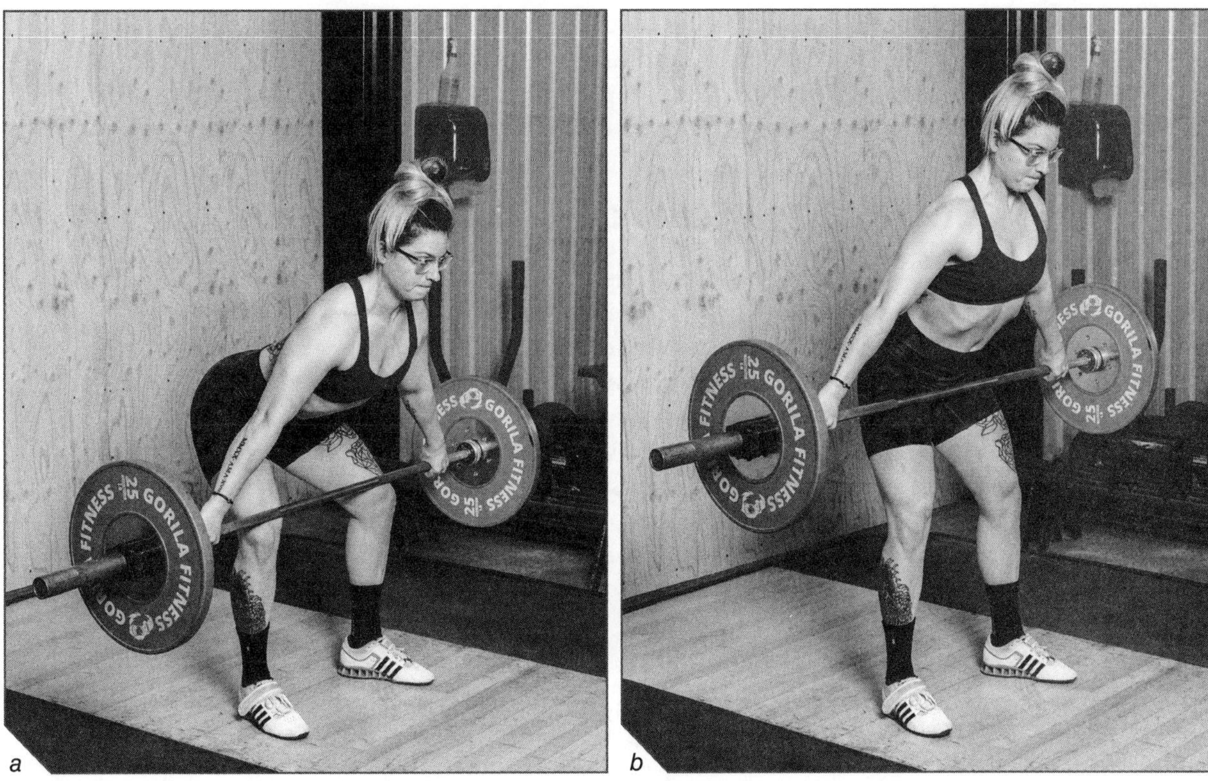

FIGURE 9.4 Getting into the power position from the hang for a power snatch.

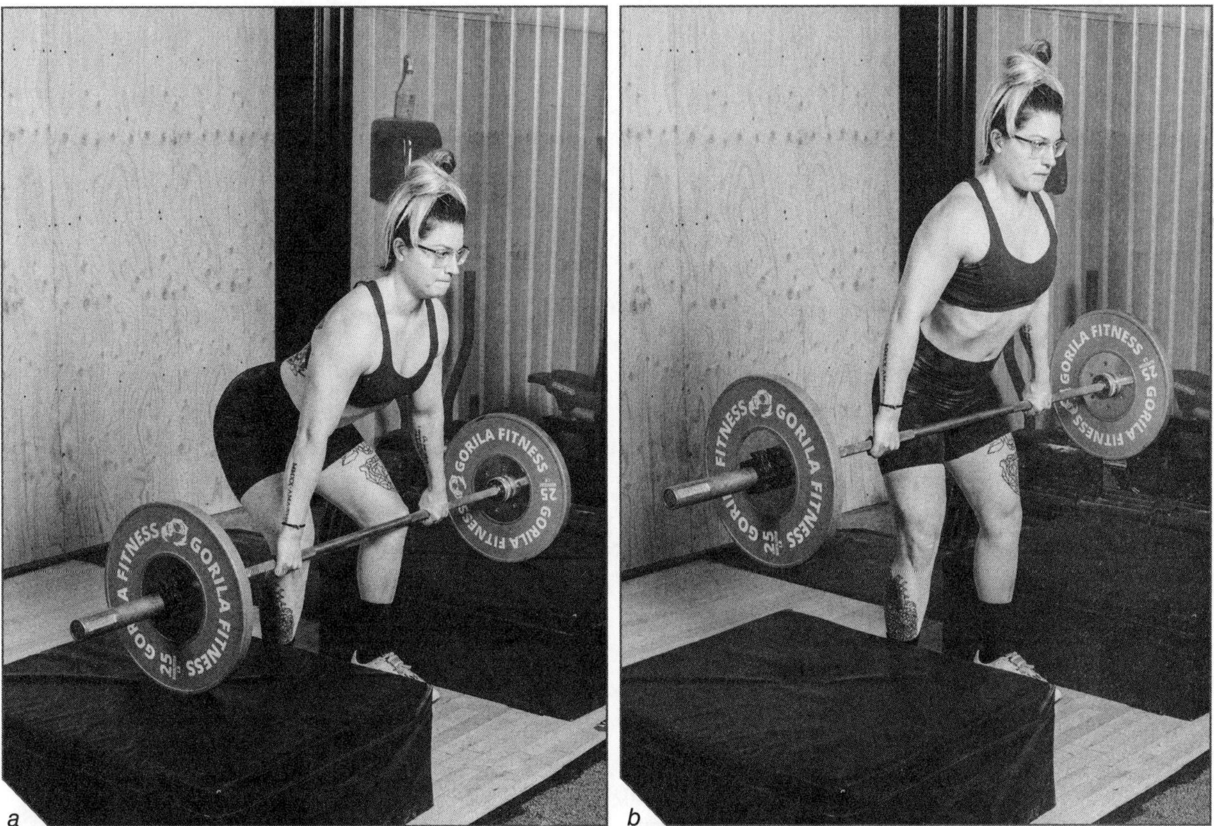

FIGURE 9.5 Getting into the power position from the blocks for a power clean.

As such, explosive pulls from the blocks are the easiest, technique-wise. Lifts from the hang are second easiest, and lifts from the floor are the most complex. Typically, even elite lifters will do 3 to 6 percent more from blocks than from the floor or hang.

Bar Path and Movement Pattern

Explosive pulls come in many varieties based on grip, pull height, start position, and so on, but they do share some key similarities. The main driving force is a powerful triple extension of the lower body (ankle, knee, and hip joint); this provides the bar with the majority of its upward momentum. Once the bar is already moving upward, the goal is then to pull aggressively with the traps and upper back to get the bar to rise higher. Regardless of grip used, the goal of the pull is for the elbows to rise as close to directly upward as possible to keep the bar close to the body.

The initial momentum imparted into the bar by the lower body allows us to perform these exercises with much more load than would be possible if we were simply using the muscles of the upper back. This overload is what can make them such an effective tool for building the upper back, along with the obvious benefits of improving lower-body strength and power.

Concentric Portion: The Motor

This is what I would call the "motor" of the lift common to all the explosive pulls—the explosive upward action of the legs, hips, calves, and traps. At this point, we are not going to talk about pulling with the arms because in a proper pull, this only happens once momentum has already been created by the motor of the lift. Early arm pull will lead to lower power production and an increased risk of injury. When people get shoulder pain from high pulls and cleans, it is usually because they arm-pull too much or too early. The pain in their shoulder is actually inflammation of the biceps tendon where it attaches to the humerus. That's why I like to start teaching explosive pulls with the power shrug. By nature, it is devoid of any arm pull and focuses on being as explosive as possible with the legs and traps.

So, how do you execute the motor of the explosive pull? It is very simple, but people make it a lot more complex than it needs to be. The key technique cue is simply *stand up fast*. Really.

It will get a bit more complex when you move on to the longer pulls, like high pulls and power clean and power snatches, but as far as the motor is concerned, it's just "stand up fast." Well, it is a bit more than that. It's actually stand up violently fast, with as much force as humanly possible. You want to stand up so fast from the power position that the bar would move up to the navel even without the use of the traps, just from the momentum created by standing up fast. The hip should move forward so fast from the power position that it should look like someone stabbed your butt with a cattle prod (this suggestion also works as an effective teaching tool, not talking from experience, of course). You can even do explosive partial Romanian deadlifts before getting into explosive pulls. If you can't stand up violently fast on this movement, you will always tend to rely more on arm pulling to compensate.

Once you are capable of standing up violently fast, you add to the motor the "finish": a fast shrug and calf action. Both happen almost at the same time. Technically, the calves fire a bit before the traps, but don't think about that. On complex movements, especially if they are explosive, you should never focus on the action of a specific muscle. Never use internal cues. Always focus on a movement. Stand up violently fast and finish by trying to punch your ears with your shoulders!

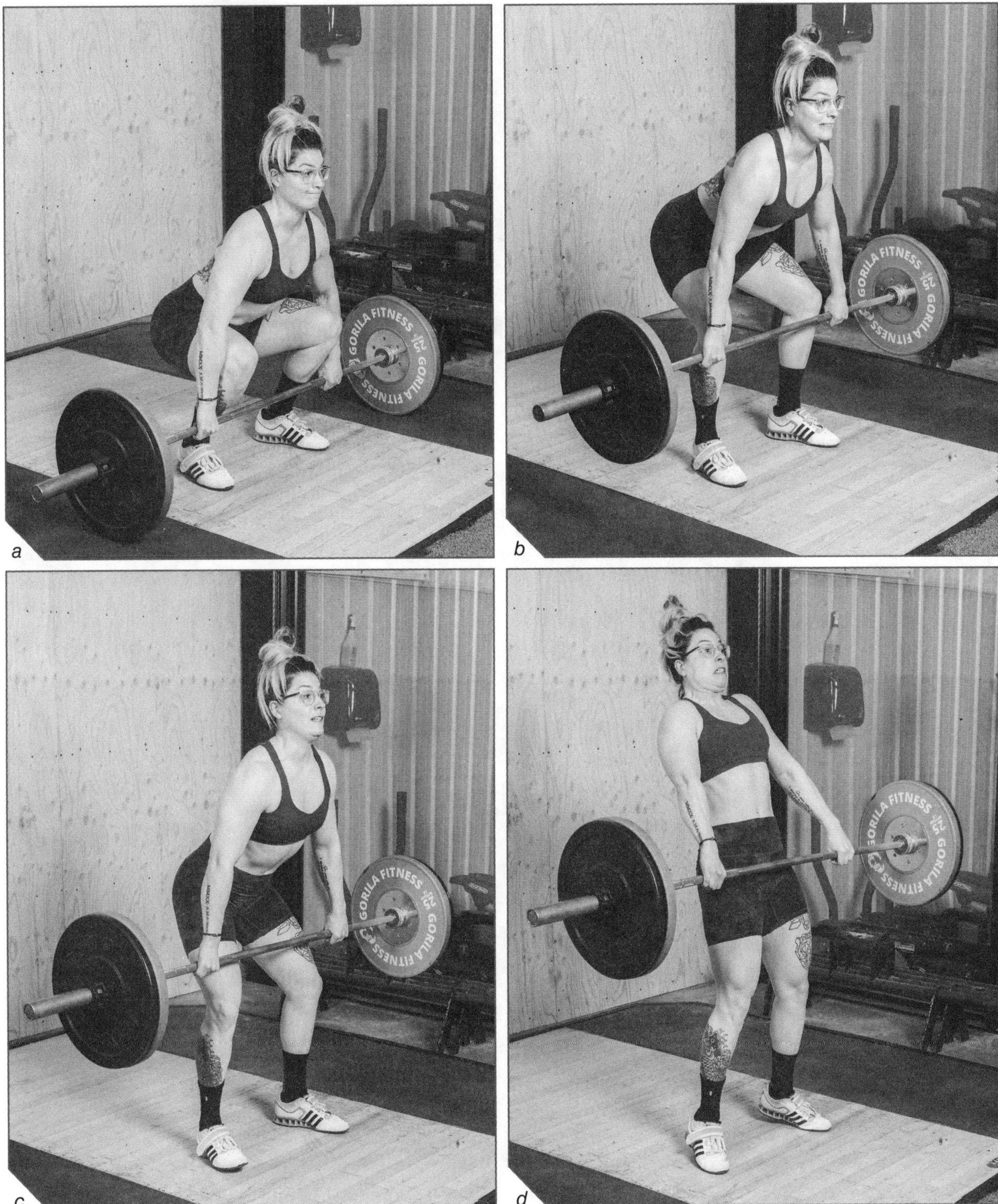

FIGURE 9.6 Motor portion of the power clean: During the motor portion of the lift, momentum is imparted into the bar through the lower body via knee and hip extension. This is where the majority of the momentum is created that is necessary for a successful lift.

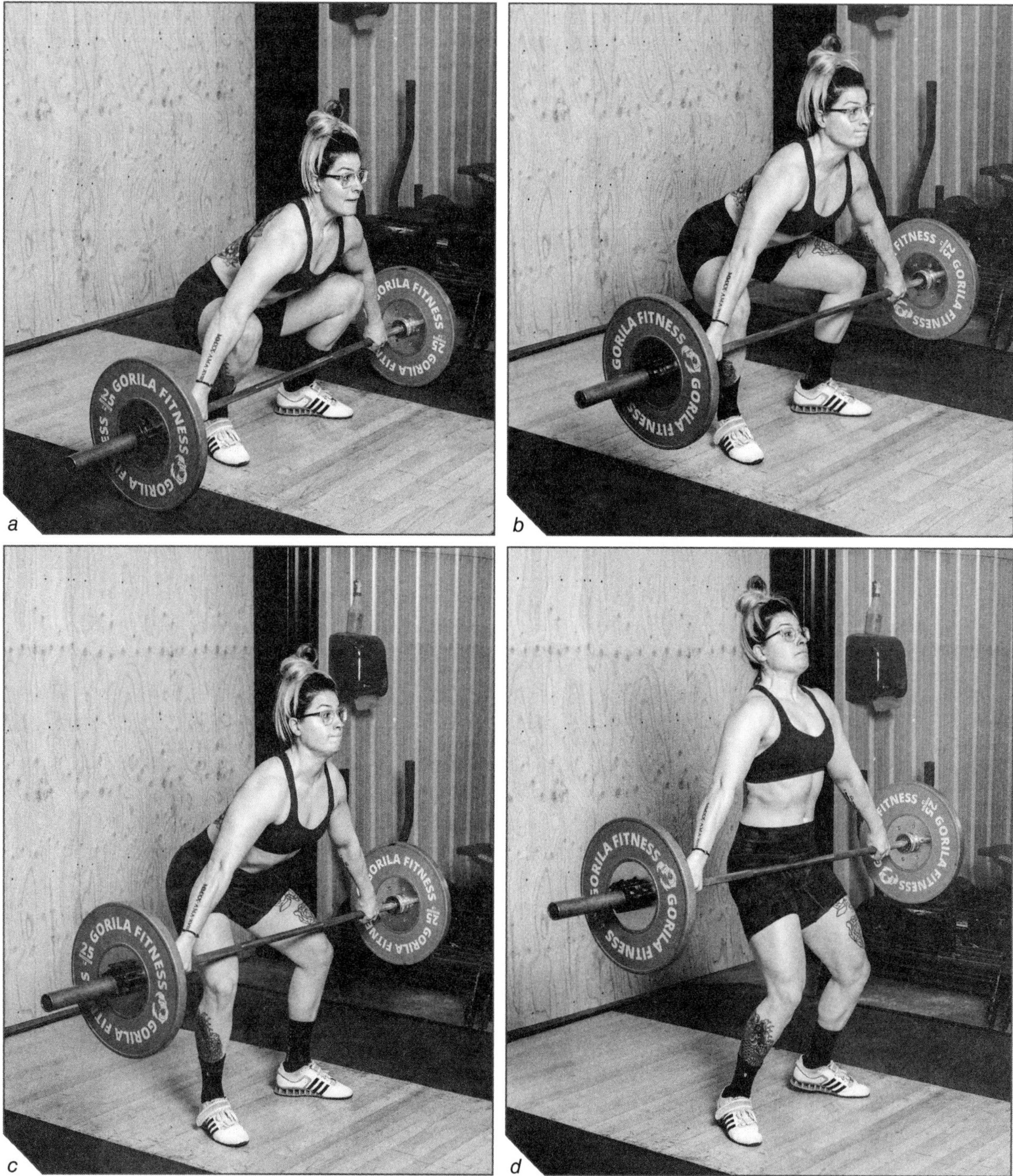

FIGURE 9.7 Motor portion of the power snatch: During the motor portion of the lift, momentum is imparted into the bar through the lower body via knee and hip extension. This is where the majority of the momentum is created that is necessary for a successful lift.

There should be no arm pull at all occurring in this motor pattern (this is the power shrug). If you do it right, there might be some arm bend. That happens not because you are pulling with your arms but because you are producing so much upward acceleration that the arms have to bend to let the bar move up on its own momentum.

Concentric Portion: Arm Pull

Once you have mastered the motor and can create a good amount of upward momentum using your legs, traps, and calves, creating more height in your pull is only a matter of finishing the pull with the arms. There are two key considerations, though:

- You have to time the arm pull so that it comes when momentum has been imparted into the bar. If you arm-pull too early, you will lose a lot of power and increase the risk of injury; but if you wait too long and momentum dies down, you will have the same issue. As soon as you have performed the powerful calves and traps action, you pull with the arms. The proper timing will leave the bar much lighter so that you need a lot less force to further accelerate a moving load than to get it moving in the first place.
- The higher the pulling target is, the less weight you can use, even if you properly time the arm pull. Having the bar cover a greater distance requires more force application. Don't expect to do the same weight on low pulls as you did on high pulls just because you throw the arms in there. For example, when I could do a 180-kilogram (397-pound) high pull, I could do a low pull with 200 to 210 kilograms (441 to 463 pounds) and a power shrug with 240 to 250 kilograms (530 to 550 pounds), and I was very efficient technically. Don't be surprised if your high pull is only 50 to 60 percent of your power shrug at first.

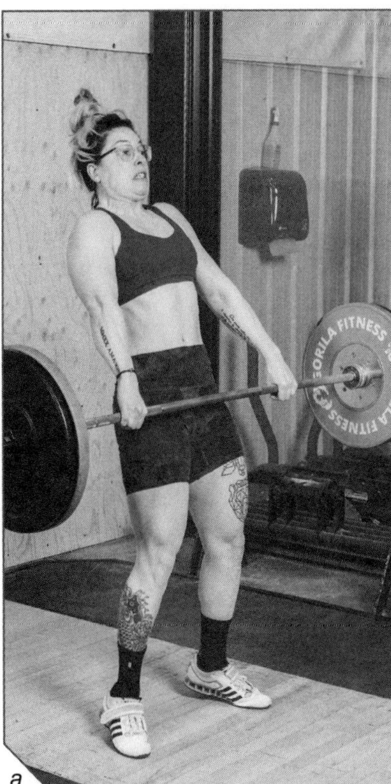
a

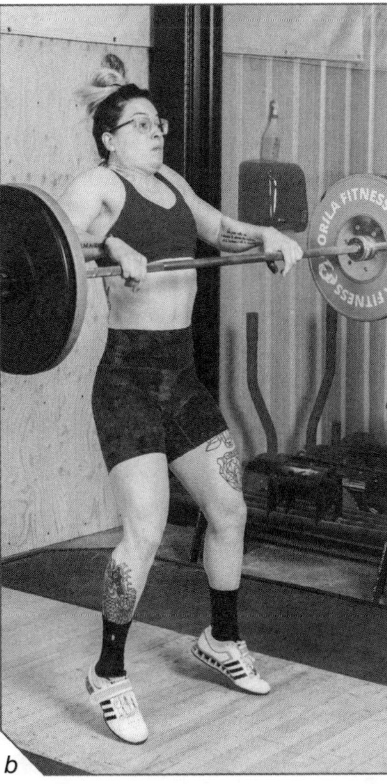
b

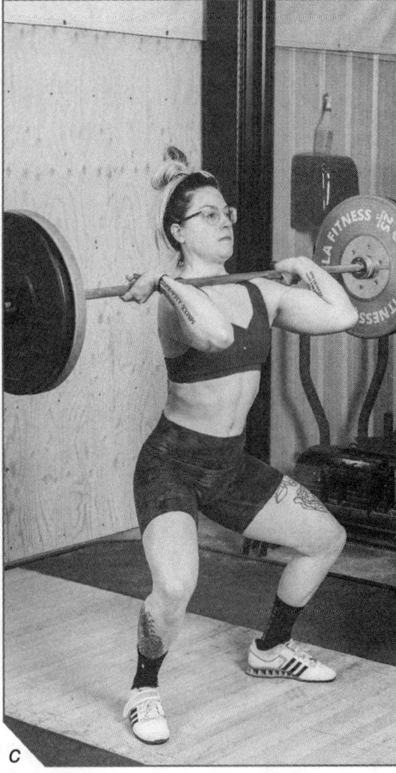
c

FIGURE 9.8 Arm pull portion of the power clean: During the arm pull portion of the lift, the upper back is used to pull and redirect the bar toward the catch position. This arm pull does impart further momentum into the bar, but not to the same degree as the lower body in the previous motor portion.

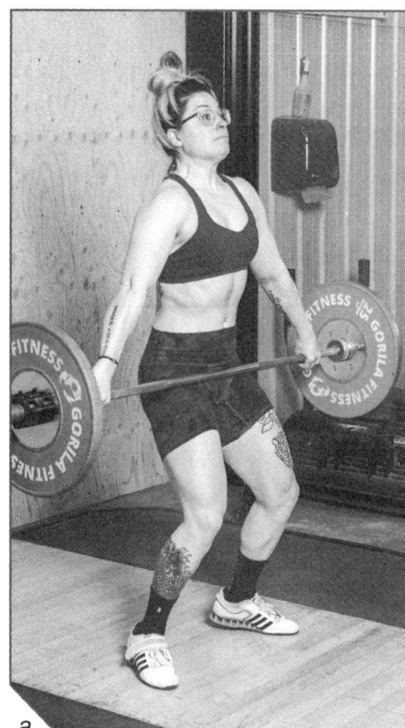
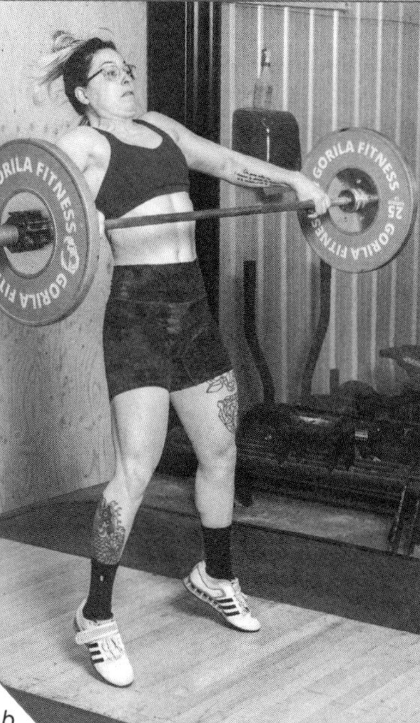
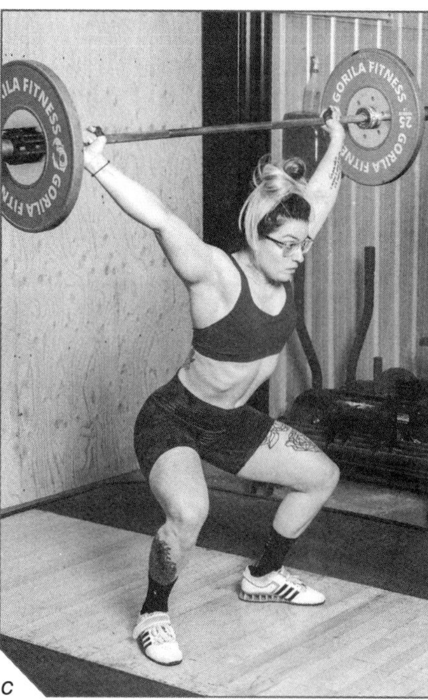

FIGURE 9.9 Arm pull portion of the power snatch: During the arm pull portion of the lift, the upper back is used to pull and redirect the bar toward the catch position. This arm pull does impart further momentum into the bar, but not to the same degree as the lower body in the previous motor portion.

Eccentric Portion

Let's not kid ourselves: There is no way that you will lower a high pull (or even low pull) under control. At least not once you are capable of using even remotely decent weights. You will have to let the bar "drop down" (although you don't let go of the bar like you do after a clean or snatch). However, it is not a free fall all the way down, and you certainly don't just let it go anywhere. The worst mistakes to avoid are:

- Letting the bar free-fall from the top and "catching" it with straight legs
- Letting the bar drop down too far away from your body
- Letting the bar pull you forward when you catch

While there are a few ways to properly lower a high pull, clean, or snatch (also applicable to a low pull or even a power shrug), they all have three things in common:

1. Keep the bar as close to your body as possible.
2. Catch it with bent legs. In fact, I personally almost mimic the "hang" position when lowering the bar.
3. Absorb the impact of the bar to some extent with the upper thighs. While the traps and arms break the fall of the bar, the bar lands on the upper third of my thighs, dramatically reducing the tug on the traps and arms. However, don't let the bar free-fall on your legs, either. Make sure you lower it toward the upper portion of the leg and not lower, where it might be too close to the knees.

KEY POINT

All explosive pulls can develop size, strength, and explosiveness. But you can bias your results slightly toward a specific goal, depending on the movement you use (provided that you are equally as efficient in all of them).

- *High pulls* are the best to develop muscle mass (especially if done from the hang).
- *Low pulls* are the best to develop strength (especially if done from blocks).
- *Power shrugs* are best suited to emphasize trap development. They can be done from the hang for sets of 5 to 8 to build maximum size or from blocks for sets of 2 to 5 to build maximum strength in the traps.

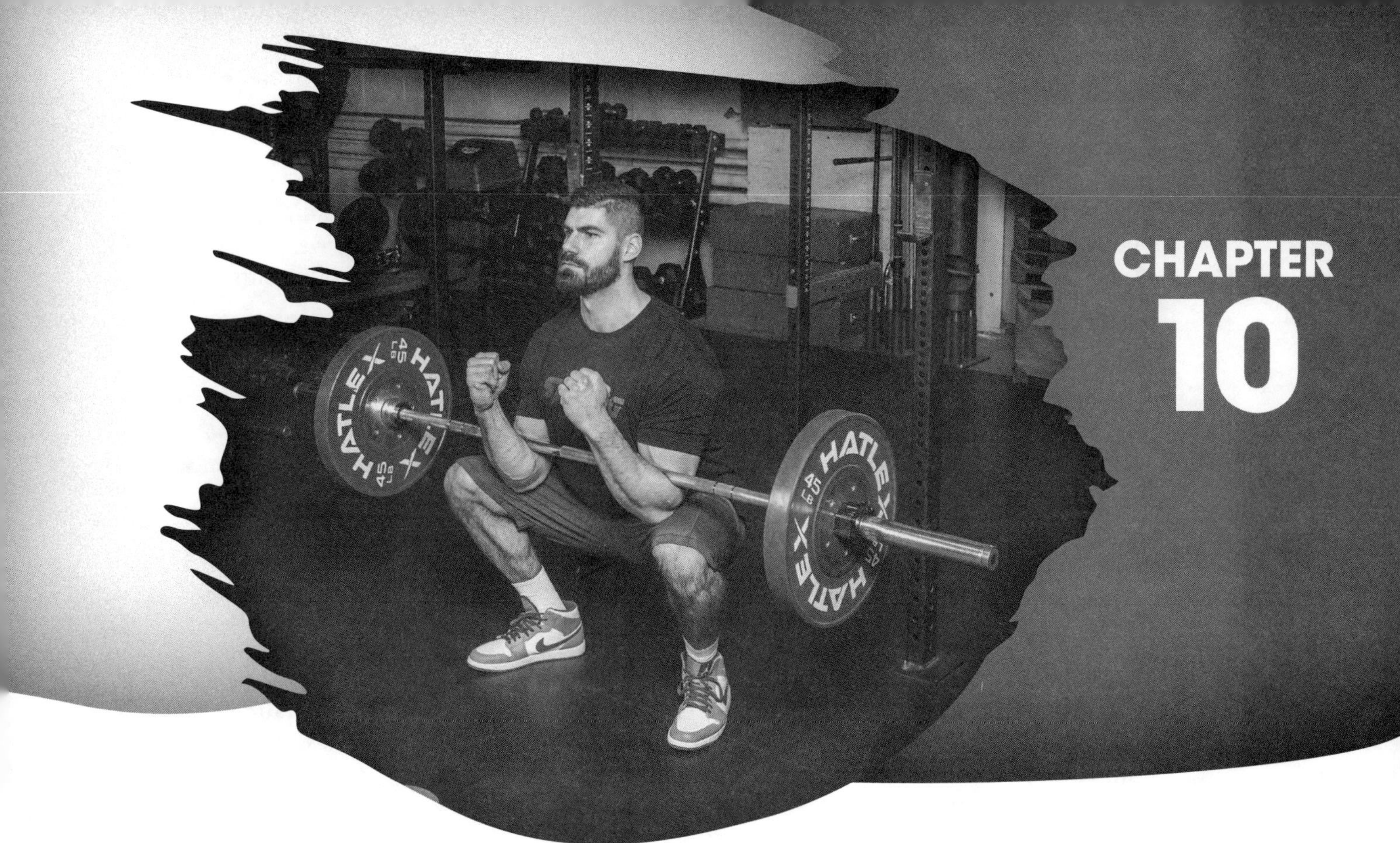

CHAPTER 10

Assistance Exercises

This chapter covers several effective assistance exercises for each foundational exercise (main lift). This is by no means an exhaustive list, but we have purposely listed exercises that have worked well historically with a broad spectrum of clients. As you learned in chapter 1, assistance exercises are exercises that will directly improve a main lift because they are structurally close to those main lifts. There are five components that make an assistance exercise structurally similar to a main lift. An assistance exercise does not have to combine all five components, but the more it has, the more effective it will be at directly improving the main lift. These components are:

- Same joints involved, moving in a similar way
- Same muscles involved, doing the same function
- Same range of motion
- Same contraction types
- Same rhythm

These assistance exercises will not be explained in as much detail as we covered the main lifts in chapters 4 to 9, but we will give you the key coaching points and explain how and why they are useful. There are, of course, many other effective assistance exercises, so if you have found some that worked great for you in the past and fit the criteria of a proper assistance exercise, feel free to use them.

Note that in the overload system, explosive pulls are used to not only build explosive power but also to stimulate and strengthen the upper back and lower body. So, they are in essence an accessory movement, but one that carries over to all the main lifts. As such, we do not add assistance work for these movements into this program.

DEADLIFT ASSISTANCE EXERCISES

Romanian Deadlift

For the Romanian deadlift, you simply perform only phase II of the deadlift (see chapter 4). This is the hip and posterior chain dominant portion of the lift. The bar is lowered from the top position just as would be done in a full deadlift, except the lowering phase is stopped between the bottom of the knee and mid-shin (depending on mobility). For maximal carryover to the full lift, I like to include a small pause in the bottom position to help eliminate the stretch reflex. After all, you don't get that on the full lift.

The hips are then driven forward toward the bar to get back to the locked-out position. The same cues and rules apply as during the deadlift: Maintain torso rigidity, bar path, and so on. The Romanian deadlift is very good for strengthening the posterior chain, especially toward the end of the range of motion. If your sticking point on deadlift is just below the knee, this is a good choice.

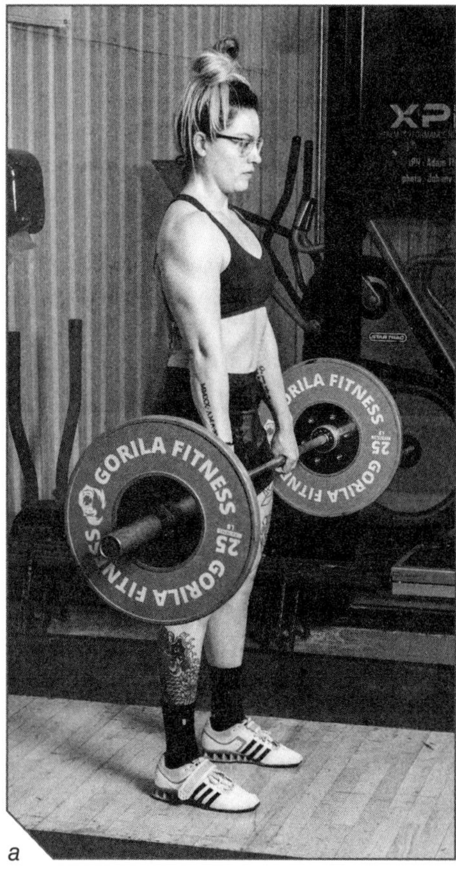

a

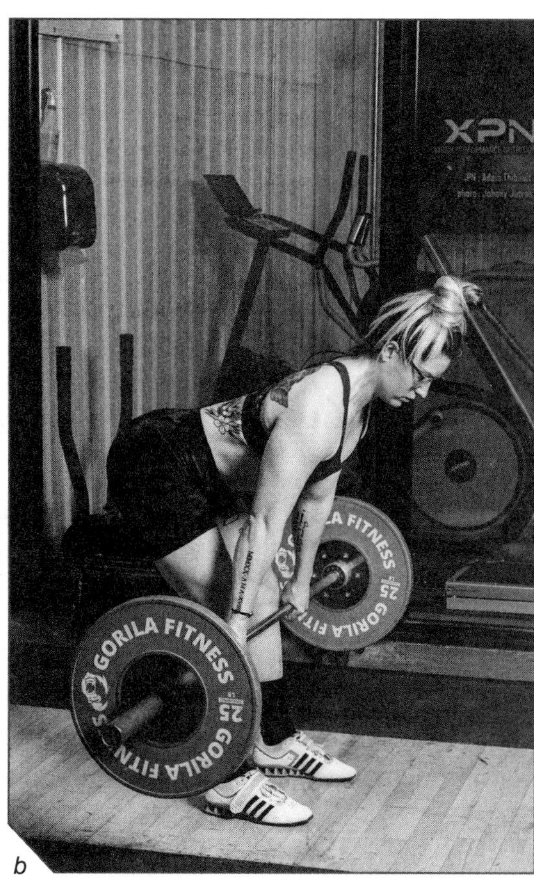

b

DEADLIFT ASSISTANCE EXERCISES

Romanian Deadlift with Band Around Waist

A Romanian deadlift is performed with a resistance band pulling backward on the hips. As the hips drive forward during the concentric, the band tension increases, which increases the difficulty of the lockout. This exercise works well with a pause at the locked-out position as your hips are still under load from the band. This is a great way of adding work for the hip extensors without adding more spinal loading. It is especially effective if your lockout is slow or weak.

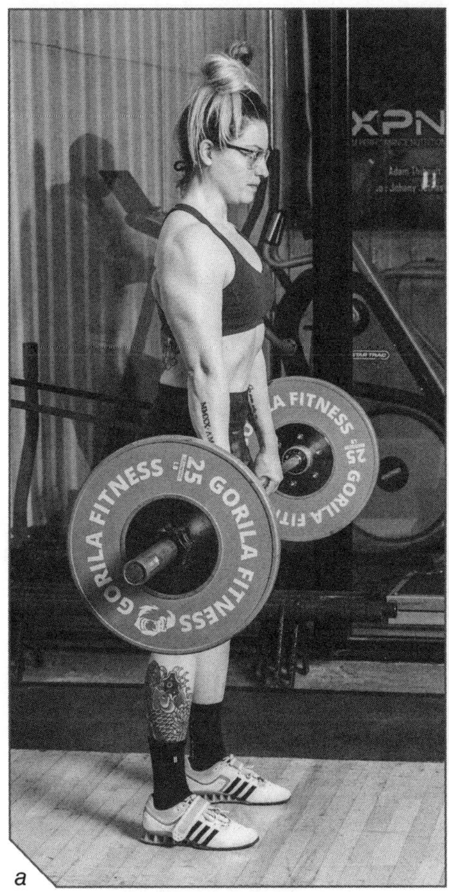

a

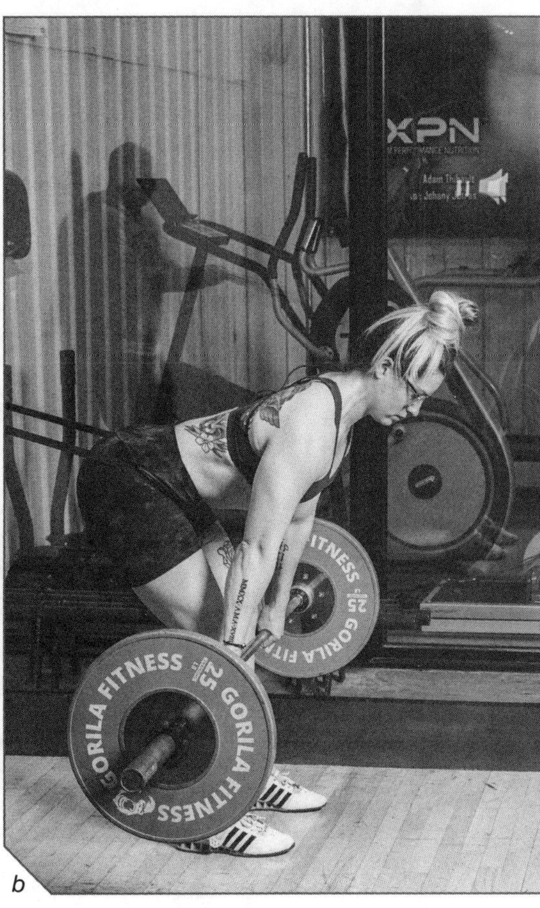

b

DEADLIFT ASSISTANCE EXERCISES

Romanian Deadlift with Front of Feet Elevated

A Romanian deadlift is performed with the front of the feet elevated, which pre-stretches the calves and hamstrings. A muscle that is stretched more during a lift is recruited and worked more, making this exercise a little more effective for targeting the hamstrings (and calves, to a lesser extent). Note, however, that you should not be doing this variation unless you have ample mobility to perform a standard Romanian deadlift to at least mid-shin level. Otherwise, you will be sacrificing position due to lack of mobility.

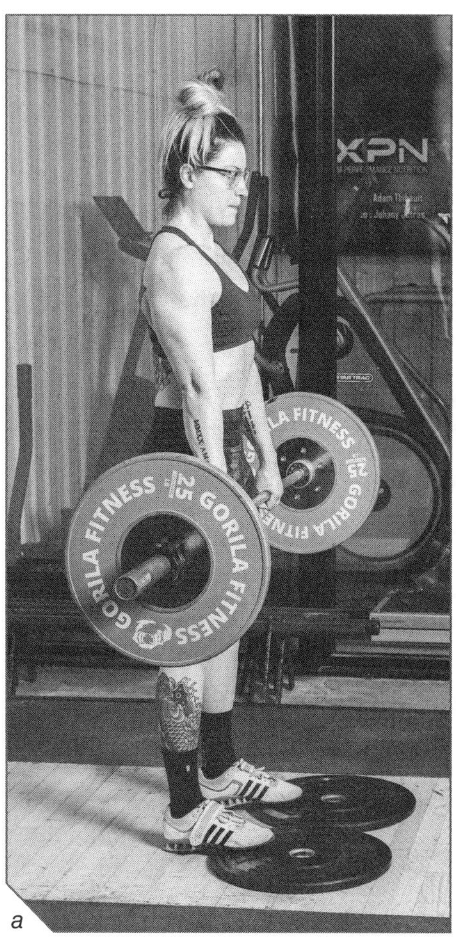

a

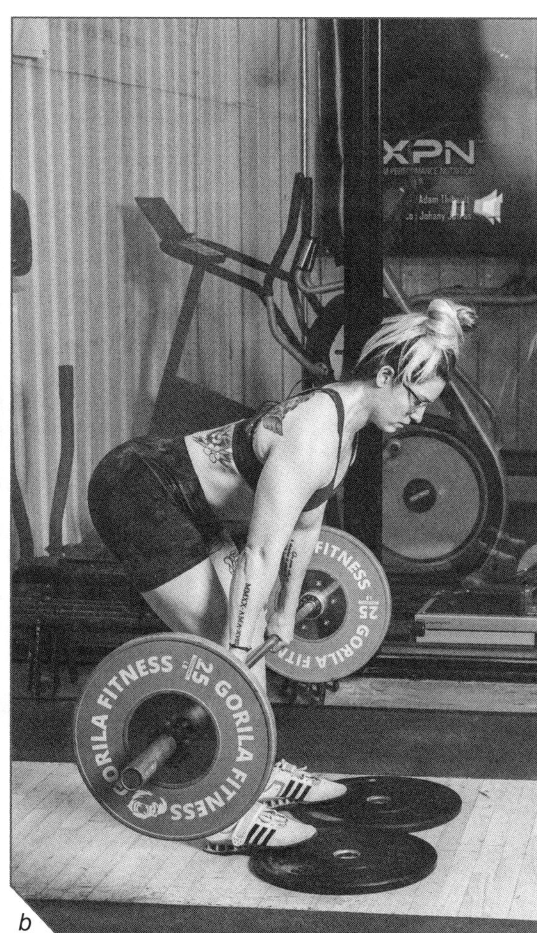

b

DEADLIFT ASSISTANCE EXERCISES

Good Morning Variations

Good morning variations are another way of targeting the posterior chain and hip-dominant portion of the deadlift. In principle, it is the same movement pattern as the Romanian deadlift, a pure hip hinge pattern. But by placing the bar on the upper back rather than in the hands, you increase the loading on the spinal erectors and thoracic extensors (as the load is placed on a long lever from these muscles). So, this exercise can be a great variation for those who are lacking in these areas. Because of the long levers involved, good morning variations will also have higher stability demands than Romanian deadlift variations (except the seated variation). While the exercise can be performed with a straight bar, the tendency for it to roll or move throughout the lift can make it awkward. As such, the use of a safety-squat bar, spider bar, cambered bar, or similar is preferable.

Arched-Back Good Morning

When we say "arched back," we actually mean neutral (the same alignment we squat and deadlift with), but this is to distinguish this variation from the often-performed "rounded back" good morning variation, which we rarely use as we find the risks often outweigh the benefits. These exercises are most effective when performed to a torso angle that matches the torso angle at the start of your deadlift. They have a very good carryover to the deadlift because the back angle and alignment matches that of the full lift.

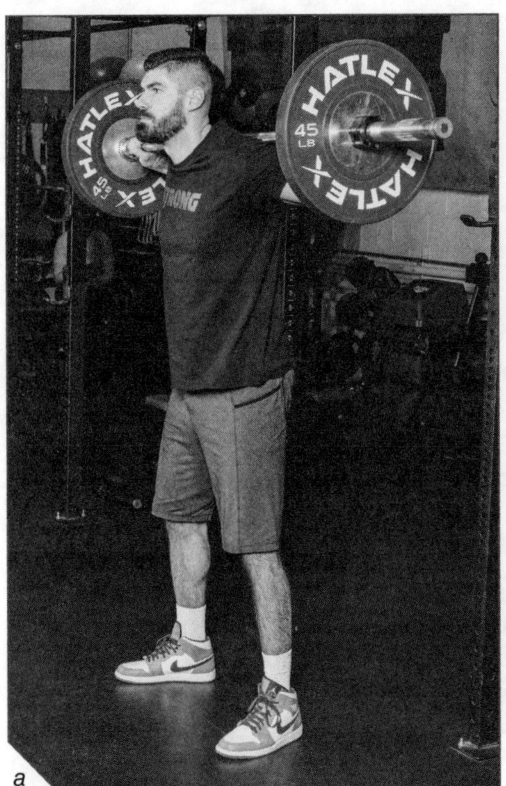

a

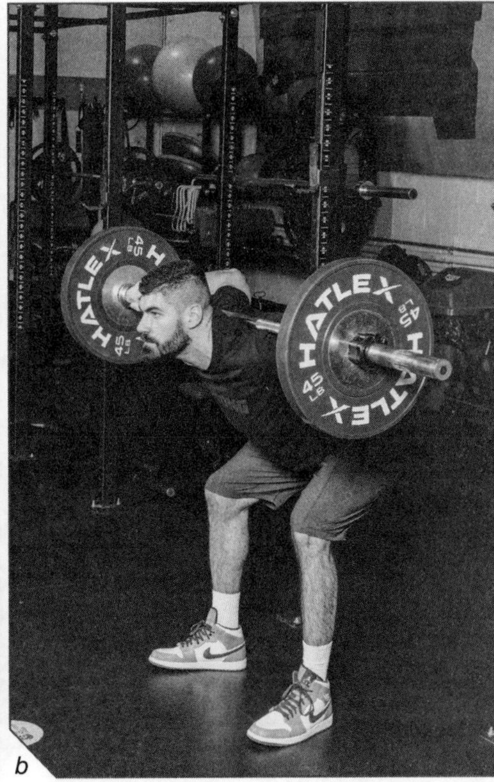

b

DEADLIFT ASSISTANCE EXERCISES

Pin Good Morning

This is my favorite variation of the good morning for several reasons. First, by setting the bar on a pin, you ensure that you are going to the correct torso angle on each rep. By beginning each rep from a dead-stop on the pin, you are also eliminating stretch reflex and developing better starting strength for this section of the lift. You are also eliminating the tendency of the spinal alignment to change during the reversal of the movement (often seen with heavy good mornings). Lastly, by starting each rep from the pin, you are able to ensure that you perform each rep with the correct alignment because you have the opportunity to fully reset each time.

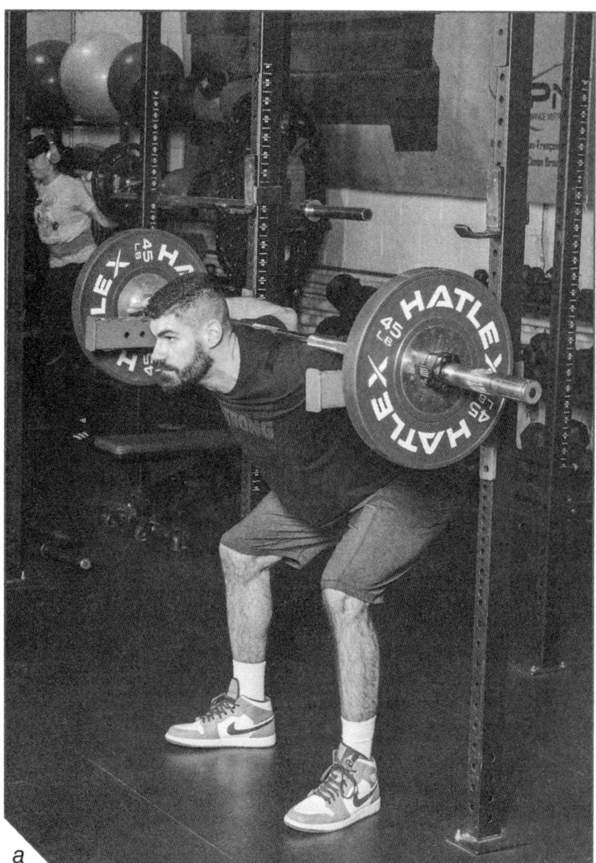

a

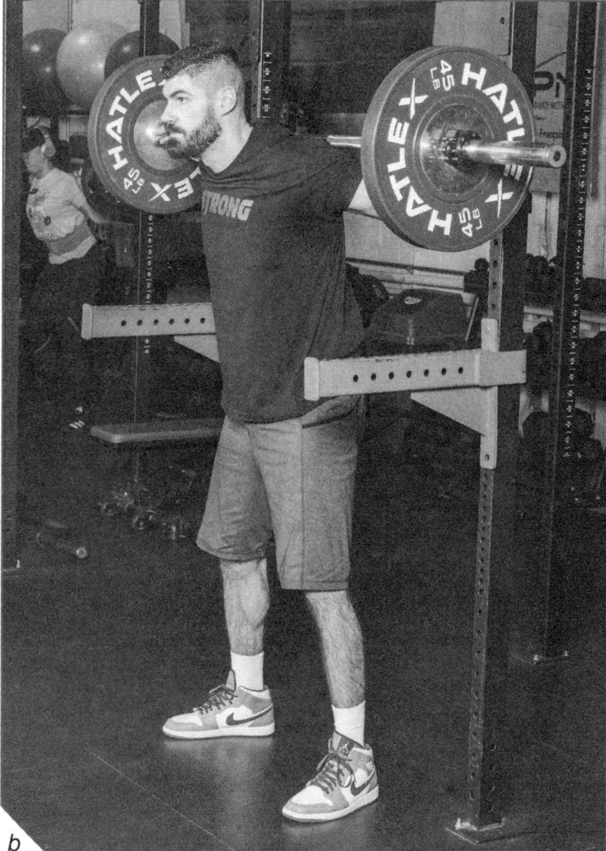

b

Seated Good Morning

This variation is very good for targeting the spinal erectors, the core, and the adductors to a greater degree because the hips are being fixed in place, meaning the prime movers can contribute less and provide less stability. This will mean that this variation can be loaded less than others, but this can be partly worked around by attaching forward bands to the bar to provide more resistance without increasing spinal loading and helping reduce the "dead zone" of little tension at the top of the lift.

DEADLIFT ASSISTANCE EXERCISES

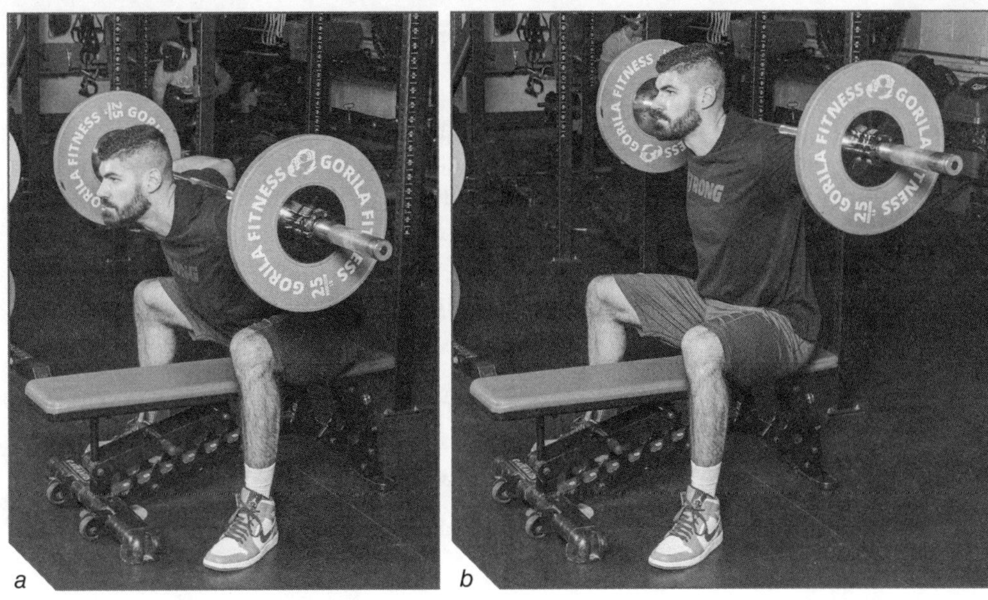

Zercher Good Morning

This is a great variation to start with if you are new to good mornings. The bar position means there is less shear stress on the spine, and it is much easier to dump the bar if you feel a rep going south. The lower loading also can make it more approachable. Zercher good mornings are not easy, however. The Zercher position brings with it a lot more loading on the abs and core and upper back; it also hinders your ability to breath (which is overrated anyway). Prepare to be humbled.

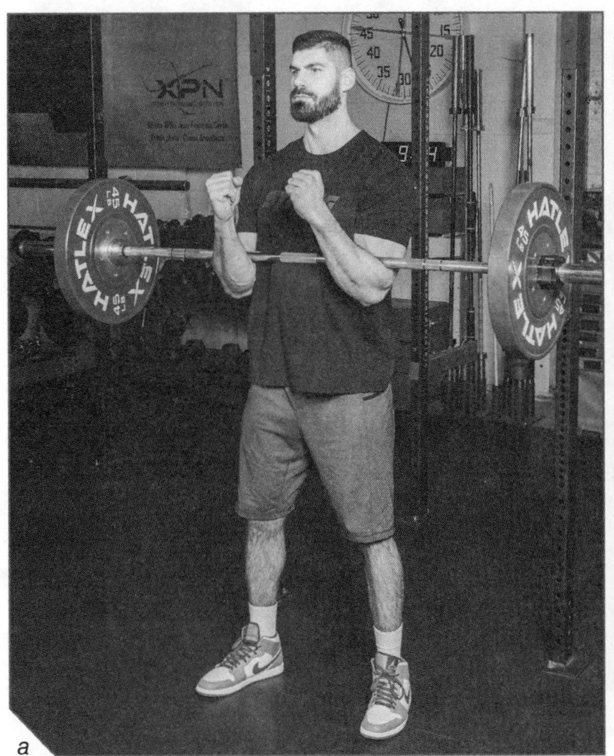

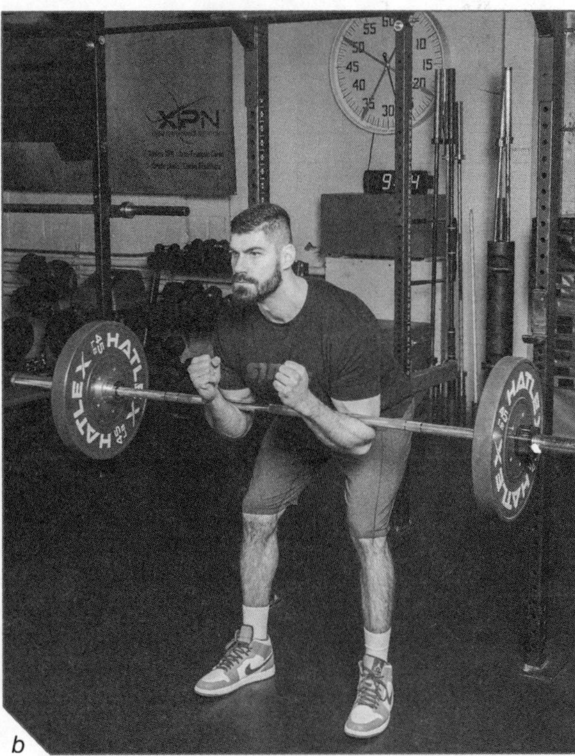

DEADLIFT ASSISTANCE EXERCISES

Floating Deadlift

The floating deadlift is performed by standing on something to elevate you an inch or two off the floor (as if you were doing a deficit deadlift), and the bar is then lifted to the top position. This is your start position. From here, the bar is lowered in the same manner as a normal deadlift until it is one to two inches from the floor (i.e., where the floor would be if you weren't standing on something). You then pause briefly before lifting back to the top.

The reason this is such a great deadlift builder is because it teaches you how to create maximal full-body tension in the start position of the lift. When done correctly, the bottom position of a floating deadlift is your start position for the full deadlift, meaning you learn to create enough tension to support the load of the bar where you normally don't have to (as the floor is kindly supporting the weight for you). This variation is fantastic for fixing all sticking points during phase I of the deadlift or just for someone who struggles maintaining correct positioning during phase I.

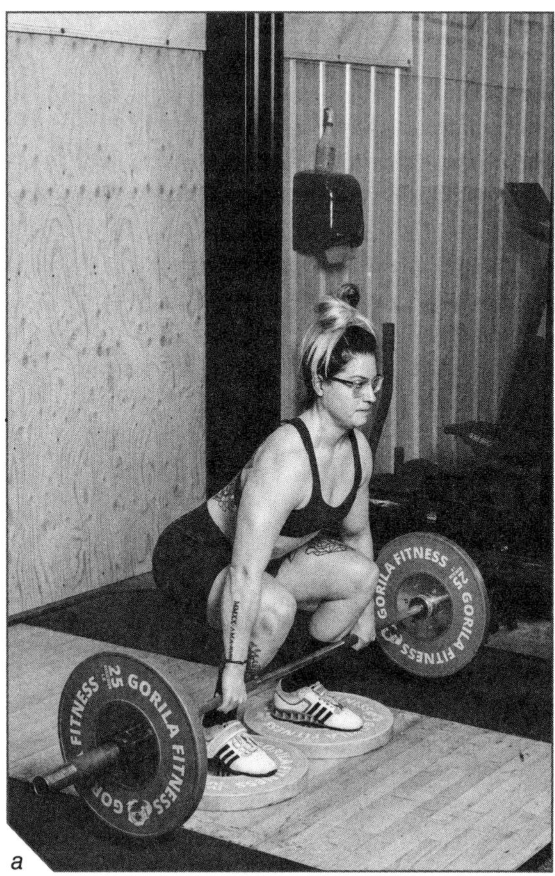

a

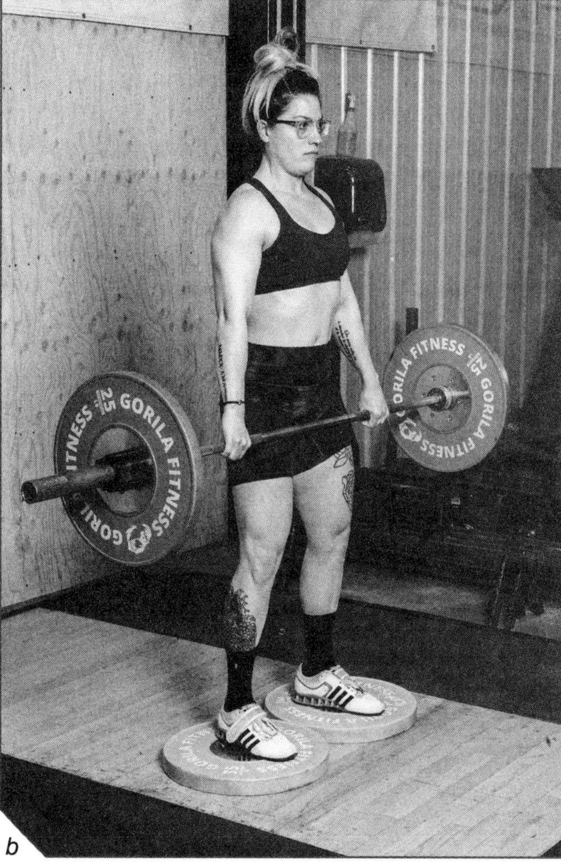

b

DEADLIFT ASSISTANCE EXERCISES

Shrugs

When done correctly, shrugs are a very effective way of strengthening the upper back's ability to maintain alignment during the deadlift. To correctly perform shrugs so that they carry over to your deadlift, perform them with a barbell to mimic the shoulder positioning of the deadlift and with the hips pushed back. From here, you want to start each rep from a stretched position, where you allow the bar to pull your shoulders forward as if you were pulled out of position by a heavy deadlift. Hold this stretched position for a second or two (to eliminate the stretch reflex) before shrugging up and backward to regain correct shoulder positioning. The goal here is not to shrug the shoulders up to the ears as high as possible but rather to regain the desired position for the deadlift (or perhaps a slightly over-retracted position). Remember, effective shrugs are all about retraction, not elevation, especially when you are looking for a carryover to the deadlift. Don't forget to hold the top position for a couple of seconds to increase time under tension before slowly lowering back down to the stretched position.

The thing to remember here is that the range of motion of shrugs is so small that if you don't perform them in this type of controlled manner and allow momentum to aid the lift, you won't accumulate enough time under tension to have a training effect. Plus, you are then training the upper back muscles in a manner that does not translate to the deadlift.

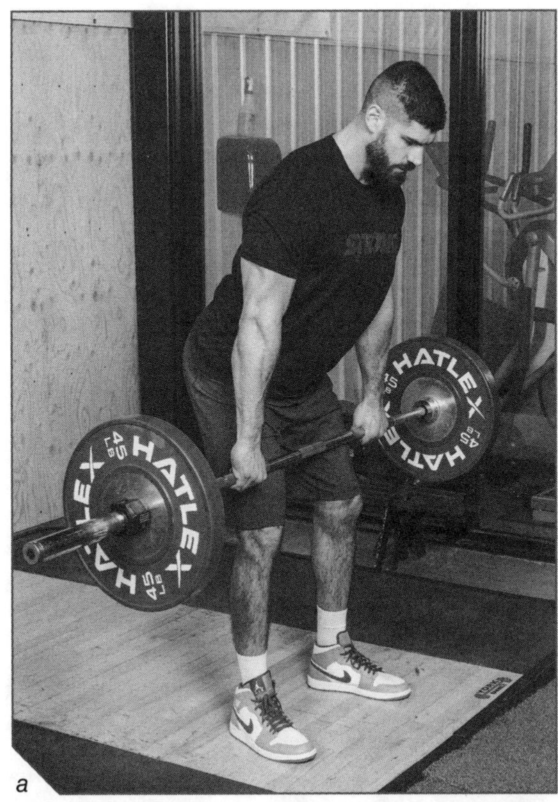

a

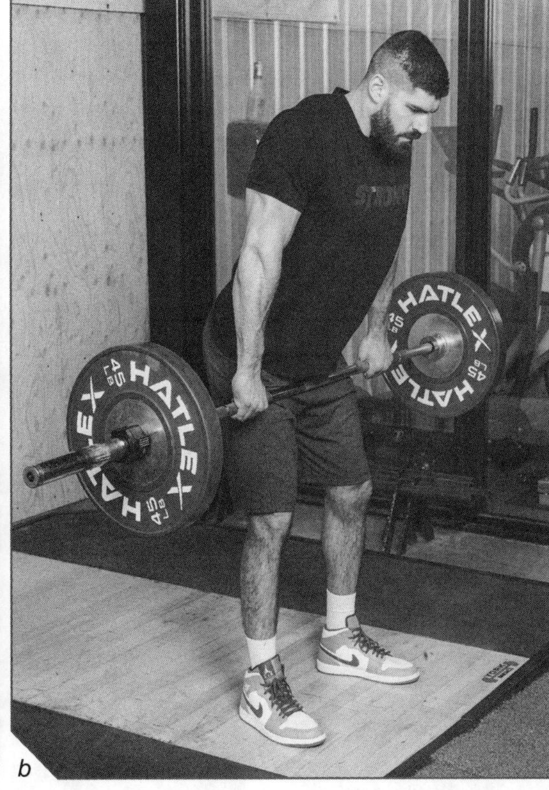

b

SQUAT ASSISTANCE EXERCISES

Front Squat

The front squat is performed with the bar held on the front side of the body (yes, I know, revolutionary) supported on the front delts. The front squat shifts the loading more to the anterior chain (quads, abs) as well as the upper back (because of the bar positioning). During a front squat, the torso will stay more upright due to a greater degree of knee flexion (and forward knee travel) and a lesser degree of hip flexion. The same ground rules still apply here as with the back squat, however. The bar should move in a vertical bar path directly over the midfoot at all times.

The front squat is the best leg strength builder for long-legged individuals and is a great choice for anyone whose leg strength is holding them back in the squat. It is also very useful for anyone who finds themselves getting "folded over" by heavier loads on the back squat due to the emphasis on upper back and ab strength created by the front rack position of the bar.

The front squat is ideally performed using a barbell in the front-rack position. If you struggle to achieve this positioning, then first try stretching your pec minors, lats, and forearms. If you still struggle to achieve a good elbow and upper arm position, then you can remove your little finger (or even little and ring finger) from underneath the bar to facilitate extra internal rotation. Failing that, the front squat can also be performed using a safety-squat bar held backward or using a front squat harness.

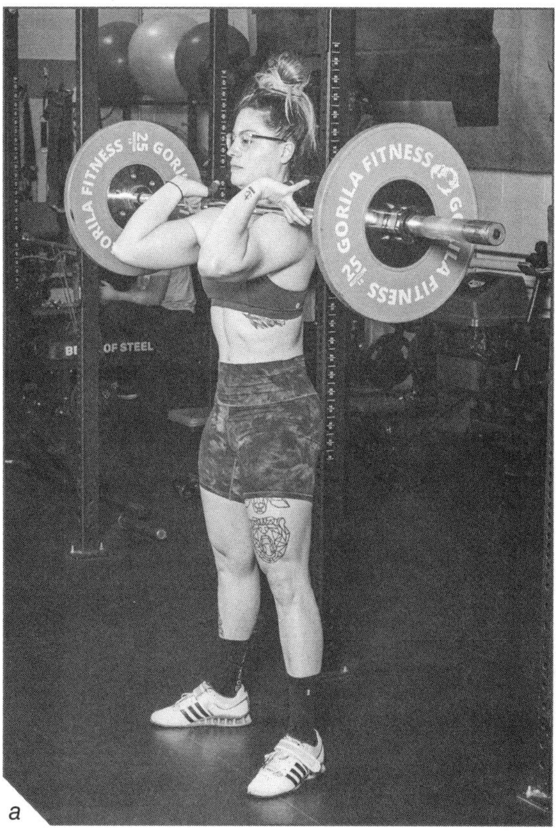

a

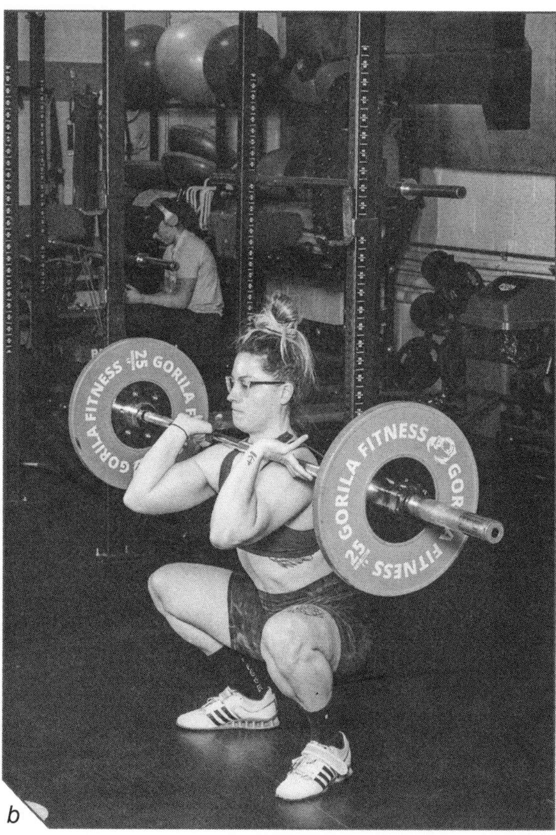

b

SQUAT ASSISTANCE EXERCISES

Zercher Squat

The Zercher squat provides similar benefits to the front squat because of the front-loaded nature of the lift. The Zercher squat, however, places more emphasis on the abdominals and upper back due to the bar positioning. Generally, most people Zercher squat less than they front squat, so it targets the legs a little less effectively (although this isn't the case for everyone). The Zercher squat is also more approachable for a lot of people because the bar position does not have the same mobility requirements as a front squat. The Zercher squat tends to punish you harder for tipping forward since the bar drifts away from the body and is very hard to rescue. So, this can be a very good option if you often find yourself turning your squat in to a good-morning (hips shooting up out of the bottom of the squat). The Zercher squat also provides a good stimulus for the biceps, making it the single most important squat variation in the universe.

The Zercher squat can be done with two different grips: hands apart or hands clenched together. The hands apart option makes the arms less stable and requires more work from the upper back to keep the bar pulled into the body. Hands together makes the bar position more stable, allowing more load to be used, meaning the legs and abs are worked harder.

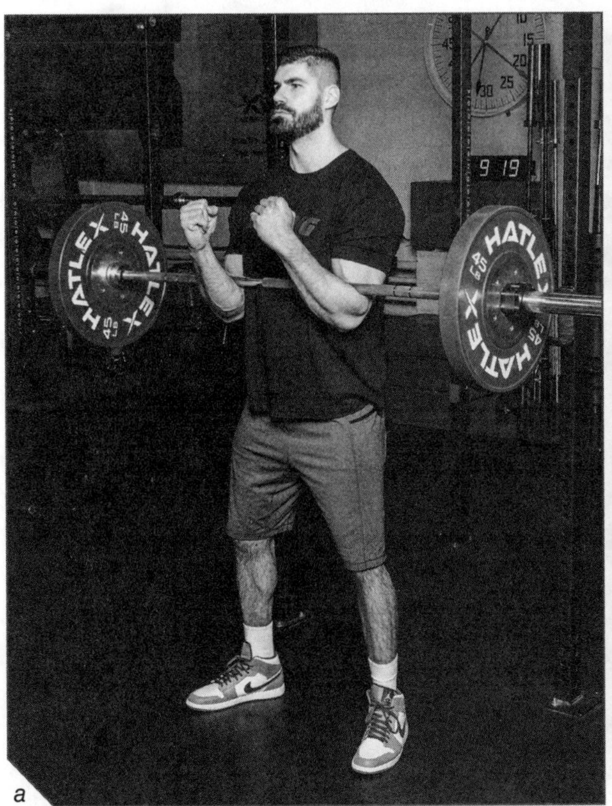

a

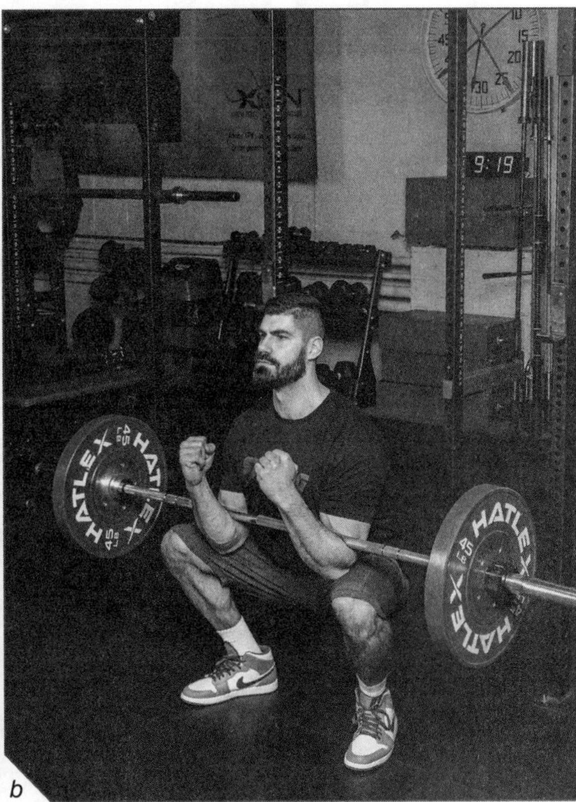

b

SQUAT ASSISTANCE EXERCISES

Squat or Front Squat with Heels Elevated

Elevating the heels is a great test of whether ankle mobility is holding back a lifter's squat. If a lifter tends to fold forward from the hip toward the bottom of the squat (usually struggling to hit depth in the process), it is often because the calves are restricting the required forward knee travel. If elevating the heels helps, then ankle mobility needs to be improved.

Elevating the heels will lead to a higher degree of forward knee travel, which, as discussed previously, will mean less hip flexion and more anterior loading. This can be a great tool for increasing the quad loading of your squat without altering the mechanics of the lift too much.

Elevating the heels can also allow lifters to achieve a greater depth in the squat, so it can be useful for improving strength out of the hole and confidence with regards to going to depth. The heels can be elevated by wearing Olympic-style lifting shoes, using a form of squat wedge or ramp, or using the good old method of sticking some (stable and flat) plates on the floor to put your heels on.

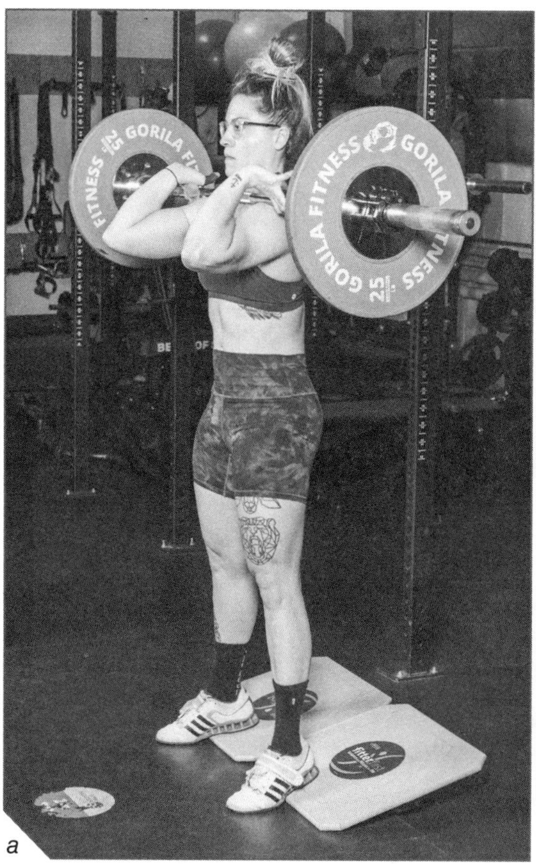

a

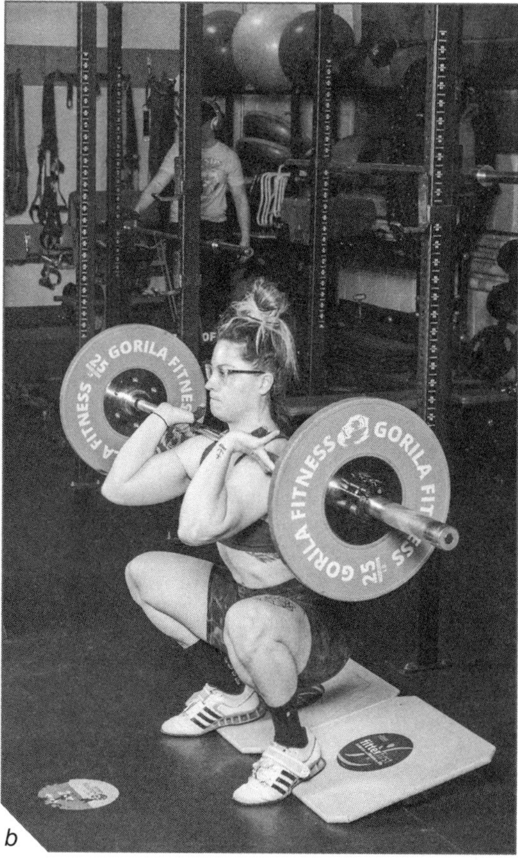

b

DEADLIFT AND SQUAT ASSISTANCE EXERCISES

In theory, most assistance exercises that help you squat will be somewhat helpful in improving your deadlift, and vice versa.

Of course, exercises like good mornings and Romanian deadlifts (as examples) will be helpful for *both* the squat and deadlift, especially if you use a low-bar powerlifting style of squatting. However, there are exercises that will be equally as effective for the squat as for the deadlift. These are heavy loaded carries, and they are the best movements to improve your capacity to stay tight under a heavy load and are especially effective at strengthening the core, which is so important on the squat and deadlift.

When it comes to loaded carries, I like to use the formula 10 meters (33 feet) = 1 repetition. If you are using them to build strength, 10 to 50 meters (33 to 164 feet) are best (1 to 5 reps); for size, 60 to 100 meters (197 to 328 feet) are recommended (6 to 10 reps); and for endurance, you can go up to 200 meters (656 feet).

Farmer's Walk

The farmer's walk is likely the first weight-training exercise ever invented. After all, people were carrying stuff thousands of years before the first gym even existed! This primitive form of resistance training is also one of the best and most useful exercises you can do: It dramatically strengthens your core and your capacity to keep your body tensed, preventing strength leaks. It does wonders for your grip strength. It is also very effective to build the traps and even the deltoids, believe it or not (the delts are used to fight the tendency of the weights to move around). It also has some effects on the calves, upper arms, and lower body.

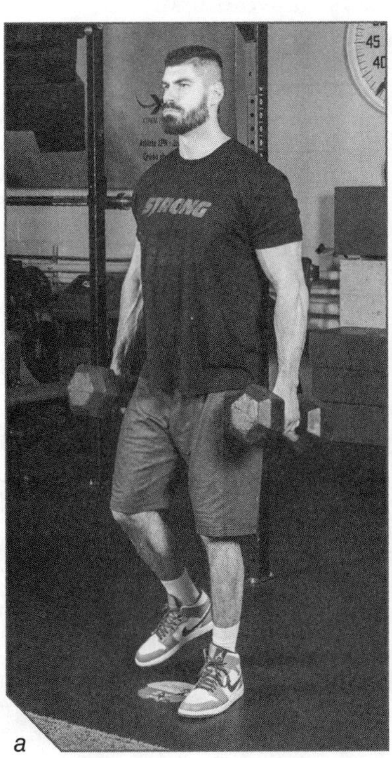

a

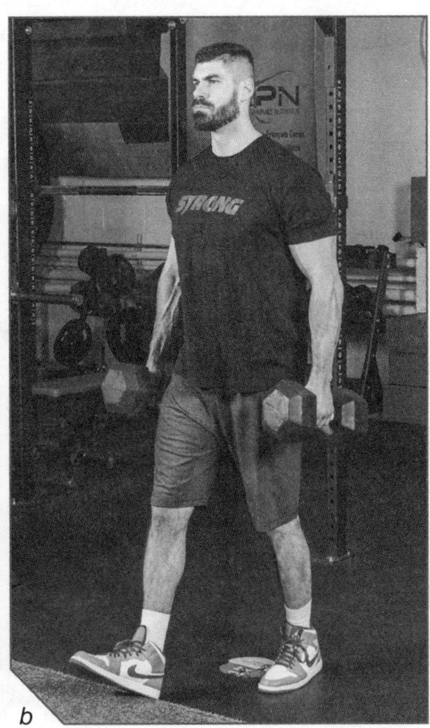

b

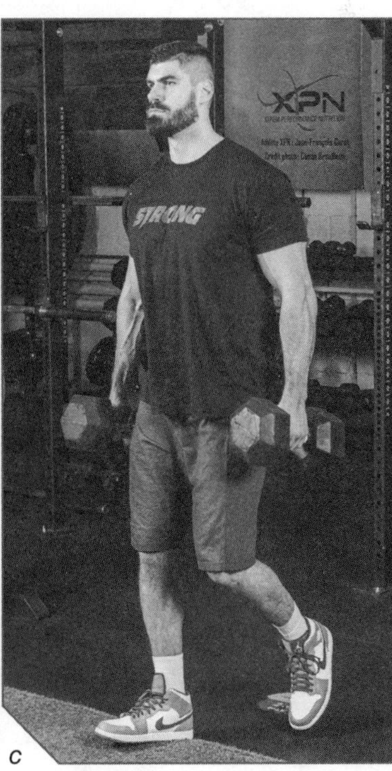

c

DEADLIFT AND SQUAT ASSISTANCE EXERCISES

You can do the farmer's walk with several implements: specific farmer's walk handles, dumbbells, a pair of regular bars, kettlebells, a wheelbarrow, or a trap bar. Generally speaking, the more unstable an implement is, the more the deltoids and core will get worked, and the more stable they are, the greater the impact on the traps, grip, and lower body (because you can use more weight). In order of stability, from the least to the most stable, you can use two regular bars, farmer's walk handles, a wheelbarrow, kettlebells, dumbbells, and a trap bar.

When using the farmer's walk as a training exercise, it is important to focus on maintaining a solid body position and good overall tightness. It is best to use a regular walking speed instead of trying to cover the distance fast. Strongmen who compete in that movement will obviously make modifications to go as fast as possible. In a way, it's like a strict pull-up versus a kipping pull-up: the latter is more effective to get better numbers, but the former is more effective at building muscle strength and size.

Zercher Carries

This is a second form of loaded carry that is highly effective to improve any lift requiring a high level of overall tightness. This exercise consists of carrying an implement in the crooks of the elbows. It could be a bar, a dumbbell (placed sideways), a heavy bag, a strongman log, or really any object that you can carry in your arms. It might actually be superior to the farmer's walk for core work and also involves the upper arm to a greater extent.

The key for the Zercher carry to be optimally productive is to avoid leaning back when you do it. This will decrease core work and could lead to lower back issues. Stay as upright as possible.

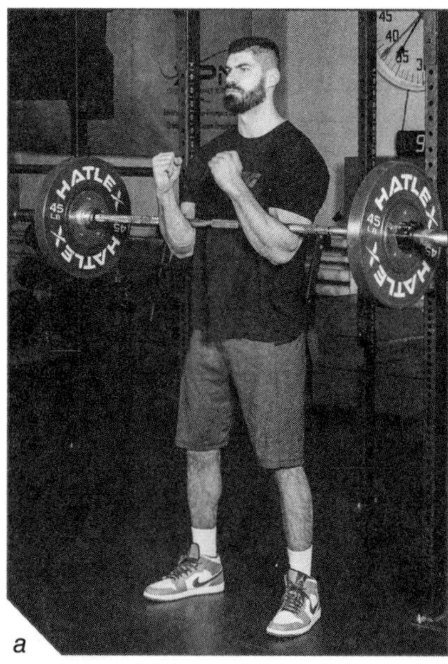
a

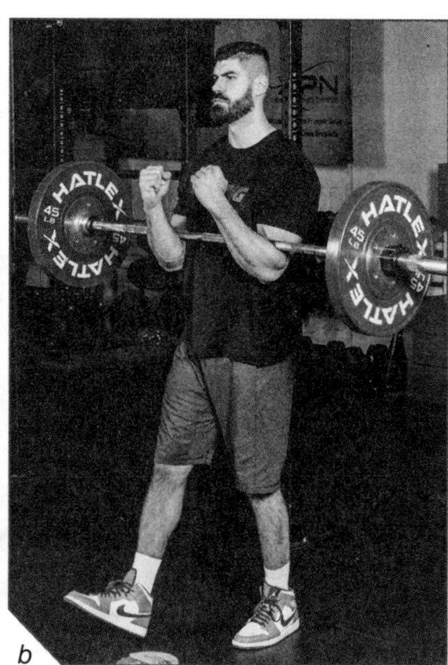
b

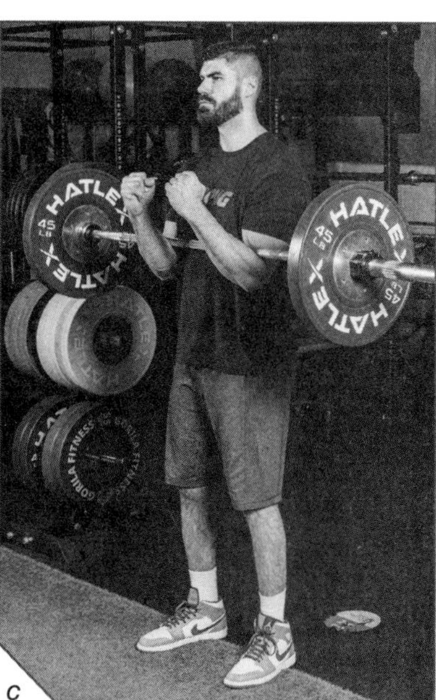
c

BENCH PRESS ASSISTANCE EXERCISES

Floor Press

For the best carryover, the floor press should be performed with the same grip and the same thoracic arch and upper back setup that you would use for the bench press. The overall arch will be less pronounced when lying on the floor, but you can still get extra stability from the legs by setting up with the knees at 90 degrees and the feet flat on the floor (as opposed to out straight). The bar path and joint alignment should be the same as your bench press until the back of the arms come into contact with the floor. At this point, pause on the floor for a second to avoid bouncing the arm off the floor, which is (a) bad for your elbows and (b) likely to throw off your bar path.

The part of the lift the floor press targets will depend to a degree on the lifter. Those with very short forearms and big rib cages can sometimes still get the bar to the chest during a floor press, whereas longer-armed lifters may only come down to around the midpoint. Therefore, whatever sticking point the floor press will target will depend on your own levers. Regardless, this exercise is a great pressing movement for improving raw pressing power because it removes the aid of leg drive as well as the ability to bounce the bar off the chest.

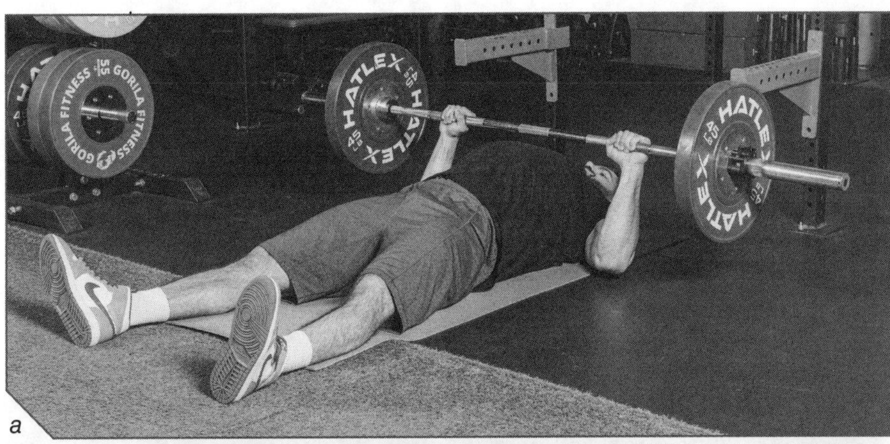

a

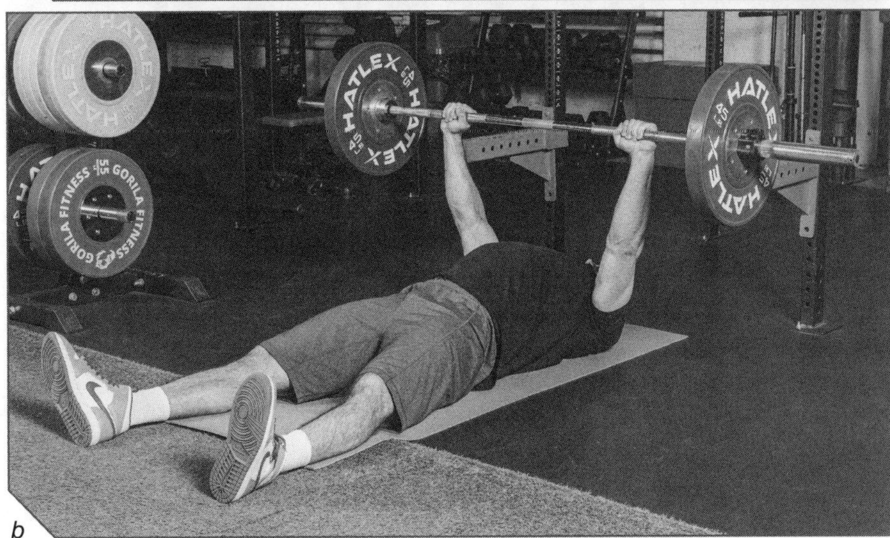

b

BENCH PRESS ASSISTANCE EXERCISES

Close-Grip Bench Press

Setting up for a close-grip bench press should be the exact same as your regular bench press with the only change being the grip width. You should bring your grip in anywhere from a half to one full hand width on each side. Anything less than this and the change in motor recruitment isn't significant enough to improve anything. Any more than this and you can take the movement pattern too far away from the main lift for it to effectively carry over. Generally, the more experienced the lifter and the more stable their technique, the bigger the difference they can have between their grips and still get a carryover.

The closer grip will mean the bar touches lower down on the torso with the elbows in closer to the sides of the body. This increases the horizontal and vertical travel distance of the bar and the degree of flexion in the elbow and the shoulder. The main result is an increase in tricep loading, but this grip also increases the work required from the front delts. As such, the close-grip bench is a good option for improving the midrange and top end of the bench press.

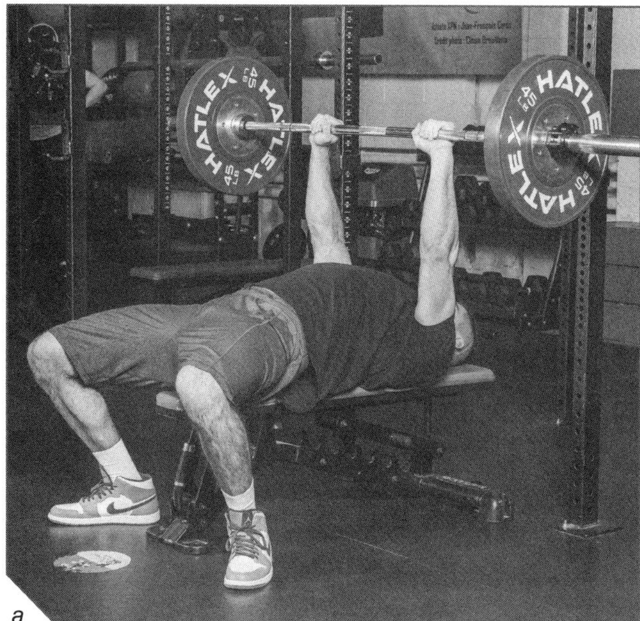

a

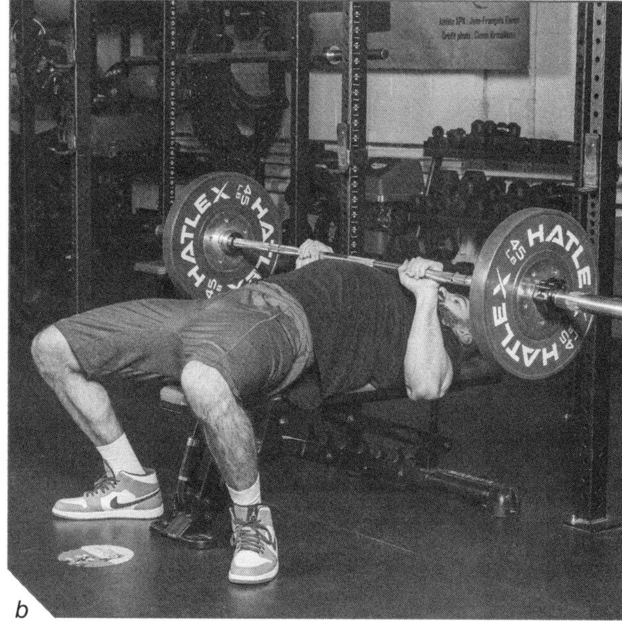

b

BENCH PRESS ASSISTANCE EXERCISES

Spoto Press

This is another great option for building raw pressing strength. In a Spoto press, everything should be the same as your regular bench press (e.g., grip, setup, bar path); the only difference will be that the bar stops one-half to one inch above the chest. Briefly pause in this position before driving back, again in the same manner as you would for a regular bench press.

The Spoto press improves just about all elements of the bottom end of the bench press. Just like the floor press, the Spoto press removes the leg drive and any potential bouncing and stretch reflex element of the lift. The pause just off the chest improves upper back stability and positioning (it's common to see lifters lose eccentric control of the lift close to the chest). Pressing from a dead-stop just above the chest also improves starting strength and fiber recruitment in the bottom range of the press, similar to a pin press. So, the Spoto press is one of the best options for improving the bottom range of the bench press, especially in lifters who are overly reliant on leg drive and momentum.

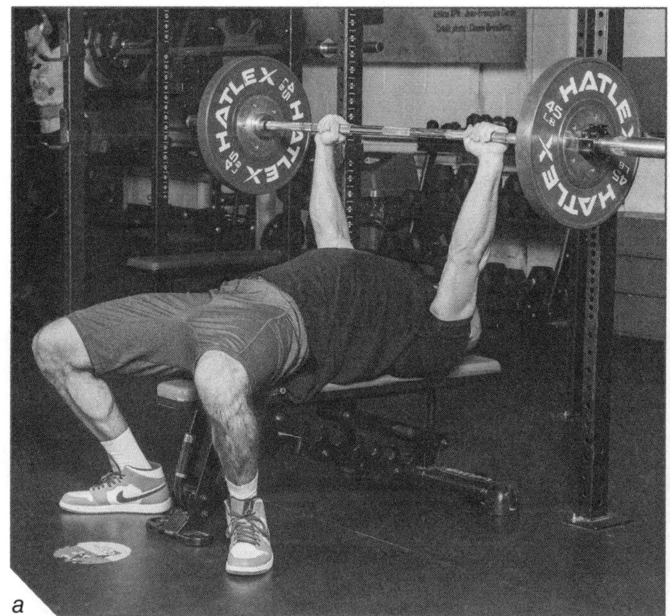

a

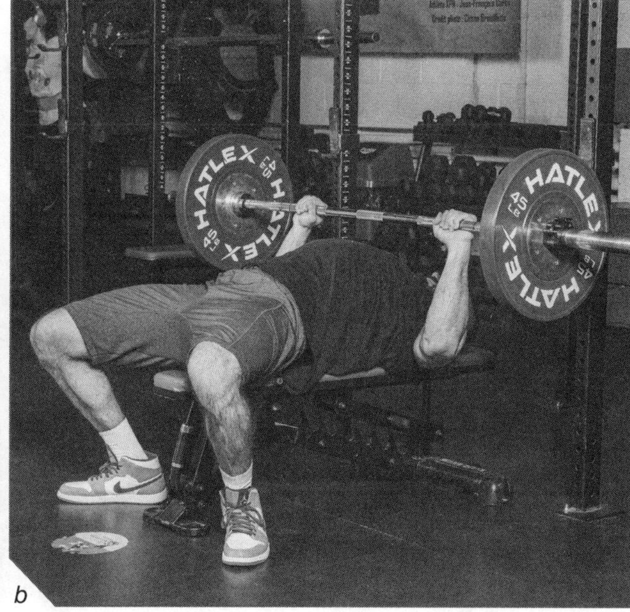

b

BENCH PRESS ASSISTANCE EXERCISES

Incline Bench Press

In terms of front delt loading and recruitment, the incline bench press is pretty much the king. It involves just as much front delt recruitment as a military press but can be loaded significantly heavier, resulting in greater stimulation. This exercise is best used for strengthening the midrange of the bench press, which is a common sticking point due to the prime mover transitioning from being the pecs to the front delts and triceps.

For improving the bench press, you want to use an incline of 15 to 30 degrees. Any more than this and you will make it too shoulder-dominant and change the recruitment pattern to a degree that it will not carry over as well. You should set up using the same thoracic arch as you do on the regular bench. If you set your feet in the same manner, you can still get decent leg drive on an incline bench. During an incline bench exercise, there is a greater degree of shoulder flexion owing to the torso angle (hence the front delt recruitment), and the bar will touch higher up the torso compared with a regular bench press (around or above the nipple line for most lifters).

The bar path on an incline bench has less horizontal travel, so it is more of a vertical line of travel. There is still a horizontal component, but it is reduced because the bar is touching higher up the torso. So, there should be a slight curve to the bar path on the eccentric and concentric but notably less than that of a regular bench press.

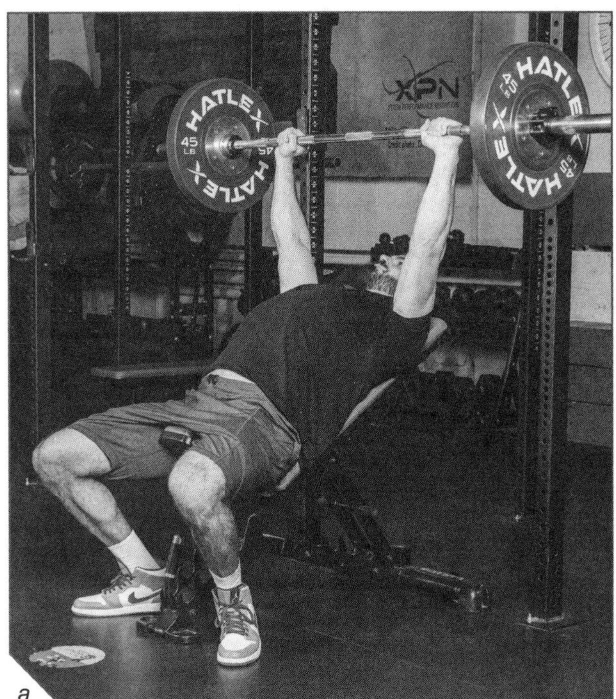

a

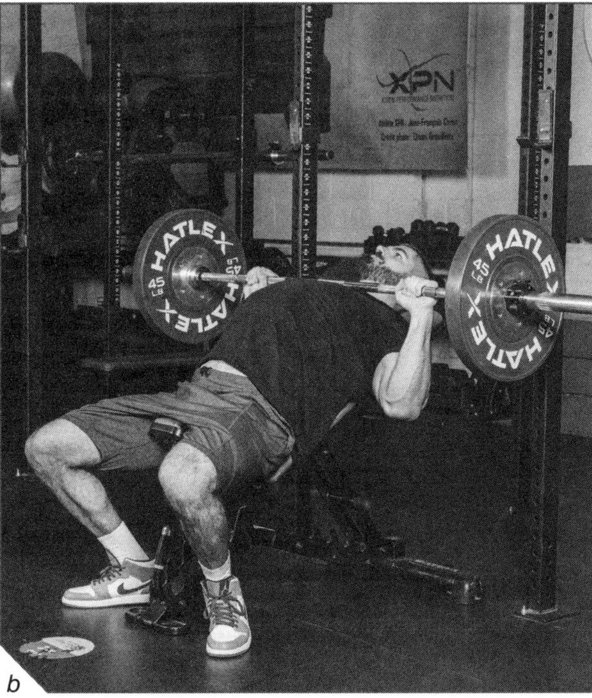

b

BENCH PRESS ASSISTANCE EXERCISES

Decline Bench Press

The decline bench press is all about strengthening the pecs and, in turn, the bottom range of the bench press. Once again, the upper back and grip should be set the same as your regular bench press. The decline torso angle means the bar will touch lower down on the torso (often around the lower ribs and upper stomach), and the bar path will be closer to vertical. This more vertical bar path, along with the mechanically advantageous position the pecs are placed in, means that you can (generally) move more load on a decline bench press even though the front delts are able to contribute less to the lift.

For that reason, the decline bench press can also work as a nice overload tool for the bench press as well as strengthening the bottom portion of the lift. Yes, mechanically speaking, the lift is quite different from the bench press, but the act of having the heavier loading in your hands is still going to have a positive impact on the nervous system, desensitizing the Golgi tendon organs (GTOs) and increasing confidence.

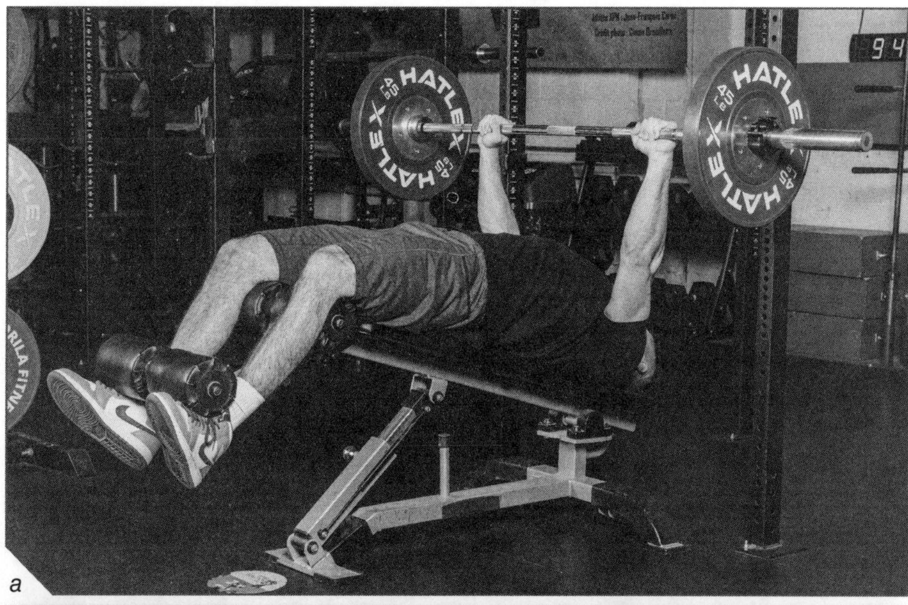

a

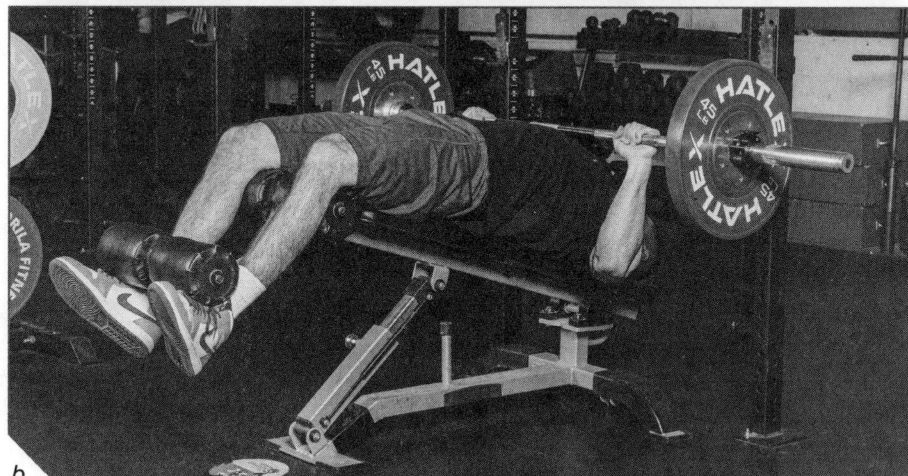
b

BENCH PRESS ASSISTANCE EXERCISES

Dips

This exercise is the original chest builder. Dips were regarded for a long time as *the* chest exercise. Dips are, in essence, an extreme decline press when you look at the arm angle relative to the torso. However, because of the plane of motion of the upper arm relative to the body, dips are actually a better front delt exercise than a pec exercise. Do they recruit the pecs? Yes, and in a stretched position also, which is great. But the workload is actually higher on the front delts than pecs. As a result, dips are decent for improving the bottom end strength of the bench press (due to the loading of the pecs in a stretched position), but they are even better for strengthening the midrange.

Setting up for dips is often done completely wrong. First, the body should be set with a slight forward lean at the hips and with the legs also placed slightly in front of the body while locked straight (imagine setting your body in a banana shape). This slight forward torso lean better places the emphasis on the pecs; more importantly, it puts the shoulders in a much better position to move freely throughout the lift. The shoulders should be set in a slightly shrugged and retracted position, which will best centrate the shoulder joint. The upper arm and elbows should be set 30 to 45 degrees away from the torso.

During the lift, the torso angle, relative to the floor, should remain constant. Throughout the lowering phase, the shoulders will retract and shrug up slightly (which is why it is important to not start in a fully retracted position) toward the bottom position, which would ideally be with the shoulder joint parallel with, or below, the elbow joint.

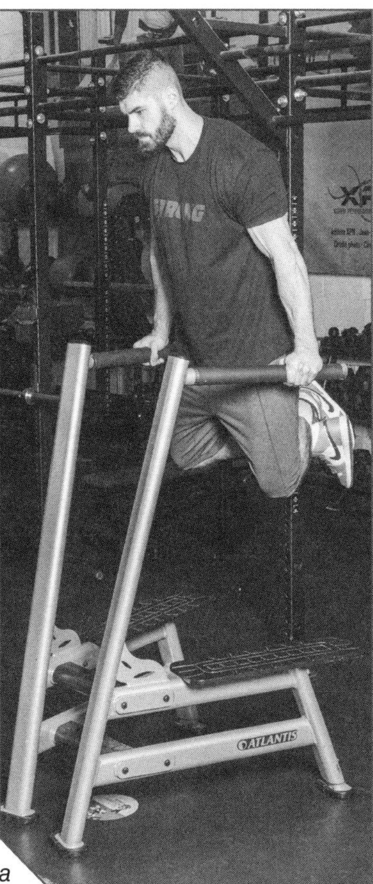

a

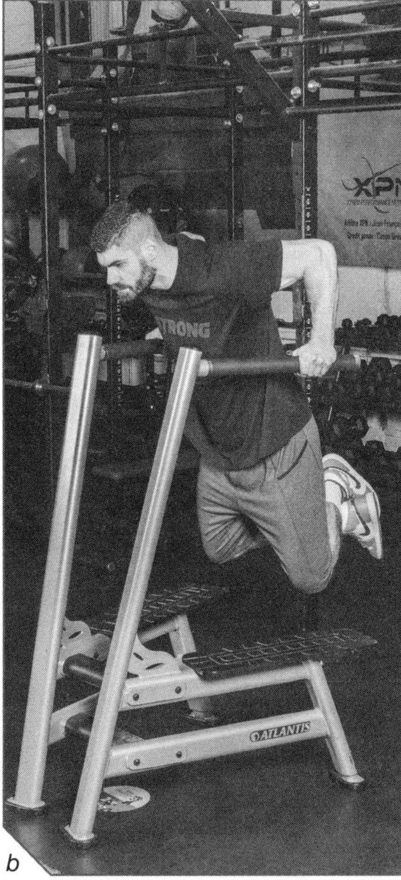

b

MILITARY PRESS ASSISTANCE EXERCISES

Overhead Press Variations

These three variations are all aimed at improving core and postural strength. All three postures will place emphasis on maintaining proper bracing and alignment during the lift and will reduce the ability to lean back throughout the lift. By stopping you from leaning back, these variations can also improve your shoulder and starting strength. In terms of the pressing mechanics, however, everything else should remain the same as your normal press.

In ascending order, in terms of emphasis on core and postural strength, they would be arranged: Tall-kneeling > Z-press > Half-kneeling. Likewise, the ability to load these movements would increase throughout that sequence. So, which posture you would choose would simply depend on how weak your core is or how much you need to improve your postural strength. These variations are good choices if you struggle with the bottom portion of the lift, especially if you lean back excessively when initiating the movement.

Tall-Kneeling Overhead Press

Tall-kneeling posture refers to you kneeling down on both knees with your hips stacked under your rib cage. Basically, think about being as tall as you can, but while on your knees. This posture is in fact more difficult than sitting on the floor because the bar (and your center of gravity) is higher from the floor, making it more unstable.

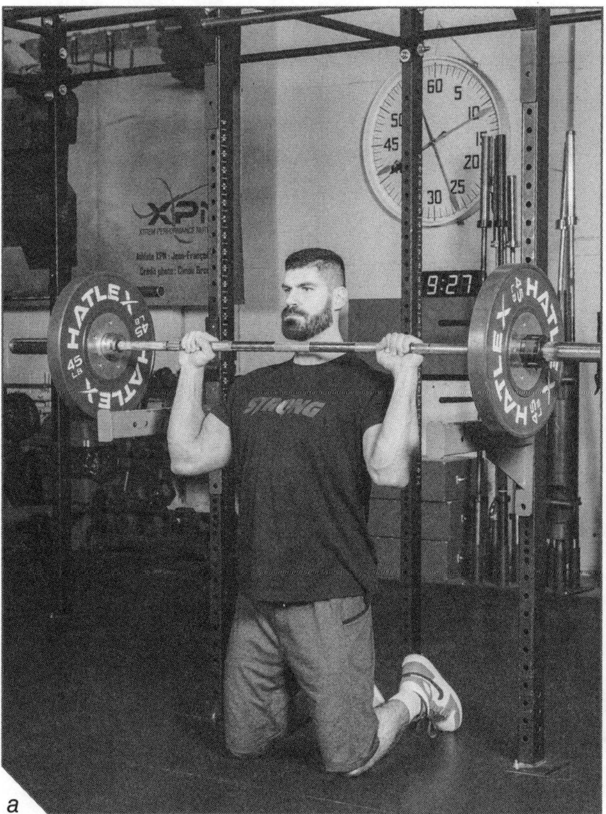

a

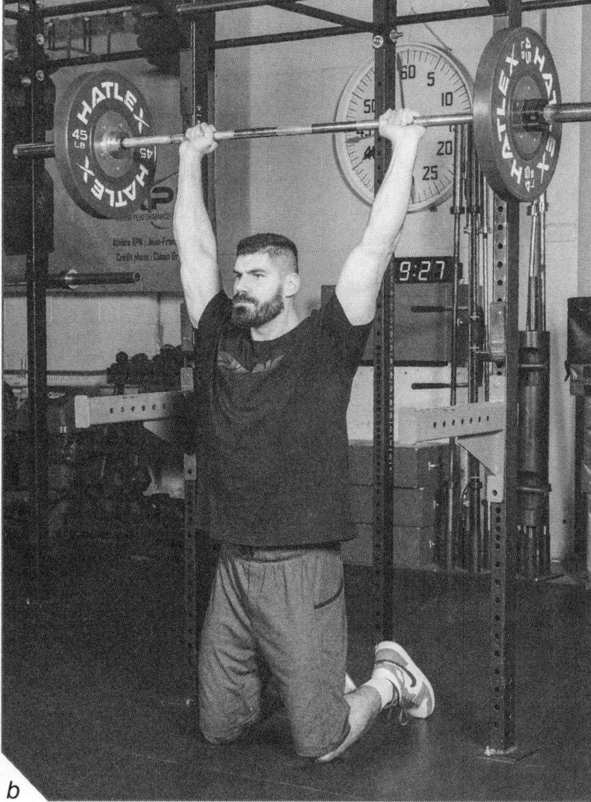

b

MILITARY PRESS ASSISTANCE EXERCISES

Z-Press

A Z-press, or Savickas press, on the other hand, is performed while you sit on the floor with your legs out straight in front of you. It is important that the legs are straight and that your feet are not placed against anything for artificial support. Just like the tall-kneeling press, this movement is great at placing demands on the core by reducing your ability to compensate through body movement. If you go into lumbar extension and lean backward, then you get punished by losing your balance backward. So, this movement teaches the lifter to stay neutral and to keep weight on their abs.

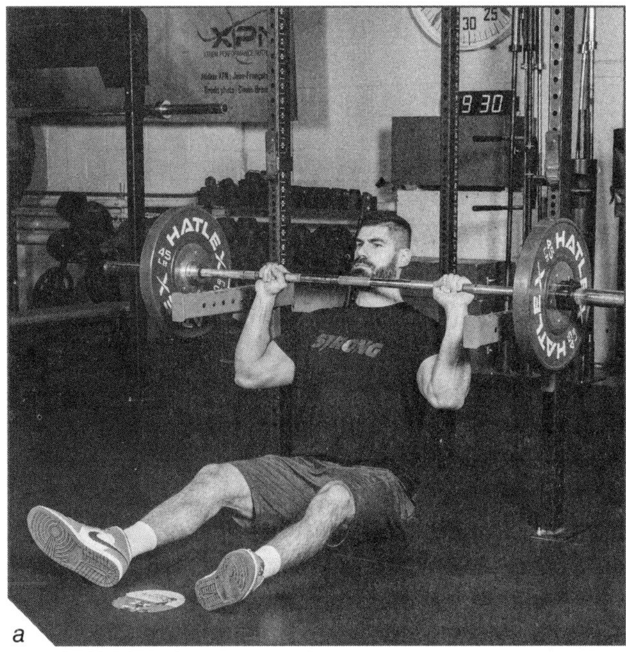

a

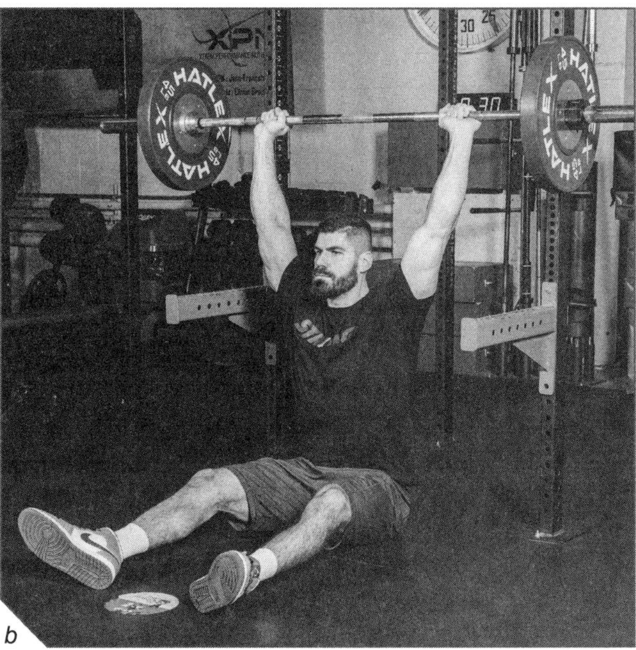

b

MILITARY PRESS ASSISTANCE EXERCISES

Half-Kneeling Overhead Press

The half-kneeling posture refers to being on your knees but having one leg out in front and one behind (almost like you got to the bottom of a split squat but then rested on the floor). Because of the larger base of support, this is the most stable of the three overhead press variations, which makes it a good choice for someone new to these exercises. It is also a good choice for those inexperienced with these variations because the half-kneeling posture in fact makes it quite difficult to go into extension (due to the hip position caused by having one leg in front and one behind). So, it actually helps lifters to stay in neutral when they may normally fall into extension.

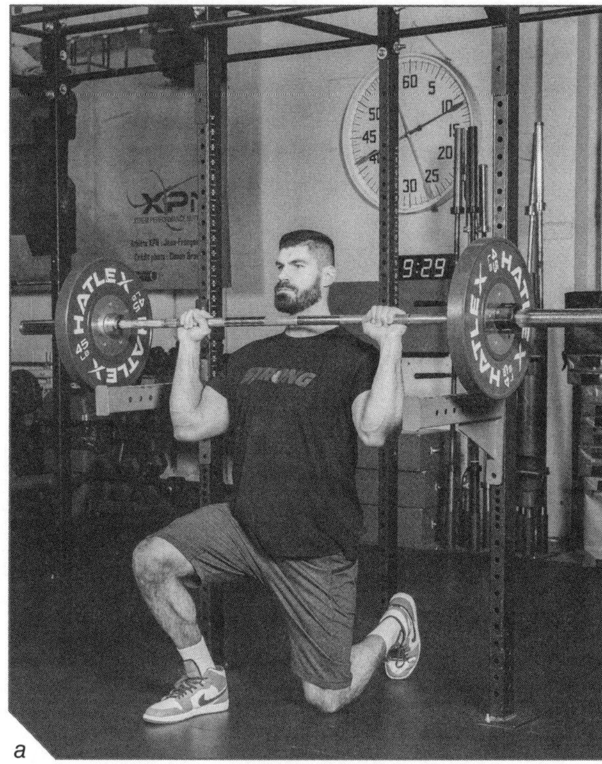

a

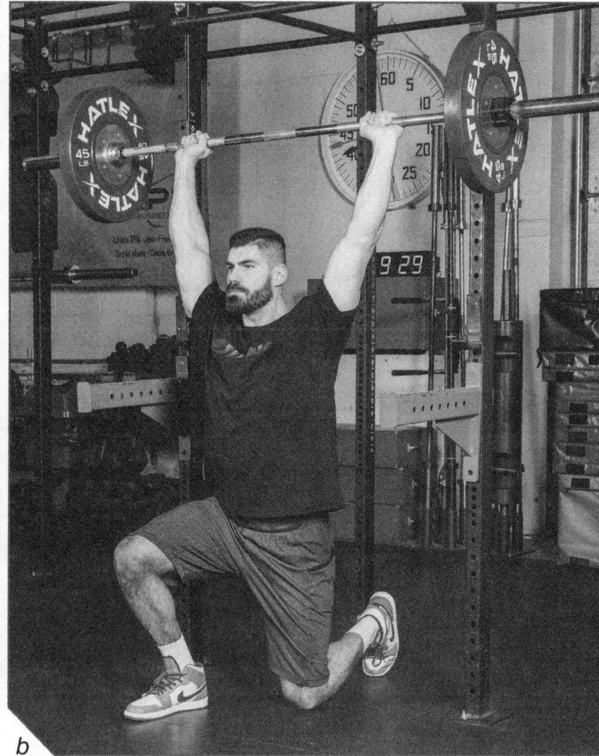

b

MILITARY PRESS ASSISTANCE EXERCISES

Push Press

The push press is simply a press in which you dip through the hip and knee joint and drive through the legs to initiate the lift. This leg drive gives a lot of momentum during the (more difficult) bottom half of the lift. This allows more load to be used and places a large workload on the triceps to lock out the lift once the momentum from the leg drive has run out. As such, the push press offers many potential benefits when it comes to improving the press: It acts as an overload exercise (e.g., improving nervous system firing, desensitizing GTOs), increases demand on the triceps (e.g., improving lockout strength in the press), and also places great stability demand on the upper back and core because of the greater load. What's not to like, right?

You can either set up for the push press using the same grip and rack position as your press (less to think about, closer to press mechanics), or you can use a full clean and front-rack position, which allows a much better transfer of force from the lower body. Whenever possible, I favor the proper front-rack position because it allows more load to be used, which amplifies all the benefits of this exercise. Other than this, the pressing mechanics are the same as for the regular press.

The dip for the push press should be just that—a dip, not a squat. Think as if you were going to do a max effort vertical jump on the spot. This is the height you dip to since it is the height that allows you to maximize upward momentum. If you perform your press with a very narrow stance, then you may want to widen it for the push press so that you do not tip forward onto your toes during the dip. The jump phase should involve proper triple extension, with the heels being slammed back down to the floor as soon as this is achieved to regain balance as quickly as possible.

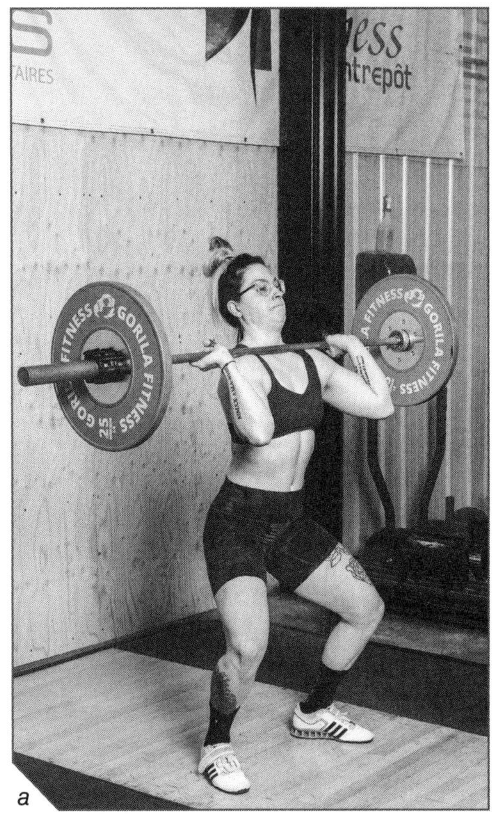

a

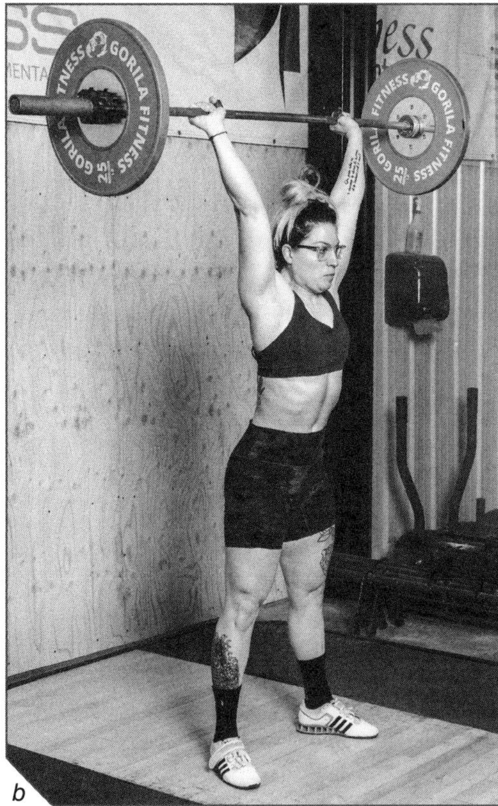

b

MILITARY PRESS ASSISTANCE EXERCISES

High-Incline Bench Press

I have already discussed the benefits of incline pressing in the section on bench press assistance exercises. Yet, when trying to improve the press, we use an even higher incline (45 to 60 degrees) to further increase front delt recruitment and better mimic the bar path of the press (a 60-degree incline press has an almost vertical bar path). Improving front delt strength (especially at high angles of shoulder extension) is a great way of improving bottom half strength in the press. In addition, here the incline press also acts as an overload exercise because of the greater loads being used.

Unlike with shallower incline presses, when using inclines of 45 to 60 degrees, I recommend you stop short of going to the chest. In fact, since we are talking about improving the press here, I like to see the bar lowered so that it is level with the same part of the body that the bar is at the bottom of your press. To further increase the carryover to the press, it is beneficial to use the same grip as your press. Yes, a wider grip would facilitate more load, but if it doesn't carry over to the main lift, then it defeats the purpose of being used as an assistance exercise.

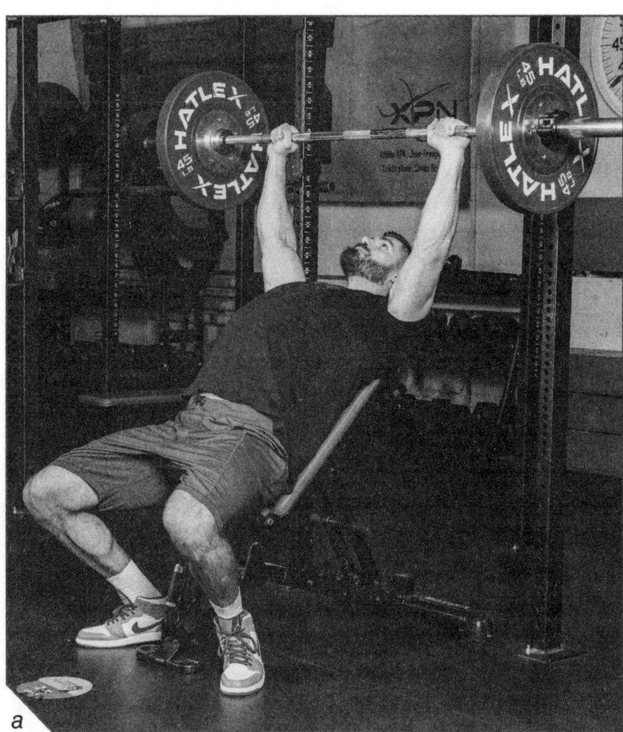

a

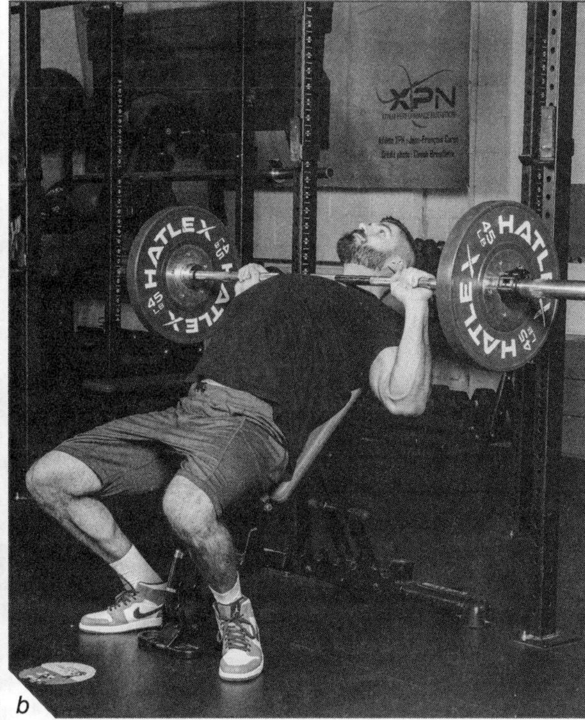

b

MILITARY PRESS ASSISTANCE EXERCISES

Bradford Press

This is an old-school shoulder builder that was really popular until behind-the-neck presses started being touted as the work of the devil that will tear your rotator cuff instantly. During a Bradford press, the bar is pressed up to just above forehead level (think back to phase I of the military press; see chapter 6); at this point, the elbows flare and the bar is moved backward over the head and then lowered behind the head. This movement is then reversed to end up back at the same start position that you use for your regular press.

What this movement does (other than illustrating you have acceptable shoulder mobility) is target the entire shoulder (not just the front delts) and keeps it under constant tension throughout the lift. From a hypertrophy perspective, this gives the Bradford press an advantage over the military press since the tension is significantly reduced after phase I is completed. So, this is a great shoulder builder all round, and bigger, stronger delts are going to lead to a bigger press. Furthermore, by targeting the lateral and rear heads of the shoulder, the Bedford press can help keep your shoulders balanced and healthy (yes, it can improve shoulder health rather than destroy it, believe it or not).

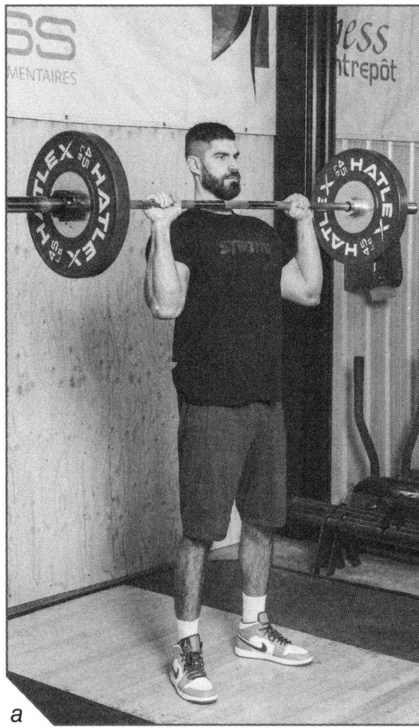

a

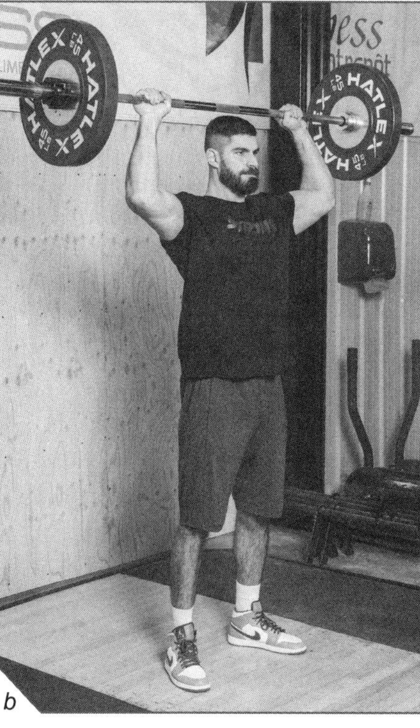

b

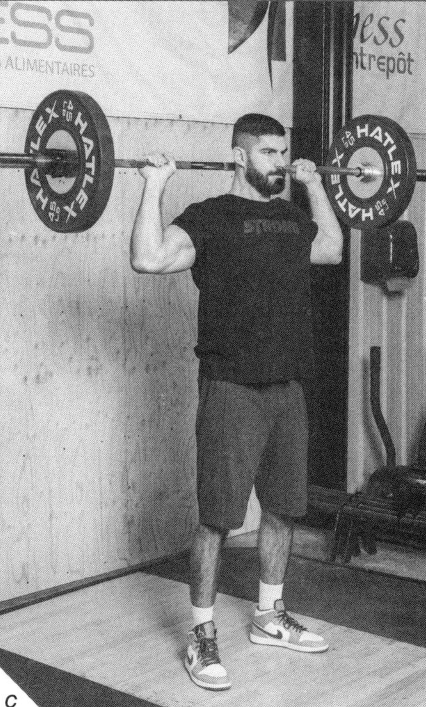

c

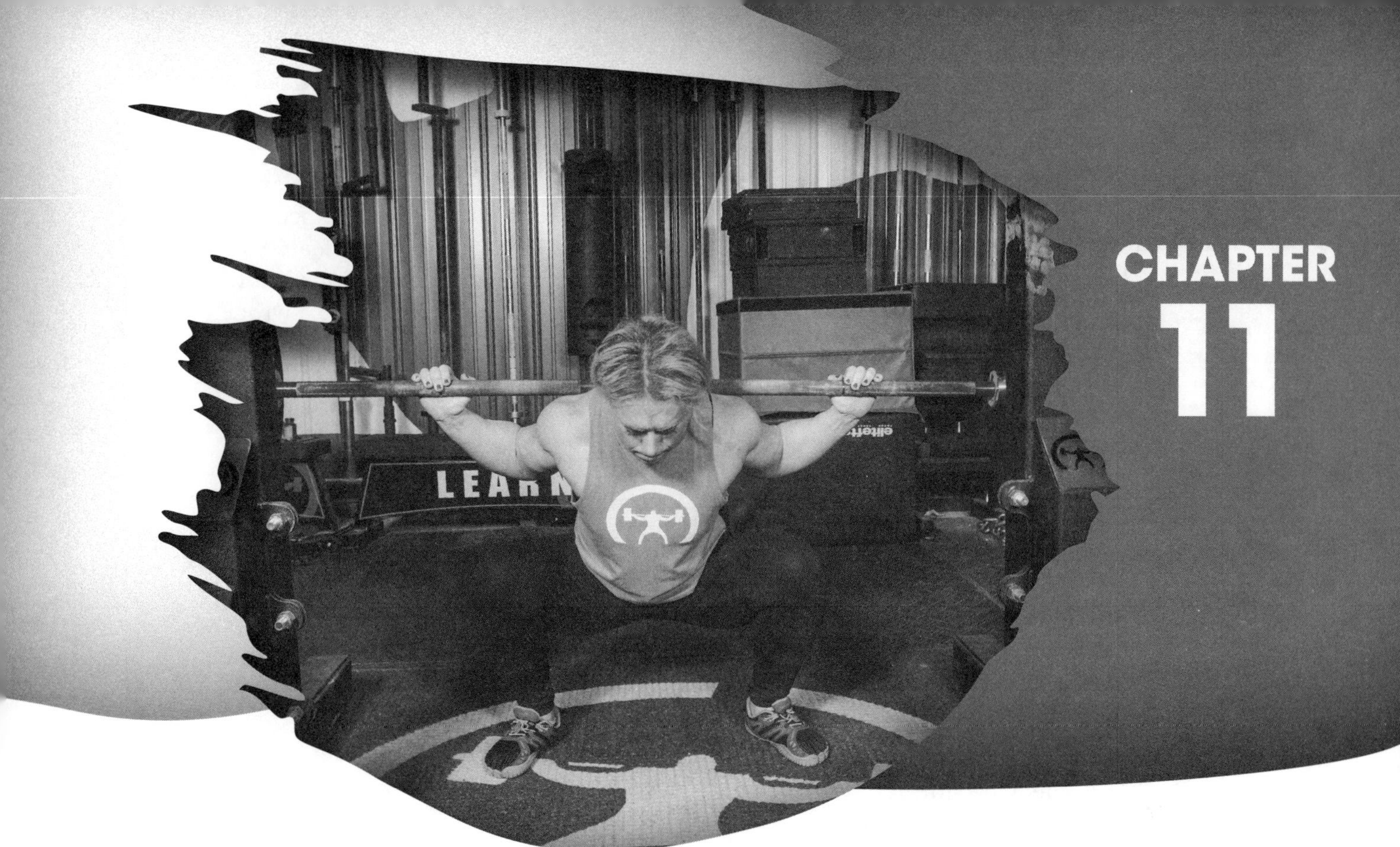

CHAPTER 11

The Overload System Programming

As you have seen throughout the previous chapters, there are a lot of methods that you can use to build an old-school overload program. It might be overwhelming at the moment, but our objective is not to give you a handout. If we were doing that, we would simply sell you a program, not write a whole book! If you bought this book, it is because you want to learn how to program using these methods or at least learn to integrate some of them in your own plans. We will therefore look at how to build a program and training strategy (linking several programs together) using this system of training.

Training Frequency and Split

The first thing to discuss is training frequency as well as schedule. I (Christian) have been all over the board when it comes to frequency in the past. Mostly because I just love to train and eventually became more addicted to the training itself than to getting results. That's why I tried (and was able) to find justifications to train 6 days a week. This led to stagnation, feeling run down, and getting injured.

Most of my clients, even pro athletes, have always lifted 3 or 4 days a week. It turns out that 3 or 4 workouts a week is what is ideal for most lifters, especially with the intensity of the work involved with this system. Let me be clear: You absolutely can train 5 or 6 days a week if the overall stress of the sessions is low enough. This normally equates to a very low volume of work. For example, I wrote a series of articles on "The Best Damn Workout for Natural Lifters" that used 6 training days a week, but the overall volume was extremely low: 4 to 5 total work sets per workout (not per exercise). I have also produced some plans based on a very high frequency of submaximal work, where you would go heavy-ish but keep 3 or more reps in reserve (e.g., sets of 3 reps at 80 to 85 percent of your max). However, a plan where you train brutally hard and do even a moderate amount of work will yield better results at 3 or 4 weekly workouts than 5 or 6 workouts. The harder you train, the less you can train. It should actually be pretty obvious to anyone who has actually trained. Just look at some examples:

- Before the 1960s, most lifters trained 3 days a week (Mon-Wed-Fri or Mon-Wed-Sat). That included strength legends like John Grimek, Steve Stanko, and the legends who came before them.
- Ed Coan, the greatest powerlifter of all time, trained 4 days a week.
- The Westside Barbell guys (if you don't know them, you don't know strength!) train 4 days a week.
- The Metal Militia lifters (who, for a while, were among the best pressers in the world) train 4 days a week.
- Hafthor Bjornsson (one of the best strongmen in the world) lifts 3 days a week and has one event day per week.
- Bill Kazmeir (strongman legend and possibly the best strongman ever) trained 4 days a week.
- Brian Shaw (one of the best strongmen in the world) trains 4 days a week.

Now, many of these men take anabolic steroids. Steroids help you recover faster. Yet they only train (or trained) 4 days a week. Why would someone without that advantage train hard 5 or 6 days a week? Granted, there are exceptions. There are guys who did train hard and often. However, you will find that the norm is 4 days a week, not more. Try not to look at what the exceptions can handle but what most lifters can do.

Before you tell me about Olympic lifters training 6 days a week, sometimes twice a day, I want to remind you that, first, most of their workouts are skill workouts and they don't push the sets hard, and second, they are essentially professional athletes who have nothing to do but train and recover. So, what I recommend with this system is hard workouts 3 days a week, on nonconsecutive days. With the possibility of adding a fourth, smaller workout to work on weak points. I call this lower stress workout a gap workout. My traditional schedule looks like this:

Monday	Tuesday	Wednesday	Thursday	Friday	Saturday	Sunday
Whole body 1	Off	Whole body 2	Off	Whole body 3	Gap workout	Off

I also sometimes use a 1-on/1-off schedule *without* a gap workout. In other words, some weeks you train 3 days a week; other weeks you train 4 days a week. For example, the schedule might look like this:

	Monday	Tuesday	Wednesday	Thursday	Friday	Saturday	Sunday
WEEK 1	Whole body 1	Off	Whole body 2	Off	Whole body 3	Off	Whole body 1
	Monday	Tuesday	Wednesday	Thursday	Friday	Saturday	Sunday
WEEK 2	Off	Whole body 2	Off	Whole body 3	Off	Whole body 1	Off

Or, I will use a 1-on/1-off schedule *with* a gap workout, which might look like this:

	Monday	Tuesday	Wednesday	Thursday	Friday	Saturday	Sunday
WEEK 1	Whole body 1	Off	Whole body 2	Off	Whole body 3	Off	Gap workout
	Monday	Tuesday	Wednesday	Thursday	Friday	Saturday	Sunday
WEEK 2	Off	Whole body 1	Off	Whole body 2	Off	Whole body 3	Off

I use the traditional schedule with 90 percent of the people I work with. The 1-on/1-off without a gap workout works well for people with a bit more stress in their life. The 1-on/1-off with a gap workout is the option that I use with people who have the most stress or a physical job.

Note that some people don't like whole-body workouts, so I do use an upper-lower split or a whole-body, upper body, and lower body split from time to time. Another option that I really like with this system is the lift-specific approach, which is also a form of upper-lower body split. A lot of people prefer that approach because it allows them to focus on one single goal per workout (improving one lift), and it also works very well with the overload system because it allows us to use several methods for each lift in the same workout (partials, functional isometrics, and holds seem to work better if they are done in the same workout as full-range exercises). In this lift-specific split, you select four lifts you want to focus on and that cover the whole body. For example, the schedule could look like this:

Monday	Tuesday	Wednesday	Thursday	Friday	Saturday	Sunday
Squat and squat assistance exercises	Off	Bench press and bench press assistance exercises	Off	Deadlift and deadlift assistance exercises	Overhead press and overhead press assistance exercises	Off

You can also use a 1-on/1-off schedule instead of the set-in-stone 4 days a week plan:

	Monday	Tuesday	Wednesday	Thursday	Friday	Saturday	Sunday
WEEK 1	Squat and squat assistance exercises	Off	Bench press and bench press assistance exercises	Off	Deadlift and deadlift assistance exercise	Off	Overhead press and overhead press assistance exercises
	Monday	Tuesday	Wednesday	Thursday	Friday	Saturday	Sunday
WEEK 2	Off	Squat and squat assistance exercises	Off	Bench press and bench press assistance exercises	Off	Deadlift and deadlift assistance exercises	Off

While there are six main lifts in this system (deadlift, squat, bench press, military press, row, explosive pull), and each will have an important impact on your physique and strength, there is another important point I want to make:

- They don't all have to be used in every program. You can rotate them.
- They don't all have to be treated as primary lifts. For example, the row or high pull can be a secondary movement on one of the training days.

Just because you are doing whole-body sessions doesn't mean you have to hit four or six main lifts in one workout. You could do two main lifts per day (e.g., overhead press and squat on day 1; bench press and deadlift on day 2; and power cleans and rows on day 3). This would allow you to use two methods and one assistance exercise per lift in each workout, or three methods. It can be a very interesting use of whole-body training. It would essentially be a cross between a whole-body and a lift-specific approach.

There really is more than one way to skin a cat. And no, I'm not saying this to take the easy way out. I always said that the split you use is just about the least important training decision you make. If you pick from one of these, it will work:

Three whole-body workouts (plus an optional gap workout)

Lift-specific split

Lift-specific and whole-body hybrid (one upper and one lower body main lift)

By now, you might be happy to know there are various ways of making this system work, but you may be confused about which split to use. I'll help you make up your mind!

First, let me say that I learned the hard way that it is *always* better to recover too much than barely enough (let alone not enough). If you train brutally hard on the methods presented in this book, there is pretty much no way to undertrain with this approach. The other training split options are mostly to fit a certain type of personality. Do not neglect the importance that liking the way you train can have on the gains you get. The more you like your training, the more motivated you will be in the gym and the better you can perform, leading to more gains. So, I'll be up front and tell you that the two approaches that I like best are the traditional schedule (whole-body workout 3 days a week split with the possibility of adding a gap workout) and the lift-specific split. Which split you choose may depend on your recovery capacities. You can go either with the static 4 days a week schedule (e.g., Mon-Wed-Fri-Sat or Sun-Tue-Thu-Fri)—that's if you have good recovery capacities—or a 1-on/1-off schedule if you need more recovery time. Table 11.1 provides a brief look at the pros and cons of these two types of schedules.

TABLE 11.1 Pros and Cons of Lift Schedules: Traditional Versus Lift-Specific Split

	Pros	Cons
Traditional (3 whole-body with possible gap workout)	• Can hit a lift or muscle 3 days a week, faster neurological improvements • A day focused on fixing weaknesses • Easy to plan by using one main method per session • Less chance of under-stimulation if you have to miss a workout (you still hit everything twice in the week) • Greater myostatin inhibition (a positive for muscle growth) • Generally, burns more "fuel" (greater caloric expenditure)	• Harder to combine several methods for a lift in one session • More draining than more concentrated sessions, even at an equal volume • Lifts performed later tend to suffer more than with another approach • Workouts tend to be longer (you need to warm up for every lift because they hit different muscles)
Lift-specific split	• Allows you to really focus on a lift • Easier to structure several methods for a lift • Greater strength transfer from partials, isometrics, and holds to the main movement because they are done in the same period • More motivational for many people because of the singleness of purpose of each workout and the feeling that everything is done to accomplish one specific goal • Workouts tend to be shorter because you don't need to warm up extensively for all exercises	• Can lead to slower progression in lifters who are less technically efficient and still building their neurological efficiency and technique • A higher frequency of practice of a lift leads to more rapid strength gains, at least for a 3- to 5-week period • Can affect your motivation mentally (i.e., when using a 1-on/1-off schedule you can have the impression of underworking a movement because you might not do it every week; in reality, this is a moot point because you do each lift every 8 days instead of every 7 days, which is not significant)

Number of Exercises

While the previous section on training split was a bit more complex (because there are several variations you can use and I wanted to explain how to make your decision), the number of exercises to use is a lot more straightforward.

First, let's make it clear that when it comes to programming, we will define an "exercise" as a movement with a specific method or loading scheme. For example, if you do 5 sets of 5 on the bench press and 3 sets of 5 on top half bench press from pins, that would be two exercises. We use three to six exercises in a workout. This refers to either the main lifts, special methods on the main lifts, or the primary assistance work. Remedial exercises (mentioned in chapter 1) can be added, but usually only one or two and only if absolutely necessary. When you hit the main lifts hard (especially with the high-impact methods described in this book), there is no need to do isolation work for all the major muscle groups. Only use a remedial exercise to fix a weak link in the chain.

There is still a lot of play between a half dozen or fewer exercises. In reality, most lifters should use four to six exercises per workout. You would go down to three exercises (even to two, in extreme cases) for three main reasons:

- *You want to do more sets for each exercise you do*. For example, if you want to do 3-2-1 wave loading for all of your movements, you can go up to 9 to 12 work sets for an exercise. Doing that on 4 to 6 lifts will be too much for most people. The same goes if you want to use the tried-and-true 10 × 3 method. Doing that on more than 3 lifts per workout is going to be way too much.
- *Your recovery capacity is low*. This could be because of genetic factors, lifestyle, work, or overall stressful period. For example, I have worked with many elite athletes in my time. One athlete, at a bodyweight of 181 pounds (82 kilograms), could bench 425 pounds (193 kilograms), squat 550 pounds (249 kilograms), power clean 335 pounds (152 kilograms), jump 40 inches (102 centimeters), and run 40 yards (37 meters) in under 4.3 seconds. Another athlete, at a bodyweight of 187 pounds (85 kilograms), could squat 575 pounds (261 kilograms), power clean 355 pounds (161 kilograms), front squat 475 pounds (215 kilograms), jump 38 inches (97 centimeters), and run 40 yards (37 meters) in 4.35 seconds. But these athletes could not perform more than 6 to 9 total work sets per workout, otherwise they would crash the next day! The most we could do was 3 work sets on three exercises or 4 to 5 work sets on two movements. Not being able to recover from a lot of work doesn't mean that you are at the bottom of the genetic pool.
- *You don't have much time to train*. When you have limited time to train, you need to be smarter about how you allocate your training time and volume. In this case, you want to put as much of your energy into the main lifts as possible and do less exercises per workout (so you don't spend half your workout warming up for five different exercises).

So, the question is: *How many exercises should I do?* The answer is this: four to six per workout, with the possibility of going even lower in certain circumstances.

Workout Structure

There are a few ways to organize how the exercises are structured in a workout. Let's take a look.

- *Horizontal*: You perform all the sets of an exercise before moving on to the next.
- *Vertical*: You perform one set of each exercise (with rest) before coming back to the first one and starting over again until you have done all your sets (called a "circuit" or circuit training).

- *Alternated*: Also known as the "A1/A2 method" and popularized by Charles Poliquin, you perform a set of one exercise, rest, perform a set of the second exercise, rest, then go back to the first one and start over until all your sets are done. Traditionally, this is either done with antagonistic movements or an upper and a lower movement.
- *Hybrid*: You use combinations of the first three approaches. For example, you might do the first two exercises as stand-alone (horizontal) then the last four exercises paired using the alternated approach.

I have used all of them at some point in my career and still do, because depending on the situation and training approach selected, they all can be the best tool for the job. However, when it comes to very heavy work, horizontal is the way to go. Pretty much all of the strongest lifters who ever lived have done all their sets on an exercise before moving on to the next. Except maybe when they did lighter work. The reason is that when you are training with near-maximal, maximal, and supramaximal weights, you want your mind to stay focused on that one task. Also, going from one motor pattern to the other makes you lose some of the repeated bout effect that makes you more neurologically efficient on a movement with every set you do. In my experience, when you do very heavy work and alternate two compound movements, one of the two will always suffer.

Coach Poliquin was a strong believer in alternating work, even for heavy lifting. He believed that doing so provided you with a "neurological advantage," although he never actually said what it was. In reality, it is easy to understand, and the advantage can quite easily become a huge drawback. What happens is that the harder the brain needs to work, the more adrenaline you release. That's because adrenaline is needed to speed up the neurons to give you the necessary "brain power." Adrenaline will also increase muscle contraction strength when binding to the beta-adrenergic receptors in the muscles. Thus, in a way, Poliquin was not wrong, at least theoretically. However, heavy lifting by itself will have the same impact on adrenaline, and too much adrenaline can lead to three main issues in this situation:

- *Increased risk of burning out:* Burning out is when you overload the beta-adrenergic receptors with too much adrenaline. As a result, they downregulate (become less sensitive), so they respond less to your own adrenaline, and you lose strength, speed, coordination, motivation, endurance, drive, and mental acuity.
- *Loss of coordination:* While adrenaline will make you stronger and faster, too much of it will negatively affect movement precision and control (that's the main reason athletes choke in competition). This could actually decrease performance by making your technique less efficient.
- *Increased risk of injury:* The more adrenaline is present, the higher your muscle tone becomes. This is useful to produce more force and speed, but if it becomes excessive, it will lead to muscle tightness instead of muscle readiness. Lifting maximal weights with tight muscles is more conducive to injuries.

Even in the best circumstances, the extra adrenaline from the alternating exercises rarely compensates for the lower efficiency increase you get from doing several sets in a row of the same motor task. While the A1/A2 method is fine when training for hypertrophy (or when strapped for time), I would avoid it as much as possible when training for strength and performance. The only time you will see an alternating set format in programs using the approach detailed in this book is when low-stress and high-rep isolation work is done. To save time on these low-impact movements, we might join two or even three together. Otherwise, stick to horizontal sets programming. Another exception, used with advanced programming, is using alternating contrasts on the same movement. For example:

A1. Top half bench press from pins × 5.

Rest 3 minutes.

A2. Bench press × 3.

Rest 3 to 4 minutes.

Alternating exercises creates a potentiation effect, and because both exercises use the same basic movement pattern, you still get a learning effect from set to set, and the motor pattern still gains efficiency.

Rest Between Sets

Sometimes your worst enemy is the one that you would never suspect. I'm a hard worker, and I'm not saying that to give myself a pat on the back or to look hardcore. I've done my fair share of completely crazy things in the gym. I once did 100 sets of bench press in a workout (okay, all sets were between 1 and 5 reps, but all were heavy). For five months, I would drive for hours (two hours to get there, two hours to come back) so that I could train for two hours in the morning and two hours in the afternoon at the national training center.

You will not be surprised to learn that I would often run myself down into the ground until I finally knew better (this took some time). I was passionate, I wanted—no, I *needed*—to be respected for my strength and was willing to do anything to get stronger. But even when I learned more about proper training and started doing a sane amount of volume, I would still hit the wall. This was despite the fact that the training parameters were all logical and worked for my clients. It took me a long while to realize that the source of my burning out was the thing I least suspected: my rest intervals!

Why would I have thought about that causing my crashes? Too much volume? Sure. Excessive frequency? I could see it. Going too heavy, too often? Possible. But *rest intervals*? Surely not.

See, I'm someone who instinctively likes to train fast. That's my default mode. Why? Probably because training faster keeps my adrenaline up, which makes me feel better during the workout. But remember what I said about adrenaline earlier: too much of it can downregulate the beta-adrenergic receptors, and when that happens, you crash.

Several variables can increase adrenaline. A high training density (short rest intervals) is just one of those variables, and it is far from being the most impactful one. However, if you add short rest intervals to using big compound movements, done with heavy weights, pushing each set hard and doing a decent amount of volume, the extra adrenaline from the short rest periods could be the straw that breaks the camel's back. Plus, when it comes to building strength and even muscle (with fairly heavy work), short rest intervals are the only adrenaline-promoting training variable that *does not* help make you stronger.

Studies are finding that you can use a greater average load and gain more strength with long versus short rest periods. When it comes to hypertrophy, it is less unanimous. While most studies find more size gains from rest periods of around 3 minutes than a minute or less, you do have some studies finding similar results with short rest intervals. However, this is mostly in beginners. The point is, except for making you feel like you are training harder, short rest periods will not work as well as longer rest periods to get you stronger and bigger. Short rests can help with conditioning and fat loss, but these are not our main goals here.

Exactly how long of a rest period are we talking about? While it can vary from movement to movement (e.g., a deadlift might require a longer rest time than a bench press, and the difference is even greater with minor movements) and how hard you push each set, there are some elements to consider that give us a pretty universal rest period range when using heavy work on the big basic lifts. For aesthetic purposes, short rest periods are often used, and there are certain advantages as far as metabolism, energy, and hormonal considerations go. However, when you train for strength and performance, the goal is to perform optimally during each set.

The level of performance depends largely on the interaction between two factors: potentiation and fatigue. Post-tetanic potentiation is a phenomenon by which the strength production potential of a muscle is increased for a brief period following a high level of force production. In other words, when you do a heavy set, your strength production potential increases slightly for some time. Potentiation normally peaks at around 2 minutes after the effort and gradually comes back down. Around 5 minutes after your effort, potentiation becomes a nonfactor.

Fatigue is caused by the set. It can affect the muscles or the nervous system and leads to a decrease in performance. Note that the level of fatigue depends on the amount of work performed in the set as well as how close to failure you went. So, take this recovery curve with a grain of salt. I took the data with the longest rest intervals to be safe. After a hard set, you still have a lot of fatigue at the 2-minute mark. After 3 to 4 minutes, fatigue is down to very low levels, and 5 minutes after your set, there is almost none left (there is still a cumulative build-up, however, over the whole workout from central fatigue, which is a different mechanism).

The key is finding the rest period that will allow you to still get some potentiation while minimizing fatigue.

- *90 to 120 seconds of rest*: Excellent post-tetanic potentiation but insufficient recovery (especially neural and phosphagens). Note that for hypertrophy workouts (isolation, machine, pulley using light weights), rest periods of 90 to 120 seconds are fine.
- *2 to 3 minutes of rest*: Excellent potentiation, with some residual fatigue. However, you should see an improvement in performance potential from set to set, especially with less demanding lifts.
- *3 to 4 minutes of rest*: You lose some potentiation, but fatigue is minimal (better neural and phosphagens recovery). The rest period will allow increase in performance.
- *4 to 5 minutes of rest*: You will experience very little or no residual fatigue, but potentiation is minimal. Within this range, strength potential will not

increase from set to set, but this rest period significantly reduces the impact on the nervous system and should be useful during deload or peaking.

As you can see, *3 to 4 minutes of rest* between work sets on the big basic lifts is the zone that will pretty much work for everyone, on any lift. Some can use as little as 2 minutes on the least demanding lifts, but I feel that it's safer to stick to 3 to 4 minutes unless you don't have much time to train.

Number of Sets per Exercise

The previous training parameters were all fairly easy to explain because, even though there will always be some individual differences, the recommendations work for pretty much everyone. However, when it comes to selecting the number of sets per exercise, there are tons of factors that can influence how many to use.

First, let's look at the total workload you should do in a session because before allocating sets to your exercises, you need to know roughly how many work sets overall you can do in your workout. In my coaching career, I have trained successful athletes who could only do 6 to 9 total work sets per workout (allocated between two or three exercises). Then there were others who could do 30 work sets (spread over four to six exercises, that's an average of 5 to 7 sets per exercise). Let's look at some factors that can affect how much work someone can do in a workout.

Work Capacity

People vary in how much work they can do without quality of execution and performance dropping off. There is a difference between work capacity and recovery capacity. Recovery capacity refers to being able to recover from the workout you just did and have positive adaptations before your next workout. Work capacity solely refers to how much work you can do before you start to tank within your session. This is dependent on many factors, including the ratio of fast-twitch fibers (the more fast-twitch fibers you have, the less capacity you'll have), how long your central nervous system can sustain sending an intense neural drive, how fast you clear adrenaline once released, your nutritional status, and your general fatigue level. There is no sense in continuing to pound the body with more sets when performance starts to drop, at least when strength and performance are the goal.

Recovery Capacity

Being able to "do the work" is one thing. Recovering and positively adapting to the work is another. It is quite possible to train so much that you cause excessive damage to the body because it doesn't have time to repair and rebuild everything before the next stimulation. Protein synthesis in the worked muscles remains elevated for 24 to 36 hours after your workout. If you have not repaired the muscle by that time, it becomes very unlikely that you will once protein synthesis and protein degradation become balanced again. If you cause so much muscle damage that after 24 to 36 hours you haven't repaired the damage, you will not progress from your session. In fact, you could even lose muscle.

There is also the fact that doing too much work can lead to systemic fatigue or what I call a "training burnout" (others call it overtraining). This happens when you produce too much cortisol and adrenaline, and so you downregulate your beta-adrenergic receptors. Your muscles, nervous system, and heart respond almost half as much as usual to adrenaline. This leads to a drop in physical and mental performance, less strength and speed, a drop in endurance, and mental apathy and loss of motivation.

I'll give you an example of excessive training. A few years ago, I was getting back into Olympic lifting, and because I had trained as a bro for a few years, I knew that I needed to regain my leg strength to be able to perform at a high level. Not being a patient person by nature, I opted for the nuclear weapon: I did a workout that consisted of a complex of three exercises, done as a circuit with around 2 minutes of rest, and I completed 10 sets:

A1. Back squat with an eccentric overload using weight releasers (80 percent on the bar with an extra 30 percent from releasers): 3 to 5 cluster reps

A2. Barbell jump squat: 5 reps with 135 pounds (61 kilograms)

A3. Depth jumps from a 40-inch (102-centimeter) box: 5 reps

I felt great afterward, convinced that I had done a great session that would bring my leg strength back up by quite a bit. What actually happened is that my legs were extremely sore for 10 days, and they were still sore enough to affect performance 14 days later. It took me 21 days to get back to being able to squat the weight I was using before that session! This is the perfect example of being able to do the work but not being able to positively adapt to the work. It is an extreme example, of course, but it's something that happens on a smaller scale all the time.

Intensiveness

There is a distinction to make between intensity and intensiveness. In strength training, intensity refers to the weight used relative to your maximum. If your max on a lift is 500 pounds (227 kilograms) and you use 400 pounds (181 kilograms) for your sets, you have an intensity level of 80 percent, regardless of how hard the sets actually are. The term can be a misnomer because it has very little to do with how intense a set is. A set with 85 percent can be very easy (e.g., doing 1 to 2 reps with 85 percent) while a set with 50 percent can be brutally hard (if you take it to failure). I use the term "intensiveness" when talking about how hard you push your set, often using the rate of perceived effort (RPE) scale. Taking a set to failure is more intensive than leaving 3 reps in the tank, regardless of the load used. Intensity (weight used) doesn't have a huge impact in and of itself on how many sets you should do; rather, it's how hard you push your sets that play a big role. The closer you go to failure on your sets, the less sets you can do. To paraphrase an old-school training adage: *You can train hard or you can train long, but not both*.

Exercises Performed

Bigger, multijoint lifts are more demanding than smaller isolated exercises. Big shock! A squat is going to take more out of you than leg presses, which are themselves more demanding than leg extensions. Bigger movements involve more muscle mass. You are causing microtrauma to more muscles, which will require a lot more resources to repair. The multijoint movements are also more complex to control (especially when done with free weights) and thus require more brain power. This means more adrenaline, which increases the risk of downregulating the beta-adrenergic receptors. It also means a greater likelihood of central nervous system fatigue.

Take these two workouts, for example:

Workout A

Squat

Romanian deadlift

Farmer's walk

Heavy prowler pushing

Workout B

Leg press

Back extension

Leg extension

Standing calf raise

Anybody who has been in a gym more than a few weeks will know that even though both have the same number of exercises and hit roughly the same muscle groups, workout A is going to be a lot more demanding at an equal effort level. Ask someone to do 5 hard sets of each exercise. Most will be able to do workout B and feel like they had a good session, but they won't feel drained. Most will not be able to do that with workout A without feeling completely trashed, and a lot just won't be able to finish it. They might be able to do 3 hard sets. That's why exercise selection matters when planning the number of sets. If all you do is isolated work or machine exercises, you can absolutely handle more volume than if you do mostly big, basic barbell lifts.

So, how many sets should you do, then? As you can see, it's not simple to answer that question. I cannot give you a universal answer that will apply to all programs and training approaches. But I can give you one when it comes to the type of training promoted in this book. Let's look at the nature of the training recommended here:

- The training uses almost exclusively multijoint movements.
- Almost all of the work is done with free weights.
- The objective is to train hard, but not to failure. The work sets range from an RPE of 7 to 9. Where there is an RPE of 9, it's usually only on the last set of an exercise.
- There is sufficient rest time between sessions (often using a 1-on/1-off schedule).
- There are fairly long rest intervals.

Some of these factors decrease how many sets you should do, and some allow you to do more (with lots of rest days, never doing hard workouts on consecutive days, and long rest intervals). Considering those factors, my recommendation for most is to do between 12 and 24 work sets per workout, and most should be around 16 to 20 sets. Again, understand that there will be individual differences. Some people will be able to do slightly more sets than what I recommend while others will need less.

Another rule is that not all of these sets are maximal effort. I have always been a proponent of ramping the weight from set to set, at least for the main lifts. This means that you might do 5 work sets on an exercise but only the last two are hard and the last one is close to or at your limit. To me, anything at an RPE of 7 or more is a work set because it will provide a training effect. So, even though out of 5 sets the first two are fairly easy, they still count as work sets. That's how old-school lifters did their workouts when using something like a 5 × 5 scheme.

The intensiveness level of each set would look something like this for 5, 4, and 3 work sets:

5 work sets	4 work sets	3 work sets
Set 1: RPE 7 (3 solid reps in the tank) *Set 2*: RPE 8 (2 solid reps in reserve) *Set 3*: RPE 8.5 (1, maybe 2 reps in the tank, but second would be a big grind) *Set 4*: RPE 9 (1 grinded rep in the tank) *Set 5*: RPE 9.5-10 (can't do another rep, *maybe* could have used a bit more weight)	*Set 1*: RPE 7 (3 solid reps in the tank) *Set 2*: RPE 8 (2 solid reps in reserve) *Set 3*: RPE 8.5 (1, maybe 2 reps in the tank, but second would be a big grind) *Set 4*: RPE 9 (1 grinded rep in the tank)	*Set 1*: RPE 7 (3 solid reps in the tank) *Set 2*: RPE 8.5 (1, maybe 2 reps in the tank, but second would be a big grind) *Set 3*: RPE 9.5-10 (can't do another rep, *maybe* could have used a bit more weight)

This is the basic approach for the loading schemes we use. We also use special loading schemes like waves, plateau loading, or ratchet loading that are a bit different. There are other special loading schemes that we use, but these are just examples to show load progression. Let's take a look:

Wave loading	Plateau loading	Ratchet loading
Set 1: 5 reps RPE 8 *Set 2*: 3 reps RPE 8 *Set 3*: 1 rep RPE 8 *Set 4*: 5 reps RPE 9 *Set 5*: 3 reps RPE 9 *Set 6*: 1 rep RPE 9	*Set 1*: 6 reps RPE 7.5 *Set 2*: 6 reps RPE 8.5 *Set 3*: 4 reps RPE 7.5 *Set 4*: 4 reps RPE 8.5 *Set 5*: 2 reps RPE 7.5 *Set 6*: 2 reps RPE 8.5	*Set 1*: 1 rep RPE 6 *Set 2*: 3 reps RPE 8 (same weight as set 1) *Set 3*: 1 rep RPE 7 *Set 4*: 3 reps RPE 9 (same weight as set 3) *Set 5*: 1 rep RPE 8 *Set 6*: 3 reps RPE 10 (same weight as set 5)

So, let's return to the question: How many sets per exercise? You have several options here. The easiest is to take the total number of sets you decide to do as well as the exercises you decide to use and spread the sets pretty much equally across the exercises. For example, if you picked four exercises and 20 sets, that gives you 5 work sets per movement. You can also decide to give more sets to exercises you want to emphasize more. In the above example of 20 sets for four exercises, you might want to put more emphasis on two main movements and have two assistance exercises or methods. In this case, you might attribute 3 work sets to the assistance movements, which leaves you 14 sets for the two main movements, so 7 work sets each. This is often used in the lift-specific and whole-body hybrid setup where you have two main lifts. You could even decide to have a lot of work for one lift, for example, in a lift-specific program. You might decide to do 9 work sets for the main lift (e.g., three 3-2-1 waves), which would leave you 11 sets for three movements. You could have 4 sets for two exercises and 3 sets for the last one.

Usually, I don't like doing fewer than 3 sets per exercise with this training approach, and up to 9 sets can be done. As long as the total set number for the workout falls in the proper range, it will work. Heck, I've done workouts with one lift done for 15 sets of 3 reps. Because this system uses mostly big compound movements that have a very similar systemic impact on the body, it doesn't really matter, from a recovery perspective, how you distribute your sets. It becomes a matter of what you want to accomplish with your session.

Exercise Variation

Changing exercises is the easiest way to include variation in your plan, and it's seductive because it also gives you the illusion of progress. But what does that mean? Well, if you haven't done a lift in a while, or at all, the first 2 to 4 weeks you do it you will have rapid strength gains simply because your intramuscular and intermuscular coordination as well as technical efficiency improves. That's why I put strength in quotation marks; you aren't so much getting stronger than you are getting more efficient at doing the exercise. It is not unusual to be able to add 10 pounds (4.5 kilograms) per week for 4 weeks when you start using a new movement or one you haven't done in a while. Certainly, adding 5 pounds (2.3 kilograms) per week will be very easy. If you have been stuck and stagnating on your lifts for weeks, this can feel like gaining 100 pounds (45 kilograms)! I'm getting stronger again! It works! Yeah, but not really.

A lot of people change their main exercises every 4 weeks, and they always have the illusion of getting stronger. And they are, to some extent. After all, if you train hard on big basic lifts, you will get stronger. It's not just about being more technically efficient, but it's not working as well as you think it is.

Now, you may be thinking, *Yeah, but the Westside Barbell guys change their main lift every week, and they are superstrong!* While that's true, you have to understand the whole story.

- They keep practicing their main lift year-round (speed squats and bench are done year-round, and many do the same with speed deadlifts).
- The variations of the main lifts are not huge variations. They will do rack pulls from various heights (a deadlift with a shortened range of motion), squats with different bars (mechanically still the same as a competition squat but with the load in a slightly different position), squats to different box heights (a squat but with a shortened range of motion), bench press to blocks of different thickness (still a bench press but with a shortened range of motion), or bench press with different bars (same movement pattern as the bench). Basically, they rarely change the movement pattern; they just reduce or increase the range of motion or use a slightly different load position. They actually keep using the same mechanics as their competition lifts, which means that they do not have the rapid gains due

to technical improvements or neurological adaptations. It's not like going from a bench press to an incline dumbbell press or from a squat to a hack squat machine, for example.

- They are extremely advanced lifters who are already efficient neurologically and technically on all the exercises they rotate in. They don't have rapid strength gains from motor learning because they don't have much motor learning left to do.

Varying the main lifts certainly does have benefits, but there are also drawbacks, as we will discuss in more detail here.

Benefits of Exercise Variation

It can make you stronger overall by making you efficient at applying strength in different movements. It can lead to fewer weak points, and it can keep training fresher and more motivating (for some). Exercise variation gives you more adrenaline when you train (which is also a drawback), and it's easier to add weight to the bar. Let's briefly look at these points individually.

Makes You Stronger Overall

Doing a lift gives you two types of strength. All the muscles involved get stronger, and you become better at applying force in that movement. With the first type of strength, you will have some carryover from one exercise to a related one. For example, if your squat goes up, your front squat should also go up (but not to the same extent). The closer in coordination structure an exercise is to the one you trained, the more of the strength will be transferred, but the transfer is never one for one. If you add 50 pounds (23 kilograms) to your squat, your front squat will not automatically go up by the same amount, too. Maybe 25 to 30 pounds (11 to 14 kilograms). The more you practice a movement, the better you become at applying force in that movement. One of the benefits of rotating your main lifts is that you get to practice more movements, and as such, you improve more on each than if you didn't train them. However, this could also mean that you improve less on a movement than if you trained it more often (more on that in the drawbacks section).

Good illustrations of this are strongmen, powerlifters, and Olympic lifters. They are all strong, but usually their strength is mostly seen in their movement of choice. Olympic lifters will use a much narrower range of "strong lifts" because of the highly technical nature of their sport (meaning they must spend a lot more time and volume on their competition lifts). For example, I've trained an Olympic lifter who could jerk 200 kilograms (440 pounds) but barely bench-press 102 kilograms (225 pounds)! Heck, a friend of mine who competed at the world championships in 1982 could clean and jerk 192.5 kilograms (424 pounds) but barely get 85 kilograms (187 pounds) on the strict overhead press. Ask an Olympic lifter, even an elite one, to curl or bench-press, and their strength level will not be anywhere near elite (except for some of the freaks or those who actually do these exercises in their training, which is rare).

Powerlifters will have strength over a broader range of exercises because their competition lifts are more varied (you need to be strong in every single muscle because you don't rely on momentum created by the lower body to make the lift). In addition, they normally use more assistance exercise variations than Olympic lifters. You will rarely have a high-level powerlifter weak in any barbell or dumbbell exercises (except the Olympic lifts).

Strongmen will have the broadest range of strong movements. Top-level strongmen will be strong on pretty much anything you can ask them to do. They can do any barbell lift, even including the Olympic lifts (it might not be pretty, but they will be able to lift a lot). My friend Jean-Francois Caron, top 5 strongman in the world, can power clean 445 pounds (202 kilograms) without efficient technique. Top-level strongmen will be strong in carries, and they can throw far. You name it, they can do it. That's because the demands of their sport have them training on the widest variety of exercises out of all the strength athletes. A side effect is that even though strongman competitors are stronger than the elite powerlifters, the powerlifters are still likely to beat them in a powerlifting meet (if both lifters are of the same level, of course). The strongman will be equal or even stronger on the deadlift because it's the foundation of strongman training, but bench and squat will favor the powerlifter.

What I'm getting at is that the more you focus on a few lifts, the stronger you will be on those lifts, but the more lifts you train, the better you will be at being pretty strong on everything.

Leads to Fewer Weak Points

Even moderate changes to a movement can bias toward certain muscle groups or sections of a muscle. For example, a wider stance in your squat will hit the glutes and adductor muscles a bit more than a narrower squat. Elevating the heels on a squat will shift more stress to the quadriceps. A narrower grip on bench press will make the triceps a bit more dominant, while a wider grip makes the pecs do more of the work. Variation can thus lead you to stimulate a wider range of different muscles.

Even using different bars can bias certain muscles. For example, using a safety bar for squats will favor the quads and have the core work harder than in a regular squat. I actually like those smaller exercise changes. I personally don't see them as true exercise changes, though: the basic motor pattern remains the same, so you don't have any of the drawbacks (which we will see shortly) of exercises changes.

Keeps Your Training Fresher and More Interesting

Some people (not all) need novelty in their training to stay motivated. These people tend to jump on a new training bandwagon as soon as they read an exciting article about a training method or system or see some cool videos on YouTube. If there is some variation built into the program through a rotation in the main lifts, which also gives them freedom to try new lifts, it can curb their need to completely drop their program to do something else. It's the lesser of two evils, if you will.

Gives You More Adrenaline When You Train

I briefly mentioned this before, but when you need more brain power (i.e., require a higher neurological activation), you produce more adrenaline to speed up your neurons. When you switch to a new exercise, especially one that you have not mastered yet, you need more brain power to execute, learn, and program the movement pattern. This means more adrenaline. In fact, it's one of the reasons why changing exercises around feels exciting to some people and can create anxiety in others. (Anxiety is nothing more than your brain going too fast and making you feel like you are losing control. Individuals who already have a high adrenaline level can thus be made anxious by major exercise changes.) This adrenaline will not solely affect your brain. It also binds to the muscle and heart and will thus increase strength, speed, and endurance. Exercise variation can therefore increase excitement, energy, and performance. This will obviously be less pronounced in very advanced lifters who have mastered most exercise variations.

Makes It Easier to Add Weight to the Bar

As I mentioned before, when you switch to a movement that you haven't done in a while (or ever), it is easy to add weight to the bar because of the rapid motor learning and technical efficiency improvements. While a lot of that is an illusion of gained strength, some of it is real. But more important, it is motivating. The more motivated you are, the harder you'll train. The harder you train, the more you gain. So again, while it can start out as illusory gains, the end result can become real gains.

Drawbacks of Exercise Variation

There are also some drawbacks to frequent changes in the main lift. It can be the enemy of technical mastery which can, in turn, limit progress in a specific lift, can increase the risk of training burnout, may make it harder to assess true progression, and can become excessive. Let's briefly look at these points individually.

The Enemy of Technical Mastery

If you want to maximize performance on an exercise, you must practice that exercise. Related movements can also improve performance on the main lift, and the closer they are in structure, the greater the positive impact will be. For example, a front squat will improve the back squat more than a leg extension. However, the best way to improve performance on a lift is to practice that lift often and for a long time. That's why competitive Olympic lifters never stray away from the snatch, clean and jerk, and the squat, and it's why a lot of powerlifters (from the East European countries mostly) rely heavily on their competition lifts, year-round.

Some people are genetically more gifted than others to transfer strength gains from one movement to a related one. Others can't do it efficiently. This is highly dependent on acetylcholine levels. Generally speaking, though, if you stick to the same big compound movements for a long time rather than change them every 3 to 6 weeks, you will get better, faster on those movements.

This is because with more practice comes better intramuscular and intermuscular coordination. Basically, your nervous system fine-tunes the motor pattern it uses to do the movement. The various muscles involved in the lift are better coordinated, and the muscle fibers within these muscles work better together to maximize force production. I'm not talking about technique. Someone could have perfect technique but poor intramuscular and intermuscular coordination, and performance wouldn't be good. Similarly, someone with seemingly poor technique can have a great performance because their intra- and intermuscular coordination is so good that their body can still use a high percentage of its potential.

If you constantly change your main lifts, it might lead to overall progress on more movements but slower progress on any given lift when compared to if you focused on that movement instead of constantly changing. It's really a matter of what is more important to you.

Potentially Increases the Risk of Training Burnout

As I explained in the benefits section, exercise variation can increase adrenaline levels, which can lead to more excitement and even better performance. While adrenaline is necessary to perform, getting too much of it is like taking out a loan at the bank. It's cool in the short term because you have more money to spend, and you feel great, but eventually you will need to pay back the loan, with interest, and that can hurt. When it comes to adrenaline, the issue when you produce too much of it, too often, or for too long, is that you can downregulate and desensitize the beta-adrenergic receptors. Essentially, you make yourself resistant to your own adrenaline.

When that happens, it becomes harder and harder for adrenaline to activate the various tissues. From the perspective of the brain and central nervous system, it means less motivation, lower drive, less competitiveness and belief in yourself, laziness, less focus and concentration, slower learning, and impaired coordination. At the muscular level, it means a decrease in muscle tone and lower strength and speed production.

It also affects your cardiovascular capacity by decreasing heart contraction strength and rate, delivering less oxygen to the muscle during an effort, and making it harder to clear out metabolites like lactate and hydrogen ions. So, endurance and work capacity also go down. What we call overtraining really is, most of the time, a downregulation of the beta-adrenergic receptors. That's why I personally call it "training burnout," and it can happen quickly—in as little as one workout. We've all had an experience where we did a monster workout one day only to wake up feeling run down, almost depressed, the very next day. That's a downregulation of the beta-adrenergic receptors.

All that diatribe is to show you that one of the potential effects of variation, especially when it means variation in big complex movements, is to spike adrenaline, which could contribute to downregulating your beta-adrenergic receptors, especially if other variables that increase adrenaline and cortisol are elevated (e.g., volume, intensiveness, psychological stress, short rest periods, high neurological demands). In most people, the variation itself is unlikely to present a big risk. But people who have a high level of stress in their lives or those who train excessively will certainly be more at risk of burning out by adding too much variation too often.

Makes It Harder to Assess True Progression

It's cool to see the weight on the bar go up, which happens more easily when you constantly change exercises. But, at one point, you need to assess whether you are truly getting stronger or if it's just gains from becoming better at lifts you were inefficient in before. One reason why I like to keep some lifts for longer in the program is to assess whether the program is working and making me stronger. If my squat keeps going up, I know that my training strategy is working. If it isn't or if it's going down, I know I need to change something in the program.

If you don't know when you are truly progressing, then it's hard to know if the program is working or if you need to change it. Relying on muscle growth is hard to do because muscle growth is really slow (it can take 6 to 8 weeks in a non-beginner to make a significant, noticeable gain in muscle). For many, it's hard to really know if the gains are purely muscle or muscle and fat or even mostly fat. If you can't assess progress, you might stay with a training strategy that just isn't really working, even though you think it is. I've seen lifters gain 30 pounds (14 kilograms) on the front squat in 3 weeks, then 30 pounds on their box squat in 3 weeks only to get back to the squat and find they are doing the exact same weight, or less, than before those 6 weeks. They sure thought they were progressing, but were they really?

Becomes Excessive (and Sometimes Illogical)

I've seen a lot of Westside Barbell wannabes put max effort exercise variation above everything else in their training. It becomes so important to them that they try to never do the same lift twice, and they come up with all kinds of crazy exercises—exercises that will have a very low carryover to the competition lifts—just to avoid repeating one they already did. I personally like conjugate training, but with a limited rotation of exercises (two to four) selected for their value and effectiveness to increase the corresponding main lift. Changing to an ineffective exercise just for the sake of variation is stupid, yet it is something I see all the time.

I like exercise variation and believe that it is a valuable tool for lifters who have already mastered technique on the big basics (squat, bench, deadlift, military press, row). But it is my opinion that a narrower variation (rotating the same two to four exercises) and sticking with them for at least 3 weeks is a better approach for most lifters.

That having been said, it is also my opinion that you should stick to the big basics (squat, bench, deadlift, military press, row) until you are at a high level of efficiency on those movements. This takes a lot longer than what most people believe (or want to believe). You can never go wrong by sticking to the big basics for longer. You can always have variation in the assistance work and the training methods used on the main lifts.

Program Variation

First, let's make it clear that when I say "program," I mean using the same exercises used with the same methods for a similar intensity zone. Note that there can be minor changes without it being considered a change in program. For example:

- You can change the reps slightly (e.g., going from 5 to 3 reps per set).
- You can add or remove sets to your exercises from week to week.
- You can substitute an assistance exercise if you feel that it's not working for you.
- You can rotate the minor remedial exercise if you use one.
- You can add an intensification technique on some weeks (e.g., doing regular sets for 2 weeks, then rest for the third week).

However, when you make major changes to the content of the program, we are talking about changing your program. This kind of change and variation is important for continuous progression, but also be aware that this doesn't mean that you have to change every variable in your new program. For example, let's say that you use the progressive range of motion (PRM) method on the bench press, squat, and deadlift. After the completion of your program, you are not yet to the point of starting from the lowest position on deadlift. In the first phase (3 weeks in this case) of your new program, you could then continue with the PRM method for deadlift while you change the other elements of the program, thereby giving you 3 more weeks. You can also keep several exercises in the plan while you change the program (e.g., by using different methods or loading schemes with those exercises).

Just like exercise variation, how often you should change your program will depend on several factors, such as experience level and personality type. But some variation is needed to keep you progressing. In other words, *stimulus variation is very important*.

Your body adapts to the training stress you place on it. That's mostly good because that's what allows you to get bigger and stronger, but there is some negative to it. Why? The better adapted you are to a certain type of stimulus, the harder it is to keep forcing your body to adapt. It's like drinking coffee and the effect of caffeine. If you've never had coffee before, then the caffeine "hit" you get from it is huge: You're full of energy for hours, and you feel awesome, so you start drinking a cup of coffee every morning. But disappointingly, after a few weeks, it doesn't have any pronounced effect. Then you become a two cups of coffee a day person, and so on, until you're remortgaging your house to pay for your Starbucks tab. You get diminishing returns as your body adapts, so you need to drink progressively more coffee to get the same effect.

It's similar with training, but the difference with training is that you can build muscle and gain strength through many different stimuli. As your body adapts to a certain type of stimulus, you can change it to prevent full adaptation and give the body a new type to adapt to. That's why you have to change your program from time to time. People will immediately think of changing exercises, but that is not necessarily the most effective way to do things. If you keep training the same way (i.e., methods, intensity zone, type of contraction), then going from a squat to a front squat is not a huge change in stimulus. It's still the same type.

I prefer to include variation in the form of training methods, loading schemes, and contraction types; ask the body to work differently, not the same but on different exercises. Don't get me wrong. Changing exercise does provide some changes to the training stress and should be used, even if only to prevent boredom and keep you motivated (as we discussed in the previous section). However, by itself, it is not sufficient with intermediate and advanced lifters to keep progressing once you near full adaptation.

Also, people vary quite a bit in their need for training variation. Some people require a new taste in their mouth quite often while others are more comfortable sticking to the same thing for a long time and hate changing their program around. With the former, you have to restrain their urge to change program too often; with the latter, you have a lot of convincing to do to get them to change their program when they stagnate. I'm a strong believer that if you lose motivation in your training, it will be hard to get maximal results from your program. Sure, you can force yourself to train hard for a few sessions even if you start losing motivation or interest in your plan, but very few people can keep giving a maximal effort on a plan that doesn't get their juices flowing anymore. I'm not saying to only pick stuff that you like doing and to avoid tough lifts like the squat and deadlift. What I'm saying is that if you start to lose interest in your program, if you are less and less excited about doing your workout, results will start to go down. This is certainly a factor to consider when deciding when to change programs.

The more advanced you are, the more often you should change your plan. That's because advanced lifters are better adapted to training and also adapt more rapidly. They therefore need more frequent stimulus changes. Depending on the individual's level, I like to use this length of time for "programs":

- *Beginners:* 6 to 8 weeks block
- *Intermediates:* 4 to 6 weeks block
- *Advanced:* 3 to 4 weeks block

Again, within those blocks, you can have small planned changes (e.g., increases or decreases in volume or load) or small unplanned changes (e.g., changing an exercise that doesn't work for the individual).

Deloading

Deloads are misunderstood, probably because we don't really talk about them much, nor do we study the best way to do them. This is probably because we like to train, so talking about training less or not training as hard for a week isn't really interesting to us, even if that means greater gains along the way. Deloading comes from the world of performance training and was originally used for two purposes:

1. Peaking for a competition or a test.

   Even in the 1950s, coaches working with competitive athletes in Olympic sports (in which an athlete trains several months to compete on a single day or two) understood that if they wanted the athlete to perform optimally in competition, they needed to dramatically reduce the training load for 7 to 14 days before the competition.

   At first, the extent of their understanding was merely that a well-rested athlete performed better. Eventually, the super-compensation theory came to be (by reducing the training workload and increasing carb intake, you could store more muscle glycogen, giving you better performance). This theory is mostly true, especially in sports that are dependent on glycogen stores (e.g., endurance and moderate distance events). But the theory isn't entirely applicable to strength and power sports. Still, deloading worked for these athletes, too (more on why it works in a minute).

2. Transitioning between two training cycles.

   This was common in competitive sports where you had two or three major competitions that were normally several months apart. For example, in track and field, you could have the national championships, indoor world championships, and outdoor world championships. For each, a training cycle of 10 to 16 weeks (sometimes more) was designed, ending in a peak for the competition. Then the preparation for the next competition would begin. However, understanding the stress of competition, you would include 1 to 3 weeks of easy training between a competition and the start of the next training cycle.

Through experimentation, coaches found that if, preceding a competition, they adopted a period of gradually harder training, followed by a "taper" (deloading) period of 7 to 14 days, it led to better results after the deload than before. It didn't take long until this started to be applied to regular training blocks, not just for competition peaking. Coaches started building blocks of 4 to 8 weeks of gradually more demanding training in which the last week was a "mini-peak," or what could be called a taper or a deload (often they included a mock competition at the end of that peak). Then they would start a new block, gradually ramping up the training demands again and peaking once again at the end of the cycle. In fact, that is still how I see a deload: it really is a peak to either test yourself at the end or to be in a peak condition to start the new training block.

I believe that words and concepts have power. "Deloading" is demotivating for a hard training athlete who always wants to do more, but "peaking" sounds a lot better. Rest for a week, then test yourself to see how effective the last block was. That's how I prefer to use planned deloads.

Of course, I also use true deloads (which is the same thing minus the test at the end of the week), especially when an athlete is showing early signs of training burnout. If you start to have several of these symptoms and keep pushing pedal to the metal, you are digging yourself into a bigger and bigger hole:

Decrease in performance
Drop in motivation
Lower level of energy
Mood swings
Sudden weight loss
Sleep issues
Decrease in muscle tone
Decreased appetite
Anhedonia (no pleasure)
Drop in libido
Apathy
Concentration and focus problems

How often you should deload really depends on the individual. I know it's an underwhelming answer, but it's the truth. Someone who trains obsessively will need more frequent deloads than someone who trains with less intensity. In fact, 95 percent of the people you see training in commercial gyms will never need a deload, at least not from their training. They simply don't work hard enough. If you train 5 to 6 days a week, you will need to deload more often than someone who trains 3 to 4 days a week. Someone who eats a caloric surplus will not need to deload as often as someone who is in a caloric deficit. You get the point. Some factors that affect deloading frequency are shown in table 11.2.

TABLE 11.2 Factors That Affect Deloading Frequency

Reduces the need for frequent deloads	Increases the need for frequent deloads
Training within your zone of comfort	Training hard
Having low life stress	Having high life stress
Having a job that is easy physically and mentally	Having a physical job
Being younger	Being older (40+)
Being a female	Being a male
Being at beginner strength levels	Being very strong
Having equal or more rest than training days	Having more training days than rest days
Being in a caloric surplus	Being in a caloric deficit
Getting 8-10 hours of sleep a night	Getting less than 8 hours of sleep a night
Taking a daily nap	Always being on the go throughout the day
Good immune system (never gets sick)	Poor immune system (gets sick easily)
Good gut health	Poor gut health

Now, you don't have to use some form of meticulous calculation to find out that you need to deload exactly every 4.35 weeks, but if you look at the table and think you tend to be more on one side than the other (or if there is a balance between the two), it gives you an idea of roughly how often you should deload. Use these guidelines (most of you will be in the first two categories):

- If more factors that apply to you are from the *right column*, you should deload every third or fourth week.
- If the factors that apply to you are *balanced between both columns*, you should deload every fifth or sixth week.
- If more factors that apply to you are from the *left column*, you could deload every seventh or eighth week, but you might not even need to deload.

To understand how to properly deload or peak, you must understand how it actually works for a lifter (as opposed to endurance athletes). As I explained earlier, in endurance or moderate distance events, a lot of the performance increase that comes from the deloading and peaking process comes from an increase in glycogen storage. This can also contribute slightly to lifting performance with better leverages as well as more pressure around the joints, increasing stability. However, the main effect that deloading has on strength sports (and other sports as well) is to re-sensitize the beta-adrenergic receptors. That's also why deloading is effective at reducing the risk of training burnout and overtraining.

We saw earlier that if you produce too much adrenaline for too long or too often, you can downregulate and desensitize the beta-adrenergic receptors. When this happens your muscles, heart, and nervous system don't respond as well to your own adrenaline, which decreases strength, speed, coordination, endurance, motivation, drive, and well-being. Yet the opposite is also true: if you produce less adrenaline, less often, you will re-sensitize your receptors and will therefore respond better to your own adrenaline, increasing strength, speed, coordination, endurance, motivation, drive, and well-being.

That's what a deload and peak does. Adrenaline is connected to cortisol. Cortisol leads to an increase in adrenaline because cortisol increases the conversion of noradrenaline into adrenaline. The more cortisol you produce, the more adrenaline you'll have too. That's why, for example, when you are stressed out, it's hard to sleep. The cortisol from the stress leads to a high adrenaline level, which speeds your brain up, making it hard to get to sleep. When you reduce training, you also lower cortisol and adrenaline. The result is that you can make your adrenergic receptors sensitive again. Yes, you can super-compensate glycogen and intramuscular fatty acid stores, but more of the increase in performance comes from the fact that you once again respond optimally to adrenaline and are able to show your full performance potential. When you train really hard for a good period of time, to use a car analogy, it's as if you removed the fifth gear on your car by overusing the transmission, and when you deload you get that back.

To get back to our question: *How should I deload?* The answer is that it really is a matter of decreasing cortisol and adrenaline. There are six main training variables that can increase cortisol release (see table 11.3). The variables are ranked in order from the largest to the smallest impact on cortisol and adrenaline levels. For example, if you significantly lower one of the first two variables (volume or intensiveness) enough, you might not have to lower anything else. In fact, these are the two most common ways to deload (cutting sets by around

50 percent or pushing your sets at an RPE of 6 to 7 instead of 8 to 9). Another common way to deload is to decrease psychological stress. In lifting sports, we are talking about lowering the weights used. This is, for example, the approach used by Jim Wendler's 5-3-1 system.

Reducing volume, intensiveness, or psychological stress are the three most popular and effective ways of deloading. Decreasing the weight is often not enough, especially if the athlete is showing signs of fatigue. You might want to decrease another variable slightly (e.g., reducing volume by 25 percent). The three other variables—neurological demands, density, and competitiveness—are rarely enough by themselves to have a successful deload, but you can manipulate them along with one of the first three variables to produce an even more effective deload. Table 11.3 also shows the strategies used to deload each variable.

TABLE 11.3 Training Variables That Can Increase Cortisol and Deload Strategies for Each

Variable	Description	Deload strategy
Volume	The amount of work being done (exercises × sets × reps)	Decrease the number of sets by around 50% (either by cutting exercises or reducing the sets per exercise)
Intensiveness	How hard you are pushing your sets	Reduce the RPE of your work sets to no more than 6-7
Psychological stress	Mild anxiousness or the need to psych yourself up (often associated with heavy weights or painful conditioning work)	Reduce the weights used for your sets by 15-30%
Neurological demands	More complex movements, combining exercises, learning new movements, more explosive work	Switch to less demanding movements (e.g., machine exercises)
Density	The length of the rest intervals (short rest = high density)	Rest longer between sets
Competitiveness	Turning each training session into a competition (against your logbook or a partner)	Try to have fun and chill during your session (basically train like an average commercial gym trainee)

So, which strategy is more effective? Honestly, I've never seen any significant difference between using one of the three main variables to deload. My recommendation is to use one of the first three variables to deload and one from the bottom three. Since the name of our sport is strength, an example to simply illustrate the concept would be:

EXAMPLE OF DELOADING BY VOLUME	
Regular session	**Deloading session**
Squat 4 × 5 at 405 lb (184 kg) Half squat from pins 3 × 5 at 505 lb (229 kg) Farmer's walk 3 × 20 m (22 yd) at 150 lb (68 kg)/hand Back extension 4 × 10 at 50 lb (23 kg)	Squat 2 × 5 at 405 lb (184 kg) Half squat from pins 1 × 5 at 505 lb (229 kg) Farmer's walk 1 × 20 m (22 yd) at 150 lb (68 kg)/hand Back extension 3 × 10 at 50 lb (23 kg)
EXAMPLE OF DELOADING BY INTENSIVENESS	
Regular session	**Deloading session**
Squat 4 × 5 at 405 lb (184 kg) Half squat from pins 3 × 5 at 505 lb (229 kg) Farmer's walk 3 × 20 m (22 yd) at 150 lb (58 kg)/hand Back extension 4 × 10 at 50 lb (23 kg)	Squat 4 × 2 at 405 lb (184 kg) Half squat from pins 3 × 2 at 505 lb (229 kg) Farmer's walk 3 × 10 m (11 yd) at 150 lb (58 kg)/hand Back extension 3 × 6 at 50 lb (23 kg)
EXAMPLE OF DELOADING BY PSYCHOLOGICAL STRESS	
Regular session	**Deloading session**
Squat 4 × 5 at 405 lb (184 kg) Half squat from pins 3 × 5 at 505 lb (229 kg) Farmer's walk 3 × 20 m (22 yd) at 150 lb (58 kg)/hand Back extension 4 × 10 at 50 lb (23 kg)	Squat 5 × 5 at 325 lb (147 kg) Half squat from pins 3 × 5 at 405 lb (184 kg) Farmer's walk 3 × 20 m (22 yd) at 120 lb (54 kg)/hand Back extension 4 × 10 at 40 lb (18 kg)

Note: To one of those strategies, you could lengthen the rest between sets by a minute or switch out some of the more demanding exercises, like the half squat from pins or farmer's walk.

These three strategies (plus a secondary one from the following table) are perfectly fine for a range of normal situations, from not showing any signs of chronic fatigue to exhibiting normal signs of fatigue accumulated from a hard training block. However, sometimes you will have an individual showing deeper signs of fatigue, even the beginning of a training burnout. This could be related to excessive training or other sources of stress. In that case, you will have to either lower volume and psychological stress (weights) or volume and intensiveness, as well as one or more from the previous table, to properly deload. Here is an example to simply illustrate this concept:

EXAMPLE OF DELOADING BY VOLUME AND PSYCHOLOGICAL STRESS	
Regular session	**Deloading session**
Squat 4 × 5 at 405 lb (184 kg) Half squat from pins 3 × 5 at 505 lb (229 kg) Farmer's walk 3 × 20 m (22 yd) at 150 lb (68 kg)/hand Back extension 4 × 10 at 50 lb (23 kg)	Squat 2 × 5 at 325 lb (147 kg) Half squat from pins 1 × 5 at 405 lb (184 kg) Farmer's walk 1 × 20 m (22 yd) at 120 lb (54 kg)/hand Back extension 3 × 10 at 40 lb (18 kg)
EXAMPLE OF DELOADING BY VOLUME AND INTENSIVENESS	
Regular session	**Deloading session**
Squat 4 × 5 at 405 lb (184 kg) Half squat from pins 3 × 5 at 505 lb (229 kg) Farmer's walk 3 × 20 m (22 yd) at 150 lb (68 kg)/hand Back extension 4 × 10 at 50 lb (23 kg)	Squat 2 × 3 at 405 lb (184 kg) Half squat from pins 1 × 3 at 505 lb (229 kg) Farmer's walk 1 × 10 m (11 yd) at 150 lb (68 kg)/hand Back extension 3 × 6 at 50 lb (23 kg)

Note: You could also either increase rest periods between sets by around one minute or substitute some of the harder exercises if you needed to further reduce training stress.

Normally, burnout should never happen because you should see it coming and do a deload before it gets too bad. Those who get there are usually people who coach themselves and are stubborn and refuse to slow down, even if their dashboard is lit up like a Christmas tree! If it ever happens to you, then you will have to dramatically reduce training stress. This means pretty much reducing every variable as well as training frequency (down to one or two sessions in the week). Some people might even need to take the week off completely.

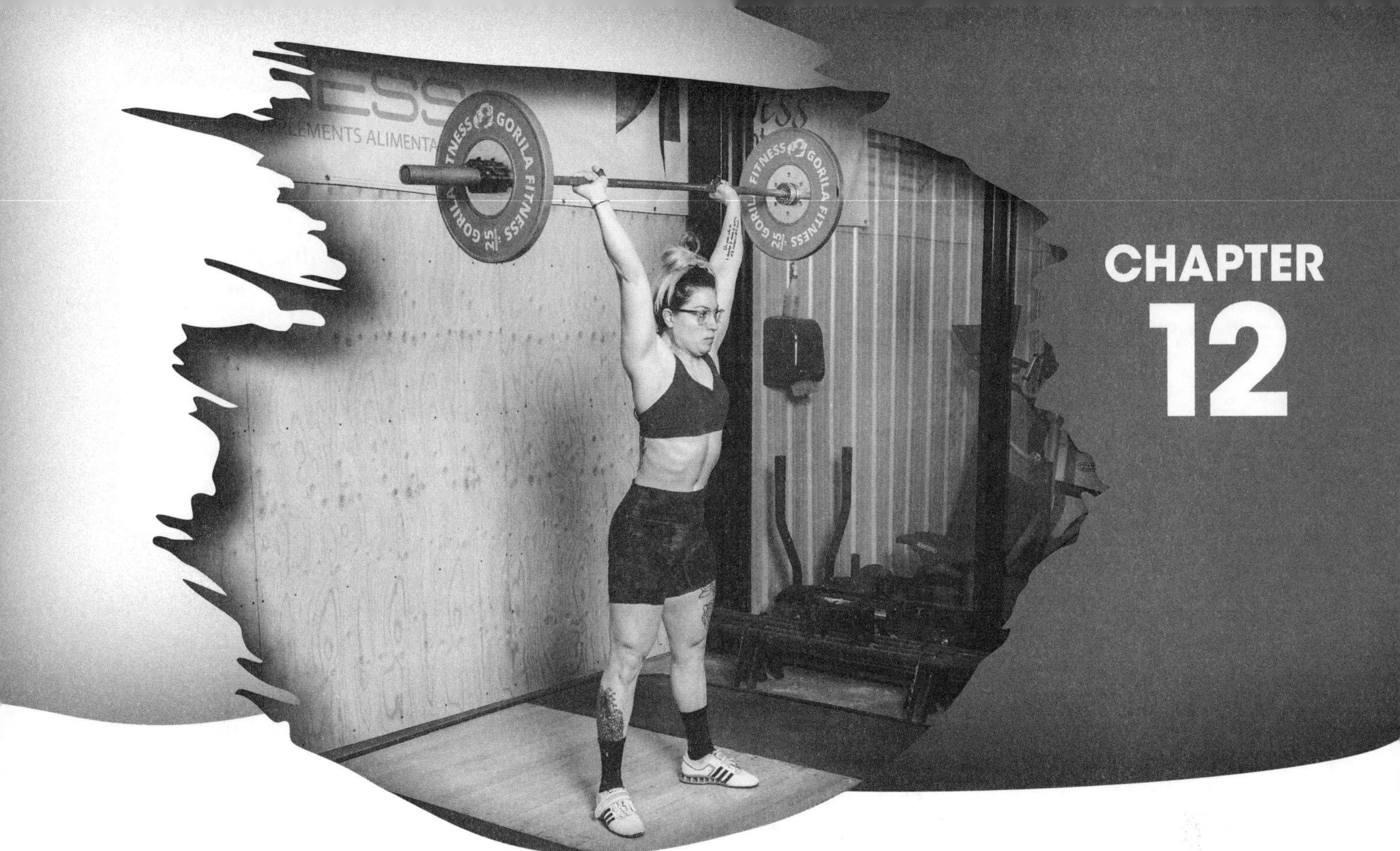

CHAPTER 12

Training Program Design

Now that we have covered the important facets of the overload system—exercise selection, training methods and their parameters, and the broad strokes of effective programming—we can start piecing everything together. The goal of this chapter is to help you design plans that make the most out of this "modern old-school" training approach.

Training Splits

This section presents three programs, each using a different training split, that are the simplest to plan and also the most effective in my experience. I would use one of these approaches for close to 90 percent of the people who want to use the overload system. I would use different options if someone wanted to focus on bringing up one or two specific lifts. But that's a whole other book! Let's master the basics first.

Lift-Specific Training Split

We will start with the easiest split to program for: the lift-specific training split (which we covered in chapter 11). In this training split, each day focuses on one main lift. The assistance exercises (chapter 10) are selected to strengthen and support that lift. Remember, even though we presented the squat, deadlift, bench press, military press, barbell row, and explosive pulls as the primary lifts, it is perfectly fine to use variations of these movements as your main lifts. For example, you might decide to use the Zercher squat or front squat as your main lift if these are better suited to your body type than squats. You can use an incline bench press instead of a bench press, a sumo deadlift, or a hybrid deadlift (narrower stance sumo) instead of a deadlift, a push press instead of a military press, or a chin-up instead of a barbell row. Just please don't use a leg press, machine bench, leg curl, or machine shoulder press as your main movements! Non-free-weight exercises simply don't have the same training effect (which we discussed earlier).

In this split, there are four training days in a training week, or what is also commonly called a microcycle. I call it a training week because if you use a 1-on/1-off approach, it will take you eight days to complete a full rotation. To begin, the first thing to do is to select four main lifts. Normally, even though it is a great exercise, the Pendlay row is not one of the main four lifts, but it is used as an assistance movement in at least one session a week (we use it in two or three sessions). It can be the same thing with the explosive pull. If it is a pull (power shrug, low pull, high pull), it is normally used as one of the assistance lifts; if it is a full Olympic lift (power clean, power snatch), it is best used as a main movement. Assuming that most people will stick to a pull and not an Olympic lift, what I like to do is put a row variation on two of the training days (bench press and squat days, usually) and the explosive pull on the two other days (deadlift and overhead lift days). The Pendlay row and explosive pulls are great exercises, but they don't function well as main lifts in this system since many of the methods we use for the main lift (e.g., progressive range of motion, partial lifts) don't work with these movements.

Considering all of this, a sample typical four-day training week would look like this:

Day 1	Day 2	Day 3	Day 4	Day 5	Day 6	Day 7
Squat	Off	Bench press	Off	Deadlift	Overhead lift	Off

Or, if you use the 1-on/1-off approach, your training week would look like this:

Day 1	Day 2	Day 3	Day 4	Day 5	Day 6	Day 7	Day 8
Squat	Off	Bench press	Off	Deadlift	Off	Overhead lift	Off

A typical workout session for the lift-specific split would look like this:

Lift-Specific Training Split: Sample Typical Four-Day Workout Session

1. Main lift (deadlift, squat, overhead lift, bench press).

2. Overload system method for main lift (supramaximal partials, accentuated eccentrics, functional isometrics, isometronics; the progressive range of motion method, which is not included in this scenario, is discussed later in this section)
3. Assistance exercise to address weak point in main lift
4. Pulling movement (explosive pull or Pendlay row)
5. Remedial exercise 1 (*optional*)
6. Remedial exercise 2 (*optional*)

The lift-specific training split is where most people will start. It is super easy to structure and will work every single time in terms of getting you stronger on your chosen lifts. Remember, the optional remedial exercises are isolation exercises targeting either a lagging muscle group (ideally related to the main lift) or a muscle you want to emphasize, or they are used for injury prevention. Whether you do them will usually depend on how fatiguing you find the main workload. If you are struggling to recover, then it's often best to leave them out.

An advanced workout session, for those who are experienced with these methods and performing at a high level, adds an activation exercise at the beginning of the session with the purpose of priming the nervous system as well as getting you ready to lift heavy weights on the main lift of the day. To allow the use of that activation movement, we also remove one remedial exercise (we don't usually want to use more than six exercises per session). An advanced workout session for the lift-specific split would look like this:

Lift-Specific Training Split: Sample Advanced Workout Session

1. Activation exercise: non-fatiguing overload (supramaximal hold or overcoming isometrics)
2. Main lift (deadlift, squat, overhead, bench press)
3. Overload system method for main lift (supramax partials, accentuated eccentrics, functional isometrics, isometronics; the progressive range of motion method, not included in this scenario, will be discussed later)
4. Assistance exercise to address weak point in main lift
5. Pulling movement (explosive pull or Pendlay row)
6. Remedial exercise 1 (*optional*)

Note that the activation exercise is either a supramaximal hold (which we covered earlier) or an overcoming isometric, where you are pushing or pulling against an immovable resistance (normally the safety pins in a power rack). Its best uses are either to strengthen a weak point in the range of motion (by positioning the pins just above your sticking point) or as an activation tool (normally positioning the pins slightly higher than the position used to address the weak point, as you will produce more force). To use an activation exercise to strengthen a weak point, position the bar just above the sticking point and push as hard as you can for 6 to 9 seconds. Do 3 to 4 sets. Or, for activation purposes, position the bar a few inches above the position you would use for strengthening the weak point and push as hard as you can for 3 seconds. Do 2 to 3 sets.

As you saw in the previous examples of the lift-specific split sessions, we noted that the progressive range of motion (PRM) method is not used. If you decide to use the PRM method, it becomes the main lift since it will eventually become the full-range lift. We also do not want to do both the regular full-range lift and the PRM method in the same training block. Performing the PRM sets as well as heavy work sets using full range of motion for the same lift is simply too taxing. Your performance would suffer in whichever exercise you did second, and you would likely end up burned out (especially if you were doing this for all your sessions). A PRM workout session for the lift-specific split would look like this:

Lift-Specific Training Split: Sample PRM Workout Session

1. PRM for the main lift (deadlift, squat, overhead lift, bench press)
2. Variation of the main lift that is not the main lift
3. Bottom partial technique (functional isometrics, overcoming isometrics, isometronics, regular partial reps) *or* accentuated eccentrics
4. Pulling movement (explosive pull or Pendlay row)
5. Remedial exercise 1 (*optional*)
6. Remedial exercise 2 (*optional*)

On exercise 2, you pick an exercise that is similar to the main lift but is not the main lift. Here are some options you can use:

Main lift	Variations of the main lift
Deadlift	Sumo deadlift, hybrid deadlift, deficit deadlift, Romanian deadlift, barbell hack squat (behind-the-back deadlift)
Squat	Zercher squat, front squat, low box squat, safety bar squat, camber bar squat, heels-elevated squat, wide-stance squat, Frankenstein squat
Military press	Bradford press, behind-the-neck press, high-incline bench press, dumbbell shoulder press (*note*: I don't recommend the push press because it does not stimulate the low portion of the range of motion), wide-grip shoulder press, reverse-grip shoulder press
Bench press	Incline bench press, decline bench press, close-grip bench press, wide-grip bench press, reverse-grip bench press, floor press

On exercise 3, you want to pick an exercise or method that will allow you to strengthen the bottom of the range of motion on the main lift. That's because for most of a PRM cycle, you don't train that part of the range in the main movement itself. While using a full-range movement that is similar to the main lift for your second exercise, it might not be enough to fully strengthen that part of the range on the main lift itself.

You can use functional isometrics or isometronics in the lower third of the range; use overcoming isometrics (which we just covered) somewhere in the lower third (it doesn't have to be at the lowest point) or simply use the main lift (squat, bench, deadlift, overhead); and then do bottom half or bottom third reps (e.g., doing deadlifts going from floor to knees). Another option (best for very advanced individuals) is to do eccentric sets. Here we don't want too much of an overload. Go with the same weight you used for your PRM and perform 3 to 4 sets of 1 rep, doing the eccentric phase only, as slowly as humanly possible for the whole range of motion.

Whole-Body Training Split

Let's now look at our second training split option: three whole-body workouts and a possible fourth session that is a gap workout (where all the remedial work is done). This option opens up a ton of possibilities, and you can play around with different workout compositions, but I'll present the simplest and most effective way to use it, in my experience. A sample typical four-day training week would look like this:

Day 1	Day 2	Day 3	Day 4	Day 5	Day 6	Day 7
Whole-body 1	Off	Whole-body 2	Off	Whole-body 3	Gap	Off

Or, if you use the 1-on/1-off approach, your training week would look like this:

Day 1	Day 2	Day 3	Day 4	Day 5	Day 6	Day 7	Day 8
Whole-body 1	Off	Whole-body 2	Off	Whole-body 3	Off	Gap	Off

Without a gap workout, here are two options for how your 1-on/1-off training week would look like this:

	Day 1	Day 2	Day 3	Day 4	Day 5	Day 6	Day 7
OPTION 1	Whole-body 1	Off	Whole-body 2	Off	Whole-body 3	Off	Off
OPTION 2	Whole-body 1	Off	Whole-body 2	Off	Off	Whole-body 3	Off

For the whole-body sessions involved in this structure, I like to use an approach in which we use a different method on every workout and we apply that method to all the lifts (i.e., eccentric focused methods in workout 1; isometric methods in workout 2; and normal or concentric methods in workout 3). Also, since a gap workout is included in this training week, you will not do any remedial work (you can do grip work) on the whole-body workout days. Sample whole-body and gap workout sessions for a typical four-day whole-body training week would look like this:

Whole-Body Training Split: Sample Typical Workout Sessions

Whole-Body 1

Note: The PRM method is not included in this scenario (more on this later).

1. Overload method for squat (partial overloads, functional isometrics, isometronics, accentuated eccentrics)
2. Overload method for bench press (partial overloads, functional isometrics, isometronics, accentuated eccentrics)
3. Overload method for deadlift (partial overloads, functional isometrics, isometronics, accentuated eccentrics)
4. Overload method for overhead lifts (partial overloads, functional isometrics, isometronics, accentuated eccentrics)

Whole-Body 2

1. Assistance exercise for squat
2. Assistance exercise for bench press
3. Assistance exercise for deadlift
4. Assistance exercise for overhead lifts

Whole-Body 3

1. Squat
2. Bench press
3. Deadlift
4. Military press

Gap Workout

1. Explosive pull
2. Pendlay row
3. Remedial exercise for squat and bench press
4. Remedial exercise for bench press and military press
5. Grip exercise (*optional*)
6. Abs exercise (*optional*)

In the previous whole-body 1 session, we noted that the PRM method is not used in this scenario because it alters the training split you would use (which I address below). If you decide to use the PRM method, it becomes the main lift because it will eventually become the full-range lift. We also do not want to do both the regular lift (performed over the full ROM) and the PRM method in the same training block. A PRM workout session for the whole-body split would look like this:

Whole-Body Training Split: Sample PRM Workout Sessions

Whole-Body 1

1. PRM for squat
2. PRM for bench press
3. PRM for deadlift
4. PRM for overhead lifts

Whole-Body 2

1. Assistance exercise for squat
2. Assistance exercise for bench press
3. Assistance exercise for deadlift
4. Assistance exercise for overhead lifts

Whole-Body 3

Note: You'll notice that we have two PRM sessions per week. The goal should be to get more reps in the second session than the first one. Usually, we use 3 work sets for the PRM method. This is what is always done on day 1. If on day 3 you can beat your best set (more reps) from day 1 on your first set, then you only do that one set and ramp up to the heaviest single you can do from the position you are at. If you get the same number of reps as on your best set of day 1 (or less), you do your 3 work sets and don't do the heavy singles.

1. PRM for squat with possible ramp up
2. PRM for bench press with possible ramp up
3. PRM for deadlift with possible ramp up
4. PRM for overhead lifts with possible ramp up

Gap Workout

1. Explosive pull
2. Pendlay row
3. Remedial exercise for squat and bench press
4. Remedial exercise for bench press and military press
5. Grip exercise (*optional*)
6. Abs exercise (*optional*)

Lift-Specific and Whole-Body Hybrid Split

Our final training split option is the lift-specific and whole-body hybrid. With this option, you pair one upper body main lift with one lower body main lift (e.g., squat or bench and deadlift or military press). There will be two workouts for each pair. This option works best with a 1-on/1-off approach because it will allow you to have a rest day after each session, which is especially relevant since we are training the whole body at each session. If you can't do that, then the second-best option is to do the following:

Day 1	Day 2	Day 3	Day 4	Day 5	Day 6	Day 7
Squat/bench press 1 (or whatever lifts you choose)	Off	Deadlift/military press 1 (or whatever lifts you choose)	Off	Squat/bench press 2 (or whatever lifts you choose)	Deadlift/military press 2 (or whatever lifts you choose)	Off

In this setup, the first two sessions are more neurologically demanding due to the overload work done on two lifts; therefore, we need to make sure those sessions have a rest day before and after them. The secondary sessions for each lift pairing are slightly less intense, so we can get away with doing them on consecutive days. I must stress, however, that this is less than ideal. Whatever lifts are done on the second day will most likely suffer because of fatigue from the previous day's workout.

Lift-Specific and Whole-Body Hybrid Split: Sample Typical Training Sessions

Squat or Bench Press 1

1. Overload method for squat
2. Overload method for bench press
3. Assistance exercise for squat
4. Assistance exercise for bench press
5. Remedial exercise for squat (*optional*)
6. Remedial exercise for bench press (*optional*)

Deadlift or Military Press 1

1. Overload method for deadlift
2. Overload method for military press
3. Assistance exercise for deadlift
4. Assistance exercise for military press
5. Remedial exercise for deadlift (*optional*)
6. Remedial exercise for military press (*optional*)

Squat or Bench Press 2

Note: The PRM method is not included in this scenario (more on this later in this section).

1. Non-fatiguing overload for squat (supramaximal hold or overcoming isometrics)
2. Squat (or the variation that suits you best)
3. Non-fatiguing overload for bench (supramaximal hold or overcoming isometrics)
4. Bench press (or the variation that suits you best)
5. Explosive pull
6. Remedial exercise for squat or bench press (*optional*)

Deadlift or Military Press 2

Note: The PRM method is not included in this scenario (more on this later).

1. Non-fatiguing overload for deadlift (supramaximal hold or overcoming isometrics)
2. Deadlift (or the variation that suits you best)
3. Non-fatiguing overload for military press (supramaximal hold or overcoming isometrics)
4. Military press (or the variation that suits you best)
5. Pendlay row
6. Remedial exercise for deadlift or military press (*optional*)

As noted previously, the PRM method is not used in the scenarios for the squat or bench press 2 and deadlift or military press 2 sessions. Once again, it means that we need to set up the split in a slightly different manner to compensate for the fact that we are not performing the full-range lift each week. If you decide to use the PRM method, it becomes the main lift because it will eventually become the full-range lift. We also do not want to do both the regular full-range lift and the PRM method in the same training block. A PRM workout session for the lift-specific and whole-body hybrid split would look like this:

Lift-Specific and Whole-Body Hybrid Training Split: Sample PRM Workout Sessions

Squat or Bench Press 1

1. PRM for squat
2. PRM for bench press
3. Assistance exercise for squat
4. Assistance exercise for bench press
5. Remedial exercise for squat (*optional*)
6. Remedial exercise for bench press (*optional*)

Deadlift or Military Press 1

1. PRM for deadlift
2. PRM for military press
3. Assistance exercise for deadlift
4. Assistance exercise for military press
5. Remedial exercise for deadlift (*optional*)
6. Remedial exercise for military press (*optional*)

Squat or Bench Press 2

1. PRM for squat
2. PRM for bench press
3. Bottom partial technique for squat (functional isometric, overcoming isometrics, isometronics, regular partial reps) *or* accentuated eccentrics
4. Bottom partial technique for bench (functional isometric, overcoming isometrics, isometronics, regular partial reps) *or* accentuated eccentrics

5. Explosive pull
6. Remedial exercise for squat or bench press (*optional*)

Deadlift or Military Press 2

1. PRM for deadlift
2. PRM for military press
3. Bottom partial technique for deadlift (functional isometric, overcoming isometrics, isometronics, regular partial reps) *or* accentuated eccentrics
4. Bottom partial technique for military press (functional isometric, overcoming isometrics, isometronics, regular partial reps) *or* accentuated eccentrics
5. Pendlay row
6. Remedial exercise for deadlift or military press (*optional*)

Loading Schemes

Old-school lifting was all about getting stronger, and while you certainly can get stronger by training with slightly higher repetitions (provided that you gradually add weight to the bar over time), training with lower reps with a higher proportion of your maximum is the most effective way to boost strength. That doesn't necessarily mean 1 to 2 sets or even 3 reps, though (which would be called the maximum effort method when using weights at or above 90 percent of your maximum), but it certainly means using weights at or above 80 percent of your maximum.

A lot of recent research shows that muscle gained from high reps and muscle gained from low reps is the same. However, the research shows that training with heavier weights leads to significantly more strength gains than when using lighter loads, even if muscle growth is the same. This is unsurprising because your capacity to produce force does not depend solely on the amount of muscle that you have. Neurological factors are at least as important as well as protective mechanisms like the Golgi tendon organs (GTOs).

Training with heavier weights has a greater impact on the neurological factors than using lighter loads. Basically, you need to lift heavy to gain as much strength as possible. This is in accordance with the specificity principle, which states that you improve the most in the type of work that you train. Or as Charles Poliquin said: "You become stronger in the rep range(s) that you train."

While doing sets of 1 to 2 reps will certainly make you stronger, it is not actually the best way to build strength by itself. Sets of 1 to 2 reps (92.5 to 100 percent of your max) are the best at improving your capacity to demonstrate the muscle strength potential that you have. It is the zone that has the greatest impact on fast-twitch fiber recruitment, firing rate, and intramuscular coordination. It is also where you have the most effect on reducing the protective force inhibition by the GTOs, but it's not the zone that is the most effective at increasing your strength potential. The reason is that, in most cases, it is not conducive to stimulating muscle growth. That's because there is not enough mechanical work per set, and if you do enough sets to get a proper amount of mechanical work, it will lead to neurological fatigue pretty quickly (it would require a good 15 sets of 1 rep or 8 sets of 2 reps with maximal weights).

The best zone to develop strength is the range of 3 to 6 reps (80 to 90 percent of your max). That's where you have enough load to have a significant impact on the neurological factors involved in force production *and* have sufficient mechanical work to trigger muscle growth. Sets of 8 to 12 reps (60 to 75 percent) provide more mechanical work per set and can thus lead to slightly more muscle growth, but the effects on the neurological factors are much lower.

That's why in this system we favor loads in the 80 to 90 percent range (for full-range movements), with occasional sets or phases in the 90 to 100 percent range.

For remedial work (targeted or isolated exercises), higher reps are to be done since they are only used to build muscle and improve tendon resilience. We actually want to minimize the neurological stress on these exercises. That's why sets of 8 to 12, as well as much higher rep work (up to 50 reps per set), are used for these movements.

For the multijoint movements (main lifts and assistance work), we want most of our sets to use 3 to 6 reps, with the occasional inclusion of sets of 1 to 2 reps (if you want to focus more on strength) or 7 to 8 reps (to focus on hypertrophy while still gaining some maximal strength). Usually, sets closer to 8 reps are only done on assistance exercises.

Here are some of the loading schemes that I find to be the most effective with this system of training:

Ramping Straight Sets

You perform 3 to 6 sets with a designated number of repetitions. You start more conservatively and add weight from set to set until you reach your top weight.

Wave Loading

Each wave consists of 3 sets (with a normal rest between sets), and each set within a wave uses more weight but less reps. The first wave is more conservative; the rate of perceived effort (RPE) is around 8. The second wave is slightly heavier than the first wave (RPE 9). Usually, I do a warm-up wave before the work waves (same 3 set progression as the work wave but with an RPE of 6 to 7). Waves work best with low to moderate reps. For example: 7-5-3 wave, 6-4-2 wave, 5-4-3 wave, 5-3-1 wave, 3-2-1 wave.

Single-Set Pyramid

Here you use a 3 to 6 set progression where you add weight from set to set but reduce the reps to keep the RPE stable (RPE 8 or 9). The more sets in a pyramid, the lower the RPE should be. For example, if a pyramid has 3 or 4 sets, you can use an RPE of 8.5 to 9, but if you have 5 to 6 sets, it is better to keep RPE at 7.5 to 8. My favorite variation of this method is the 5-4-3-2-1 countdown, but you can use pretty much any variation where you reduce the number of reps per set by 1 from set to set. You can even use a 2 rep decrease if you use less sets—for example, 6-4-2; 5-3-1; 7-5-3; or 8-6-4.

Double-Set Pyramid

Here you perform 4 to 8 work sets for an exercise, adding weight on every set but only decreasing the reps every 2 sets. The first set with a weight is easier (RPE 7 or 8) while the second is harder (8 or 9). You can do something like this: 8-8-6-6; 6-6-4-4; 5-5-3-3; 3-3-1-1; 8-8-6-6-4-4; 6-6-4-4-2-2; 5-5-3-3-1-1; or 4-4-2-2-1-1.

Double Pyramid

This is very similar to wave loading. In the ascending portion of the pyramid, you add weight while decreasing reps; then, in the descending portion of the pyramid, you do the opposite. Normally, the ascending portion is considered easier (RPE 8), and the descending portion uses a bit more weight (RPE 9). Here is an example:

- *3-sets double pyramid*: 8-6-8; 7-5-7; 6-4-6; 4-2-4; 3-1-3
- *4-sets double pyramid*: 8-6-6-8; 7-5-5-7; 6-4-4-6; 5-3-3-5; 4-2-2-4; 3-1-1-3
- *5-sets double pyramid*: 8-6-4-6-8; 7-5-3-5-7; 6-4-2-4-6; 5-3-1-3-5; 3-2-1-2-3
- *6-sets double pyramid*: 8-8-6-6-8-8; 7-7-5-5-7-7; 6-6-4-4-6-6; 5-5-3-3-5-5; 4-4-2-2-4-4, 3-3-1-1-3-3

Clusters

These were already explained in-depth in chapter 1, but as a reminder, clusters are sets of 3 to 6 reps where you perform each repetition as a single and have 20 to 60 seconds of rest between repetitions. Typically, we do only 1 to 2 work sets when using clusters.

Rest and Pause

I really love heavy rests and pauses to develop strength while getting more hypertrophy than with regular low-rep sets. You start by doing a normal set, then rest anywhere between 10 and 30 seconds (depending on the movement), and you get as many solid additional reps as you can with the same load. This counts as *one* set. While for pure hypertrophy plans you can start with 8 to 12 reps then do your additional reps, in the scope of this program, the initial portion of your set should use 4 to 6 reps, after which you shoot for an additional 2 to 3 reps. The initial portion of the set should be challenging, but you shouldn't reach failure or the point where you have to significantly grind the weight (RPE of around 8.5); on the second part of the set, you get as many solid reps as you can (RPE 9 or 9.5). Just like clusters, I prefer to do only 1 to 2 sets like this for an exercise, but you can do 1 to 2 normal sets before your rest and pause set.

Contrast Sets

In this method, you perform 2 to 3 pairs of sets. The first set in a pair is done for 1 or 2 reps with a heavy but not maximal load (RPE of around 8); the second set is done for moderate reps (for us), or 3 to 7 reps. Three rules apply when using this method:

1. The first set of the pair (1 to 2 reps at roughly 87.5 to 92.5 percent) remains the same for all the pairs.
2. The second set of the pair should get heavier from wave to wave.
3. Rest 2 minutes between the sets in a pair and 3 to 4 minutes between pairs.

Good examples would be 1-6; 1-5; 1-4; 1-3; 2-8; 2-7; 2-6; and 2-5 pairs.

These are examples of my preferred loading schemes. Feel free to use different ones as long as they fall in the proper rep range and you don't exceed your overall set allocation for the day.

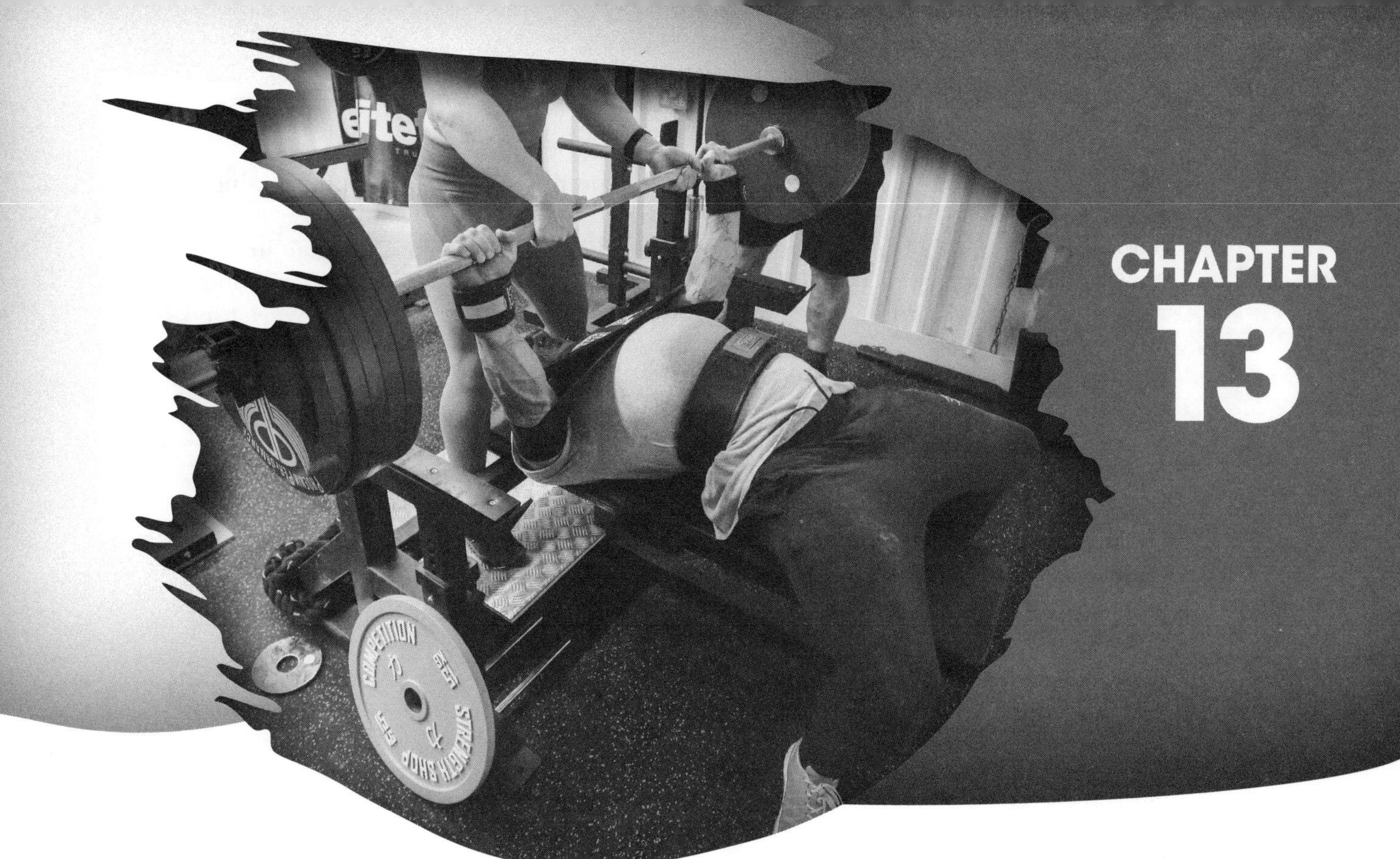

CHAPTER 13

Specialization Training

Specialization training—defined as focusing on one to two body parts or one lift by using a concentrated training approach for a brief period—was a lot more common among old-school lifters than it is today. It's a shame, really, because specialization training is one of the most powerful and effective ways to train. If done right.

Specialization used to be one of the main strategies in the 1930s up to the 1960s. People were doing "arm courses," "chest courses," or focusing on maximizing a single lift. I can personally attest to how effective that approach is. I got my biggest bench press improvements—working up to a max of 445 pounds (202 kilograms)—by specializing on the bench press. I also increased my snatch-grip high pull by 132 pounds (60 kilograms)—that's not a typo—in around 4 weeks by training almost exclusively on it. Recently, I got back to a squat of more than 500 pounds (227 kilograms) for the first time in 20 years by specializing on my squat for 7 weeks. I took it from 425 to 505 pounds (193 to 229 kilograms) at 44 years of age.

It is my honest belief that specialization training is the best way for an advanced lifter to keep progressing, and it is also a very effective approach for fairly qualified intermediate lifters. It can even be turned into a whole training system by rotating the specialization focus every 4 to 6 weeks. I find specialization to be the fastest way to boost your performance on a lift and to bring up a lagging muscle group—provided that you do it properly.

Most people understand and like the basic premise of specialization training: You increase the frequency and amount of work performed on a lift or for one or two muscles. Most of us love to train and doing more (too much) is often in our nature. The problem is that most of us are not as much on board with the second part of the specialization equation: You need to reduce the amount of work for the lifts or muscles you are not specializing on. Specialization training will not work if you don't do both. The more work you add for the specialized work, the more you must decrease it for everything else. That's because training has both local and systemic effects that lead to targeted and overall fatigue:

Local Fatigue Effects

Muscle damage to the trained muscles

Glycogen depletion

ATP-CP depletion

Loss of intramuscular triglycerides

Local inflammation

Desensitization of the neuromuscular junction

Decreased firing rate of muscle spindles, leading to decreased motoneurons firing

Systemic Fatigue Effects

Decreased excitatory drive from the motor cortex

Downregulation of the beta-adrenergic receptors

Changes in neurotransmitter levels, leading to central fatigue

Increased demands on the immune system

Increased cortisol, which affects whole-body protein synthesis

Increased brain glutamate levels, decreasing one's pain threshold (you feel pain more easily)

Essentially, the muscles themselves have a limit in terms of the stress and damage that they can recover from. Your whole body also has a limited amount of overall work that it can withstand and positively adapt to in order to maintain an optimal performance level and state of well-being. That is why it's important to maintain pretty much the same overall training volume when you do a specialization routine as when you do your normal training. For example, suppose that in a training week, you do 4 sessions with 5 exercises each for a total of 20 work sets per workout. That gives you 80 total work sets per week. Usually, those 80 work sets might be divided pretty much equally among the main lifts and their assistance work, but during a specialization routine, you might decide to invest 40 of those sets to the bench press and its assistance work. That would leave you 40 work sets to spend on deadlifts, squats, rowing, and overhead work (and their assistance exercises) during the week. Your volume distribution might now look like this (this is *not* a specific recommendation but is meant to illustrate that you must decrease volume for the nonspecialized work during a specialization phase):

Bench press	20-25 sets per week
Bench press assistance exercise	20-25 sets per week
Squat	3-5 sets per week
Deadlift	3-5 sets per week
Squat and deadlift assistance exercise	8-10 total sets per week (ideally, pick exercises that improve both)
Military press	3-5 sets per week
Military press assistance exercise	None (there is already a lot of pressing volume in this phase)
Rowing	10-15 sets per week

Once you get your head around the fact that you need to keep the overall training volume the same, planning a specialization phase is not that complicated. Likewise, once you can do that, then it is quite easy to plan out a whole specialization cycle where you line up several different specialization phases, focusing on different lifts, to create a whole training system.

Frequency

When you use a specialized approach, it is important to increase the frequency of training for the lift or muscle(s) you are focusing on. This is crucial for several reasons:

- Doing all the extra volume in one session is not going to be productive. At least half of the work will be of poor quality because of fatigue, and you will have a hard time recovering after the session.
- A higher frequency leads to a faster neurological improvement, which is critical for strength and skill development.
- Each session stimulates protein synthesis in the trained muscle. The more often you can hit a muscle, the more bouts of increased protein synthesis you get, the more growth you are likely to stimulate.
- Spreading the volume for the specialized lift or muscle(s) over more sessions allows you to be able to recover from more overall volume for that lift or muscle(s).

I find that it is best to spread the weekly volume for the specialization lift or muscle(s) over three workouts and put the rest of the work either on a fourth workout or put a small amount in each of the three weekly workouts. In our example on page 169, I would put the small amount of overhead work on one of the bench press workouts, spread the rowing work over the three bench sessions, and do the squat and deadlift work on their own day so that it looks like this (again, this is not a specific recommendation, just an illustration of a weekly schedule):

Monday	Tuesday	Wednesday	Thursday	Friday	Saturday	Sunday
Bench press and assistance exercise: 20 total sets *Rowing*: 5 sets	Off	*Bench press and assistance exercise*: 20 total sets *Rowing*: 5 sets	Off	*Squat*: 3-5 sets *Deadlift*: 3-5 sets *Squat and deadlift assistance exercise*: 8-10 sets	*Bench press and assistance exercise*: 10 total sets *Military press*: 3-5 sets *Rowing*: 2-3 sets	Off

Structure

There are several ways of setting up specialization work. We will start with the premise that we include work for the specialized lift or muscle(s) 3 days a week. There are quite a few options, and you can even combine more than one approach. In reality, they will all work pretty well, but which one is optimal depends on the person you are using the specialization program with as well as the main goal. Here are some guidelines you can use to choose your loading scheme:

Uniform Loading

Essentially, you perform the same type of work (exercises, methods, intensity zone) and similar volume on all three of the workouts. Beginners should use this scheme because it has the least variation. They need to focus on mastering the main lifts and using their body properly. The more variation you have, the harder it will be to accomplish those goals. Not to mention that, at their level, they do not need to vary the stimulus to keep progressing.

Daily Undulating Periodization

In this approach, you keep using the same exercises and methods, but you vary the loading schemes. You could have one very heavy day (sets of 1 to 3 reps), a volume day (sets of 8 to 12 reps), and a mixed strength and hypertrophy day (sets of 4 to 6 reps). This is a suitable approach for intermediate lifters, once they have a better foundation of technique on their main lift(s) because it introduces a little variation without changing too many variables. Daily undulating periodization is also a good approach when someone wants to build strength but also needs or wants to add a significant amount of muscle mass.

Exercise Variation

Here you use different exercises on each day. This could mean doing one workout where you do mostly work on the specialized lift itself and assistance movements on the two other days. Exercise variation works better for someone who has a lot of experience and is already very technically efficient on the main lifts. The more stable and efficient your technique is, the more exercise variation you can use.

Method Variation

You can also use different training methods on each training day. This could mean full-range on one day, partial overloads or eccentric overloads on another, and isometronics and functional isometrics on the third (or other methods). The method variation is the approach that best uses the full teachings contained in this book. I personally prefer to use variation in the form of methods than exercises. It is more effective for most individuals.

Physical Capacity Variation

This is similar to the daily undulating periodization, but we not only change the intensity zone but also the way the sets and reps are performed. For example, we could have a limit-strength day (sets of 1 to 3 reps in the 90 to 100 percent range), a strength-speed day (sets of 3-5 reps with 60-70 percent done explosively), and a strength-skill day (where we do a high number of sets of 2-3 reps with 80-85 percent). Physical capacity variation is best suited for athletes who not only need to be strong but also explosive and have good endurance (e.g., you could use strength, strength-speed, and resistance and endurance days).

Contraction Type Variation

This is the approach used in my OCTS programming (Omni-Contraction Training System). Day 1 uses eccentric-emphasis methods (slow eccentrics or eccentric overloads); day 2 uses isometric methods (stato-dynamic, functional isometrics, isometronics); and day 3 uses concentric methods (regular lifting, partials). Contraction type variation is very similar to the method variation approach. I've used this as a full system with a variety of clients, ranging from beginners to elite athletes, and it never fails to deliver great results, mostly because the vast majority of people undertrain eccentric and isometric actions and when you start focusing on them, you have rapid gains. Of course, with beginners, you stay with the lower stress methods like slow eccentrics and stato-dynamic sets instead of the overload methods.

Duration

It can be tempting to stay on a specialization phase for a long time because it works! When done properly, it works very well. Chances are that when you decide to specialize on a certain lift or muscle(s), it is either because it is lagging or not progressing as rapidly as you would like, or it is because it is a lift or muscle that you really love to emphasize. In other words, seeing significant progress somewhere you haven't been able to make progress on before (or on something you put a high value on) can become addictive.

The reality is that the longer you stay on a specialization routine, the less you will progress. But that's not the bad thing. The worst thing is that by staying on a specialization phase for a long time, you reduce the responsiveness of the muscle(s) you are focusing on. Getting stronger or adding muscle is part of a process called *adaptation*. Your body makes structural and functional changes in response to a physiological or physical (or psychological) stress so that it will be better suited to face that stress if it comes back again. The stronger the stress is, the greater and faster the adaptations will be. That's the whole premise behind specialization training: increasing the magnitude to the stress imposed on certain muscles so that they have a greater amount and rate of adaptation.

However, this also means that your muscles rapidly become well adapted (habituated) to the stress presented. When a muscle is well adapted to a stress, it becomes very hard to force further changes because they are not seen as needed. In previous chapters, I gave suntanning and coffee drinking as analogies; at some point your body desensitizes to the stimulus, and you are doing a bunch of extra work for no benefit.

Building muscle and strength, however, is a little more complex. For one thing, there are several mechanisms and pathways that allow you to gain size or strength, but the basic premise still largely applies: doing a high-stress specialization for a lift or muscle(s) for too long will make it more complicated to keep the lift or muscle(s) progressing when you go back to regular training.

However, ironically, doing a shorter specialization phase can make regular training more effective. That's because more frequent stimulation of a muscle improves your capacity to recruit and contract that muscle. This makes your future training for that muscle group more effective.

If you can do that without reaching a point where the muscle(s) you are focused on become habituated (desensitized to training), you will get faster gains when you go back to regular training. However, if you keep up the specialization for too long, it can backfire—although there are strategies you can use to keep a muscle responsive after a longer specialization phase (see table 13.1).

TABLE 13.1 Risk of Habituation with Specialization and Strategies to Avoid Issues

Duration	Risk of habituation	Strategy to use
2-3 weeks	Beginners: low Intermediate: low Advanced: low	None needed, but you might want to do an overall deload week.
4-6 weeks	Beginners: low Intermediate: moderate Advanced: moderate	Intermediate and advanced lifters should *dramatically* reduce the amount of volume for the lift or muscle(s) they specialized on for 2-4 weeks to resensitize.
7 weeks +	Beginners: moderate Intermediate: high Advanced: high	Beginners should dramatically reduce the amount of work for the lift or muscle they specialized on (maintenance level) for 2-4 weeks. Intermediate and advanced lifters should try to avoid stimulating the lift or muscle(s) they specialized on completely for 2-4 weeks to resensitize.

Rotation

Due to the fact that we need to reestablish sensitivity to training stress, an effective approach, especially for advanced lifters, is to use a specialization rotation as your baseline training philosophy. Basically, all you do is specialization training (except for maintenance and deload phases), and you rotate the lift or muscle(s) you are specializing on every 3-4 weeks (advanced) or 4-6 weeks (intermediate).

Why is it effective? Because when you reach a certain stage of development and training experience, your body is well adapted to regular training stress, so you need a much higher level of training stress to keep progressing at a significant rate. However, as we saw, the body has a limited capacity to adapt to training stress, so you can't just do more of everything and expect to progress. Especially since, as you get stronger, the same relative intensity of work (percent of your maximum) becomes more stressful to your body. Consider that squatting 500 pounds (227 kilograms) is more stressful on your body than squatting 250 pounds (113 kilograms), even if both represent 80 percent of your maximum.

Specialization rotation can become a viable and effective strategy to provide a strong growth stimulus for certain muscles without exceeding your capacity to recover. Sure, it means that you'll get rapid progress only on one lift or one or two muscles at a time while the rest are maintained, but isn't that better than getting excruciatingly slow progress everywhere? Here are some guidelines to make specialization rotation work optimally:

Do not specialize on two related lifts or muscles in a row.

For example, when you do pectoral work, the deltoids and triceps will also be involved in many of the exercises you use. Same thing with the bench and overhead press or deadlift and squat; they will hit similar muscles. If you specialize on pectorals (or bench) for 4 weeks, then on triceps and delts (or overhead press) for 4 weeks, the pressing muscles (pectorals, deltoids, triceps) are essentially being trained at specialization levels for 8 weeks, and you will run into trouble.

In the phase directly following a specialization for a lift or muscle(s), reduce direct work for that lift or muscle(s) as much as possible.

You can bring it back up in the second phase after the specialization phase, but in the phase immediately following a specialization, reduce it as much as you are comfortable doing. This is both to quickly resensitize the muscle(s) involved and to get a rebound growth effect (a lot of time you get the most growth in the lift or muscle you specialized in the 1-2 weeks after the cessation of the specialization phase).

Gradually ramp up the training stress over 3 weeks.

Going from normal (or maintenance) volume to maximum specialization volume right from the start might be too much for the body to positively adapt to. It is best to gradually increase the amount of work for the specific lift or muscle(s) over the first 3 weeks of the block. Week 3 should be the highest sustainable training stress, and then do a *deload* for week 4. In this situation, the deload should simply be going back to the amount of work you did in week 1. It's not really a deload in the purest sense of the word, but a reduction in stress relative to week 3. This allows you to go all in on that third week (the shock week).

Avoid special overload methods when you are not specializing on a lift or muscle(s).

It is tempting to keep using powerful methods like partial overloads, progressive range of motion, eccentrics overload, or clusters (as examples) when you stop specializing on a lift. I might reason that since my volume will be much lower, I might as well use the most powerful methods to get as much progress as I can from the minimal volume I'm doing. That's missing the whole point of the system! This will just make it harder to keep the involved muscles maximally responsive and will reduce the gains you will get from your next specialization phase for that lift or muscle(s). When you are not specializing on a lift or muscle(s), you still want to train hard on the sets you are doing, but use regular lifting, not special methods.

Personally, specialization rotation as a training system is my favorite approach with advanced lifters. It is unconventional and even a bit scary because of the dramatic reduction in volume when you are not specializing on a lift or muscle(s). That worry is the reason people fail on this approach: They just do too much for the nonspecialized lift or muscle(s), and they both burn out and fail to reestablish the sensitivity of their muscles. But if you do it right, it is one of the most powerful approaches you can use.

EPILOGUE

We hope you enjoyed this book and, more importantly, took away a few ideas that will make your own training or, if you are a coach, the training of your clients better.

It's true that in our world of pump and tone for the 'gram (I fantasize that people reading this book in 20 years will have absolutely no idea what Instagram is), the ideas promoted in this book might actually sound like heresy.

Lift uncomfortably heavy weights only on barbell exercises? What kind of nonsense is that? What about isolating my medial deltoid and the long head of my biceps?

Sadly, we see more and more people content to be a 2005 Honda Civic with a $30,000 body kit and the same 105-horsepower engine: all show and no go. But if you bought this book (thank you, by the way, because you are contributing toward that Porsche that Christian has been waiting to get), it is because you are attracted to hard, effective training and value developing the capacity to perform as much as look good.

Thank you for being part of the same dying breed as we are. Now, go out and show them what it means to be a hard worker.

Be less bad tomorrow.

APPENDIX: STRENGTH STANDARDS

With the increasing popularity of strength training and strength sports, the upper limit seems to be getting pushed higher at a fast rate. World records are climbing, and more freaks are appearing every year. This makes it hard for us to decipher what constitutes "strong" for us mortals. Luckily, we can use strength standards as our guide. We have laid out some fair standards for most of the population to shoot for in the main lifts used in this system. And depending on where your numbers are within those standards, you will fall into one of the following categories:

Gold standard—This is considered the beginning of the very strong or freak zone.

Killin' it—You are among the strongest in most regular gyms.

Good—Respectable. You've done good, kid.

Less bad—Keep working at it.

Seek help—Do it now.

Bench Press

Gold standard—2.0 × bodyweight (male); 1.5 × bodyweight (female)

Killin' it—Over 1.5 × bodyweight (male); over 1.0 × bodyweight (female)

Good—1.25 to 1.5 × bodyweight (male); 0.75 to 1.0 × bodyweight (female)

Less bad—1.0 to 1.25 × bodyweight (male); 0.5 to 0.75 × bodyweight (female)

Seek help—1.0 × bodyweight or less (male); 0.5 × bodyweight or less (female)

Squat and Deadlift

Since people are usually built for one or the other, go with your strongest method.

Gold standard—3.0 × bodyweight

Killin' it—Over 2.5 × bodyweight

Good—2.0 to 2.5 × bodyweight

Less bad—1.5 to 2.0 × bodyweight

Seek help—Less than 1.5 × bodyweight

Military Press

Gold standard—1.5 × bodyweight (male); 1.25 × bodyweight (female)

Killin' it—Over 1.0 × bodyweight (male); over 0.75 × bodyweight (female)

Good—0.75 to 1.0 × bodyweight (male); 0.5 to 0.75 × bodyweight (female)

Less bad—0.5 to 0.75 × bodyweight (male); 0.35 to 0.5 × bodyweight (female)

Seek help—0.5 × bodyweight or less (male); 0.35 × bodyweight or less (female)

Importantly, these are standards to help evaluate where you are at in your strength development and which lift you might want to focus more efforts on. Many of you will already be above the killin' it category in some lifts, but that doesn't mean that you should be content with your level of strength. Far from it. We are just providing an objective measure to evaluate your strength, weaknesses, and progression. With enough proper work, most fully functional, uninjured adults of a normal body-fat level can hope to achieve the killin' it category (although, if you are 65 and just starting training, it might not be in the cards). That would make you stronger than 90 percent of the gym population of the world.

INDEX

Note: The italicized *f* and *t* following page numbers refer to figures and tables, respectively.

ABOUT THE AUTHORS

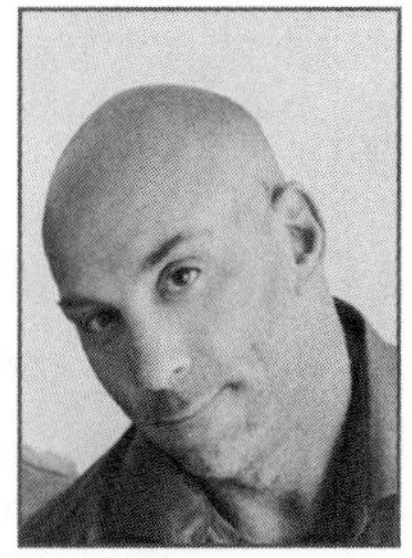

Christian Thibaudeau is a strength and conditioning coach with over 22 years of experience. He has taught seminars in over 20 different countries and has worked with athletes in 28 sports at all levels—high school to professional and Olympic athletes—as well as the everyday lifter. His training has also led him to work with competitors in the CrossFit Games and the Mr. Olympia bodybuilding competition. An athlete himself, competing in football, rugby, golf, weightlifting, and bodybuilding, Thibaudeau is the author of several strength and conditioning books, including *The Black Book of Training Secrets*, *Theory and Application of Modern Strength and Power Methods*, *High Threshold Muscle Building*, and *The Maximum Muscle Bible*, in addition to multiple training DVDs. He earned his bachelor of science degree in exercise science from Quebec University, where he also worked as a research assistant before moving on to full-time coaching.

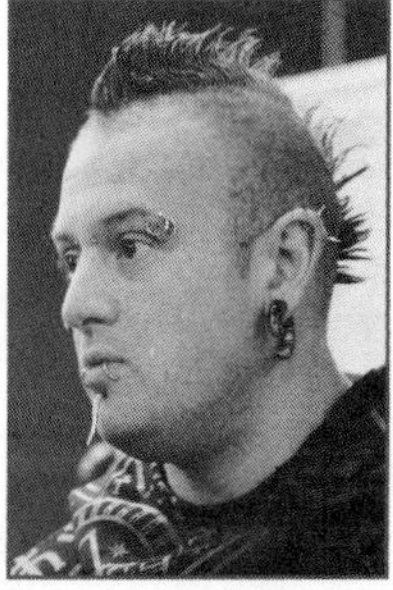

Tom Sheppard is head coach at Thibarmy and works with a wide variety of high-level athletes from all backgrounds. His philosophy is based on learning how to use the body as one integrated unit and optimizing athletes' lifting mechanics based on their body type. This approach has brought him particular success in the sport of powerlifting, where he has produced countless British, European, and world champions and record holders. In addition to his role at Thibarmy, he also works closely with EliteFTS, creating educational material, working with high-level lifters to improve their performance, and delivering seminars on the international stage, including the 2022 SWIS Symposium.

HUMAN KINETICS
CONTINUING EDUCATION
Now that you've read the book, complete the companion exam to **earn continuing education credit!**
Find your CE exam here:
US & International: US.HumanKinetics.com/collections/Continuing-Education
Canada: Canada.HumanKinetics.com/collections/Continuing-Education
Subscribe to our newsletters today!
US
Canada
Get exclusive offers and stay apprised of CE opportunities.

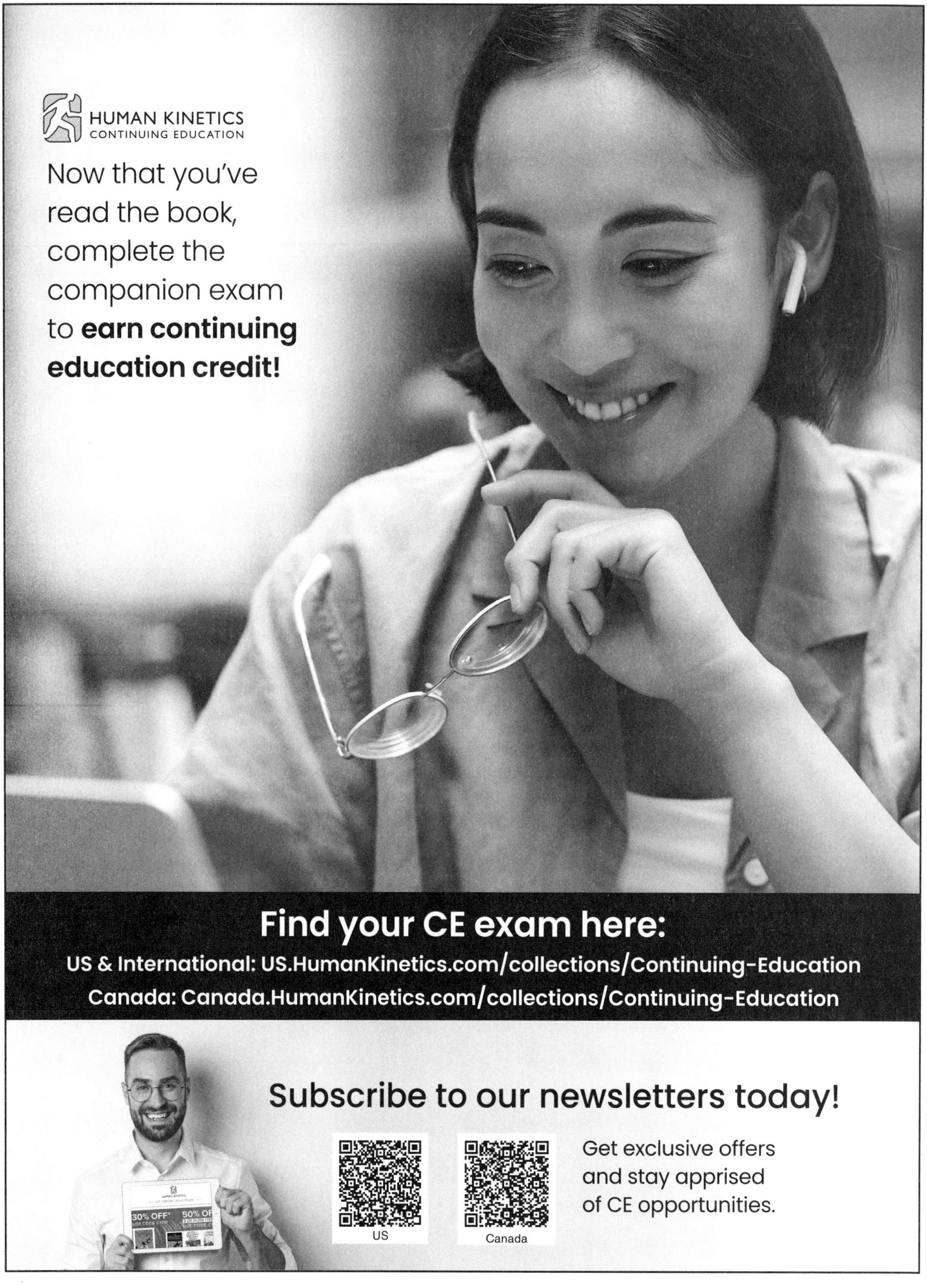